Infectious Diseases: Pathology and Treatment

Infectious Diseases: Pathology and Treatment

Editor: Cameron Harris

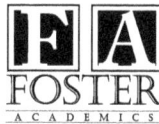

FA
FOSTER
ACADEMICS

www.fosteracademics.com

www.fosteracademics.com

FA FOSTER ACADEMICS

Cataloging-in-Publication Data

Infectious diseases : pathology and treatment / edited by Cameron Harris.
    p. cm.
Includes bibliographical references and index.
ISBN 978-1-63242-550-8
1. Communicable diseases. 2. Communicable diseases--Etiology. 3. Communicable diseases--Diagnosis.
4. Communicable diseases--Treatment. I. Harris, Cameron.
RC111 .I54 2018
616.9--dc23

Foster Academics,
118-35 Queens Blvd., Suite 400,
Forest Hills, NY 11375, USA

ISBN 978-1-63242-550-8 (Hardback)

Contents

Preface

Infectious diseases are those, which are caused by the toxins released by harmful organisms. They are also called transmissible diseases or communicable diseases. Some of the organisms causing infections are bacteria, viruses, pinworms, fungi, tapeworms, fleas, and lice, etc. The topics included in this book on infectious diseases are of utmost significance and bound to provide incredible insights to readers. It elucidates the contemporary approaches towards the pathology and treatment of infectious diseases. It is an essential guide for all academicians, researchers and those who wish to pursue this discipline further.

After months of intensive research and writing, this book is the end result of all who devoted their time and efforts in the initiation and progress of this book. It will surely be a source of reference in enhancing the required knowledge of the new developments in the area. During the course of developing this book, certain measures such as accuracy, authenticity and research focused analytical studies were given preference in order to produce a comprehensive book in the area of study.

This book would not have been possible without the efforts of the authors and the publisher. I extend my sincere thanks to them. Secondly, I express my gratitude to my family and well-wishers. And most importantly, I thank my students for constantly expressing their willingness and curiosity in enhancing their knowledge in the field, which encourages me to take up further research projects for the advancement of the area.

Editor

Central Venous Catheter-Related Bloodstream Infection with *Kocuria kristinae* in a Patient with Propionic Acidemia

Masato Kimura, Eichiro Kawai, Hisao Yaoita, Natsuko Ichinoi, Osamu Sakamoto, and Shigeo Kure

Department of Pediatrics, Tohoku University Graduate School of Medicine, Sendai, Miyagi 980-8574, Japan

Correspondence should be addressed to Masato Kimura; mkimura774@med.tohoku.ac.jp

Academic Editor: Alexandre Rodrigues Marra

Kocuria kristinae is a catalase-positive, coagulase-negative, Gram-positive coccus found in the environment and in normal skin and mucosa in humans; however, it is rarely isolated from clinical specimens and is considered a nonpathogenic bacterium. We describe a case of catheter-related bacteremia due to *K. kristinae* in a young adult with propionic acidemia undergoing periodic hemodialysis. The patient had a central venous catheter implanted for total parenteral nutrition approximately 6 months prior to the onset of symptoms because of repeated acute pancreatitis. *K. kristinae* was isolated from two sets of blood cultures collected from the catheter. Vancomycin followed by cefazolin for 16 days and 5-day ethanol lock therapy successfully eradicated the *K. kristinae* bacteremia. Although human infections with this organism appear to be rare and are sometimes considered to result from contamination, physicians should not underestimate its significance when it is isolated in clinical specimens.

1. Introduction

Patients with indwelling foreign materials are known to be at considerable risk of bloodstream infections. Early diagnoses and effective treatments for intravascular catheter-related infections are therefore crucial. *Kocuria* species are widely distributed in nature and can be found in normal skin and among oral cavity flora in humans and other animals [1, 2]. *K. kristinae* was first described in 1974 [3] and is an uncommon pathogenic organism in humans. However, some case reports indicate its emergence as a significant human pathogen [4–8]. We report a case of central venous catheter-related bacteremia with *K. kristinae* and a review of the literature.

2. Case Report

A 31-year-old Japanese man with propionic acidemia undergoing total parenteral nutrition presented with a high fever (39.5°C) after routine hemodialysis at his regional hospital. Although laboratory investigations revealed a slight elevation (1.2 mg/dL) of C-reactive protein (CRP), he was referred to our university hospital because Gram-positive cocci were

detected in blood cultures from the dialysis circuit. He had been undergoing periodic hemodialysis three times a week for 4 years and had received total parenteral nutrition (TPN) for 6 months because of repeated acute pancreatitis.

The patient was originally diagnosed with propionic acidemia following plasma and urinary amino acid analysis in the neonatal period. He developed normally after commencement of a low-protein diet supplemented with L-carnitine, but he has mild mental retardation. Immunological abnormalities were not diagnosed until admission. At the age of 27 years, he developed cardiomyopathy with a low ejection fraction (EF = 22.2%) and oliguria and was treated by cardiac resynchronization with defibrillation therapy (CRTD) and hemodialysis (HD). On admission, his height was 1.57 m, weight was 56.5 kg, and body temperature was 36.7°C, and he was fully conscious. There was no evidence of abnormalities in the cardiovascular and pulmonary systems. Blood samples for culture were obtained from one peripheral venipuncture site and one central venous catheter (CVC). They were analyzed by VITEK® MS system (bioMérieux S.A., Marcy-l'Étoile, France) and both of them were only identified with *K. kristinae* (blood culture from the dialysis circuit was also

TABLE 1: The results of antimicrobial susceptibility testing.

Antimicrobial agent	MIC (mg/L)
Ampicillin	≤0.12
Cefazolin	≤2
Cefotiam	≤2
Cefpirome	≤2
Clindamycin	≤0.5
Erythromycin	≤0.25
Gentamicin	≤1
Imipenem/cilastatin	≤1
Levofloxacin	1
Teicoplanin	≤2
Vancomycin	1

MIC, minimum inhibitory concentration.

identified with *K. kristinae* in regional hospital). Laboratory data were normal except for increased CRP levels (4.4 mg/dL). The CVC was left in place, antibiotic therapy with vancomycin was started, and the CVC was locked with ethanol for 5 days. Vancomycin was changed to cefazolin after *K. kristinae* was found in both blood cultures and its susceptibility to antibiotics was reported (Table 1). Antibiotics were administered for 16 days and the patient was discharged without complications after two serial negative blood cultures from CVC on another day. There was no reinfection after 3 months without antibiotic medication.

3. Microbiology

Two sets of blood cultures were obtained from one peripheral venipuncture site and one CVC. The blood samples were added into BacT/Alert® FA Plus and FN Plus resin bottles (bioMérieux S.A., Marcy-l'Étoile, France) and cultured BacT/Alert 3D automated microbial detection systems (bioMérieux S.A., Marcy-l'Étoile, France). Specimens were cultured on chocolate agar plate and were processed by VITEK MS system (bioMérieux S.A., Marcy-l'Étoile, France). VITEK MS is an automated microbial identification system that uses matrix assisted laser desorption ionization time-of-flight mass spectrometry (MALDI-TOF MS) technology to provide identification of microorganisms. Antimicrobial susceptibility tests are performed by Microscan WalkAway 96 Plus System (Beckman Coulter, Inc., CA, USA) and used Microscan Pos MIC 3.3 J panel (Beckman Coulter, Inc., CA, USA). Final molecular identification of microorganism was not carried out.

4. Discussion

Kocuria species are catalase-positive, coagulase-negative, Gram-positive coccoid actinobacteria belonging to the Micrococcus family. *To date, twenty-two* species have been classified in the genus: *K. kristinae, K. rosea, K. varians, K. palustris, K. rhizophila, K. marina, K. aegyptia,* and others [1, 2]. They are widely distributed in nature and have been found in normal skin and among oral cavity flora in humans and other animals. *K. kristinae* was first described by Kloos et al. in 1974 [3] and was not considered to be a human pathogen until about a decade ago. However, some case reports indicate the emergence of *K. kristinae* as a significant human pathogen, mostly in immunocompromised hosts [4], in patients with continuous ambulatory peritoneal dialysis (CAPD) [5], and in central venous catheter infections [4, 6–8].

We reviewed the literature on central venous catheter-related bloodstream infections (CRBSIs) with *K. kristinae* from 1974 to 2015. We identified 14 cases (including 7 nosocomial infections) and investigated the clinical backgrounds (Table 2 [4, 6–8]). Apart from hospital-acquired infections, there was female predominance (males, 2; females, 5) and the mean age was 44 years (range: 2–89). Long-term catheters are reported to have a lower risk of bloodstream infections than short-term catheters and almost all catheters were long-term types (long-term, 6; peripheral, 1) [9]. The revised guidelines from the IDSA (Infectious Diseases Society of America) published in 2011 recommend combination therapy with antibiotic administration through the colonized catheter for 10–14 days and antibiotic lock therapy in cases of uncomplicated CRBSI [10]. A review of the literature indicated that only one case was treated with combination therapy and the catheter was finally removed [4]. To the best of our knowledge, our patient represents the first successful treatment using combination therapy with antibiotics and antibiotic lock therapy to preserve the central venous catheter.

In conclusion, we have described a case of *K. kristinae* bacteremia in a patient with a central venous catheter and reviewed the literature. Although *K. kristinae* infections in humans appear to be rare and the organism was previously considered harmless, medical practitioners should be aware of the significance of this little recognized pathogen when it is isolated in clinical specimens.

Competing Interests

The authors declare that there are no competing interests regarding the publication of this paper.

TABLE 2: Published cases of central venous catheter-related bloodstream infections with *Kocuria kristinae*.

Year	Age	Sex	Type of catheter	Removal of catheter	Medical condition or underlying disease	Treatment regimens	Reference
2002	51	F	Long-term	Yes	Ovarian cancer, three times recurrence	Meropenem, glycopeptide-ciprofloxacin, clindamycin	[4]
2010	89	F	Long-term	Yes	Infective endocarditis, short bowel syndrome	Vancomycin → teicoplanin → oxacillin	[6]
	37	F	Long-term	Yes	Gastric cancer	Piperacillin + tazobactam → ciprofloxacin	[6]
	2	M	Long-term	Yes	Congenital short bowel syndrome	Oxacillin + lock therapy with vancomycin	[6]
	68	F	Long-term	Yes	Gastric cancer	Oxacillin	[6]
2011	29	F	Peripheral	Yes	Pregnancy	Vancomycin + clindamycin	[7]
	1 m	M	Peripheral	Yes	Prematurity, healthcare-associated	Vancomycin, ceftazidime	[8]
	0.6 m	M	Peripheral	Yes	Prematurity, healthcare-associated	Vancomycin	[8]
	0.7 m	F	Peripheral	Yes	Prematurity, healthcare-associated	Vancomycin, ceftazidime	[8]
2015	1	F	Peripheral	Yes	Prematurity, healthcare-associated	Vancomycin, oxacillin	[8]
	0.6 m	F	Peripheral	Yes	Prematurity, healthcare-associated	Vancomycin, cefotaxime	[8]
	0.6 m	F	Peripheral	Yes	Prematurity, healthcare-associated	Vancomycin, cefotaxime	[8]
	2 m	F	Long-term	Yes	Leukemia, healthcare-associated	Vancomycin, piperacillin/tazobactam	[8]

References

[1] E. Stackebrandt, C. Koch, O. Gvozdiak, and P. Schumann, "Taxonomic dissection of the genus Micrococcus: Kocuria gen. nov., Nesterenkonia gen. nov., Kytococcus gen. nov., Dermacoccus gen. nov., and Micrococcus cohn 1872 gen. emend," *International Journal of Systematic Bacteriology*, vol. 45, no. 4, pp. 682–692, 1995.

[2] V. Savini, C. Catavitello, G. Masciarelli et al., "Drug sensitivity and clinical impact of members of the genus Kocuria," *Journal of Medical Microbiology*, vol. 59, no. 12, pp. 1395–1402, 2010.

[3] W. E. Kloos, T. G. Tornabene, and K. H. Schleifer, "Isolation and characterization of micrococci from human skin, including two new species: *Micrococcus lylae* and *Micrococcus kristinae*," *International Journal of Systematic Bacteriology*, vol. 24, no. 1, pp. 79–101, 1974.

[4] G. Basaglia, E. Carretto, D. Barbarini et al., "Catheter-related bacteremia due to Kocuria kristinae in a patient with ovarian cancer," *Journal of Clinical Microbiology*, vol. 40, no. 1, pp. 311–313, 2002.

[5] A. Carlini, R. Mattei, I. Lucarotti, A. Bartelloni, and A. Rosati, "Kocuria kristinae: an unusual cause of acute peritoneal dialysis-related infection," *Peritoneal Dialysis International*, vol. 31, no. 1, pp. 105–107, 2011.

[6] C. C. Lai, J. Y. Wang, S. H. Lin et al., "Catheter-related bacteraemia and infective endocarditis caused by *Kocuria* species," *Clinical Microbiology and Infection*, vol. 17, no. 2, pp. 190–192, 2011.

[7] R. Dunn, S. Bares, and M. Z. David, "Central venous catheter-related bacteremia caused by Kocuria kristinae: case report and review of the literature," *Annals of Clinical Microbiology and Antimicrobials*, vol. 10, article 31, 2011.

[8] H.-M. Chen, H. Chi, N.-C. Chiu, and F.-Y. Huang, "*Kocuria kristinae*: a true pathogen in pediatric patients," *Journal of Microbiology, Immunology and Infection*, vol. 48, no. 1, pp. 80–84, 2015.

[9] D. G. Maki, D. M. Kluger, and C. J. Crnich, "The risk of bloodstream infection in adults with different intravascular devices: a systematic review of 200 published prospective studies," *Mayo Clinic Proceedings*, vol. 81, no. 9, pp. 1159–1171, 2006.

[10] N. P. O'Grady, M. Alexander, L. A. Burns et al., "Guidelines for the prevention of intravascular catheter-related infections," *American Journal of Infection Control*, vol. 39, no. 4, pp. S1–S34, 2011.

Typical Facial Lesions: A Window of Suspicion for Progressive Disseminated Histoplasmosis—A Case of Asian Prototype

Prasan K. Panda,[1] Siddharth Jain,[1] Rita Sood,[1] Rajni Yadav,[2] and Naval K. Vikram[1]

[1]Department of Internal Medicine, All India Institute of Medical Sciences, New Delhi 110029, India
[2]Department of Pathology, All India Institute of Medical Sciences, New Delhi 110029, India

Correspondence should be addressed to Naval K. Vikram; navalvikram@gmail.com

Academic Editor: Larry M. Bush

Histoplasmosis is caused by a dimorphic fungus *Histoplasma capsulatum* in endemic areas, mainly America, Africa, and Asia. In India, it is being reported from most states; however, it is endemic along the Ganges belt. We report a case of an apparently immunocompetent male who presented with 3-month history of fever, cough, and weight loss with recent onset odynophagia and had hepatosplenomegaly and mucocutaneous lesions over the face. The differential diagnosis of leishmaniasis, tuberculosis, leprosy, fungal infection, lymphoproliferative malignancy, and other granulomatous disorders was considered, but he succumbed to his illness. Antemortem skin biopsy and bone marrow aspiration along with postmortem liver, lung, and spleen biopsy showed disseminated histoplasmosis. This case highlights the need for an early suspicion of progressive disseminated histoplasmosis in the presence of classical mucocutaneous lesions even in an immunocompetent patient suffering from a febrile illness. Cure rate approaches almost 100% with early treatment, whereas it is universally fatal if left untreated.

1. Introduction

Classical histoplasmosis, also known as Darling disease, was first discovered in 1906 [1]. It is an endemic mycosis, caused by two species known to be pathogenic to man (*H. capsulatum* var. *capsulatum* and *H. capsulatum* var. *duboisii*). *H. capsulatum* is highly endemic in North America along the rivers Ohio and Mississippi, but Southeast and Southern Asia have focal endemicity, which is underrecognized due to the low awareness of the disease, misdiagnosis of the disease often as tuberculosis or leishmaniasis, and lack of proper diagnostic facilities [2]. "Asian histoplasmosis" as proposed differs from the American or African type, in having more mucocutaneous manifestations and a propensity for acute adrenal insufficiency, but the latter fact is disputed in many recent studies [3]. In India, the first case of histoplasmosis was reported in 1954, following which many case reports, two successive systematic reviews, and three large hospital based retrospective studies have been published in the literature [4–6]. A majority of cases have been reported from the eastern parts of the country, especially along the belt of Ganges and Brahmaputra, which may be related to the climate, humidity level, and soil characteristics. Due to migration and increased urbanization, cases are being reported from all over the country. Clinical suspicion should be high to diagnose cases in nonendemic areas.

This fungus grows in soil enriched with bird droppings, reaches human alveoli through inhalation, and causes varied clinical presentations ranging from self-limiting flu-like illness or acute or chronic pulmonary histoplasmosis to progressive disseminated histoplasmosis, depending on the quantity of antigen exposure and immune status of the individual [6]. All organs can be involved during the process of dissemination, but the reticuloendothelial system, skin, adrenals, gastrointestinal tract, and lungs are the most commonly involved sites [7]. Henceforth, skin may act as a window for early diagnosis of disseminated histoplasmosis.

We report an immunocompetent patient with disseminated histoplasmosis in whom an early suspicion of the disease may have improved the prognosis.

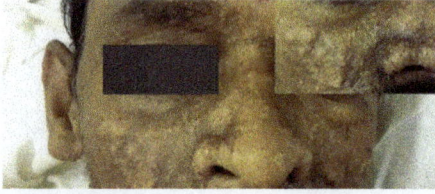

FIGURE 1: Face monograph showing skin colored, nonpruritic, nontender, papulonodular lesions (few umbilicated). Inset showing close-up view of right side facial lesions. Gray bar was used to mask face recognition.

2. Case Presentation

A 50-year-old male, resident of an area in the Ganges belt of Uttar Pradesh, India, presented with complaints of cough with scanty whitish expectoration, intermittent low grade fever, generalized weakness, and weight loss for three months. He also complained of abdominal pain, nonbilious vomiting, and progressive swelling over both legs for one month. Additionally, he noticed appearance of gradually progressive nonpruritic skin eruptions over the face and painful oral ulcers with odynophagia for the last three weeks. He also reported a history of melena for the last 10 days. There was no history of chest pain, hemoptysis, breathlessness, or urinary complaints. He was a tea vendor by occupation with no known prior illness.

On examination, he was conscious and hemodynamically stable. There was moderate to severe pallor, mild icterus, and bilateral pedal pitting-edema. He had oral nonaphthous ulcers with bleeding spots and multiple skin colored papulonodular lesions (with few showing central umbilication) over the face and bilateral ear lobes (Figure 1). There were no peripheral lymph nodes palpable. Cardiorespiratory examination was unremarkable except for occasional basal crackles. Abdominal examination revealed 4 cm, nontender, firm hepatomegaly and 3 cm, nontender, firm splenomegaly below the costal margin. Examination of other systems was unremarkable.

The different diagnoses considered at admission were post-kala-azar dermal leishmaniasis, disseminated tuberculosis, leprosy, invasive fungal infection, lymphoproliferative malignancy, and other granulomatous disorders.

The blood picture revealed Hb of 86 g/L, platelet count of 49×10^9/L, WBC count of 7.1×10^9/L with neutrophilic predominance (80%), and ESR of 50 mm/hr. Liver function tests (LFT) showed total bilirubin of 29.08 μmol/L (direct fraction, 23.95 μmol/L), AST of 0.83 μkat/L, and ALT of 0.60 μkat/L. The serum alkaline phosphatase (ALP) was very high (41.00 μkat/L), but LDH was in the upper normal range (4.43 μkat/L). There was hypoproteinemia (serum total proteins 45 g/L) with reversal of albumin/globulin ratio (1.6 : 2.9). Prothrombin time and thrombin time were deranged, and D-dimer levels were found to be very high. Kidney function tests and urine examination were normal. In view of fever, hepatosplenomegaly, bicytopenia, and deranged LFT, a possibility of secondary hemophagocytic lymphohistiocytosis

was also considered. Serologies for kala-azar, HIV, and viral hepatitis B and hepatitis C were negative.

Chest X-ray was essentially normal. Contrast-enhanced CT scan of the thorax and abdomen revealed hepatosplenomegaly with a splenic infarct, multiple calcified mediastinal nodes, fibrotic opacities in the bilateral lung apices (suggesting sequelae of old infection), minimal bilateral pleural effusion and ascites, and no lymphadenopathy. The pleural fluid was exudative with lymphocytic predominance. GeneXpert MTB/RIF of the fluid was negative. Punch biopsy was taken from the skin lesions on the face. A bone marrow biopsy was subsequently done. An upper GI endoscopy was performed which showed features suggestive of diffuse gastritis with punctate submucosal hemorrhages but biopsy could not be taken due to increased risk of bleeding.

The patient was managed with broad spectrum intravenous antibiotics, intravenous albumin, multivitamins, platelet concentrates, and packed RBC transfusions while awaiting the aforementioned biopsy reports. The patient developed altered sensorium and required endotracheal intubation and mechanical ventilation. Repeat LFT showed rising bilirubin levels with deranged PT/INR and aPTT suggestive of disseminated intravascular coagulation. A day later, the patient developed shock requiring inotropic support. Meanwhile, the provisional report of bone marrow aspirate indicated possibility of histoplasmosis. Skin biopsy showed a dense dermal infiltrate composed mainly of histiocytes and a few lymphocytes (Figure 2). The histiocytes showed numerous intracellular 2–5 μm oval to round organisms surrounded by a halo, which stained positive with periodic acid Schiff and silver methenamine stains, thus confirming Histoplasma. He was thus started on conventional intravenous Amphotericin-B at a dose of 1 mg/kg/day. However, on the same day, he succumbed to his illness. Postmortem biopsies of lung, liver, and spleen were taken (with consent of the relatives) all of which showed numerous intracellular spherical organisms in the histiocytes present in the lung interstitium, sinusoidal Kupffer cells of liver, and splenic macrophages, morphologically compatible with Histoplasma (Figure 3). The final diagnosis of chronic progressive disseminated histoplasmosis, involving liver, spleen, lung, GIT, bone marrow, and skin, was made.

3. Discussion

Histoplasmosis, caused by the dimorphic fungus H. capsulatum, has a spectrum of manifestations ranging from asymptomatic disease (>99% of cases) to progressive disseminated histoplasmosis (PDH) depending upon the intensity of exposure and immune status of the patient [7]. Further, onset of PDH may be as follows [8]:

  (i) Acute, seen in infants or immunocompromised people with certain risk factors, having high mortality where the risk factors for progressive disseminated histoplasmosis are as follows:

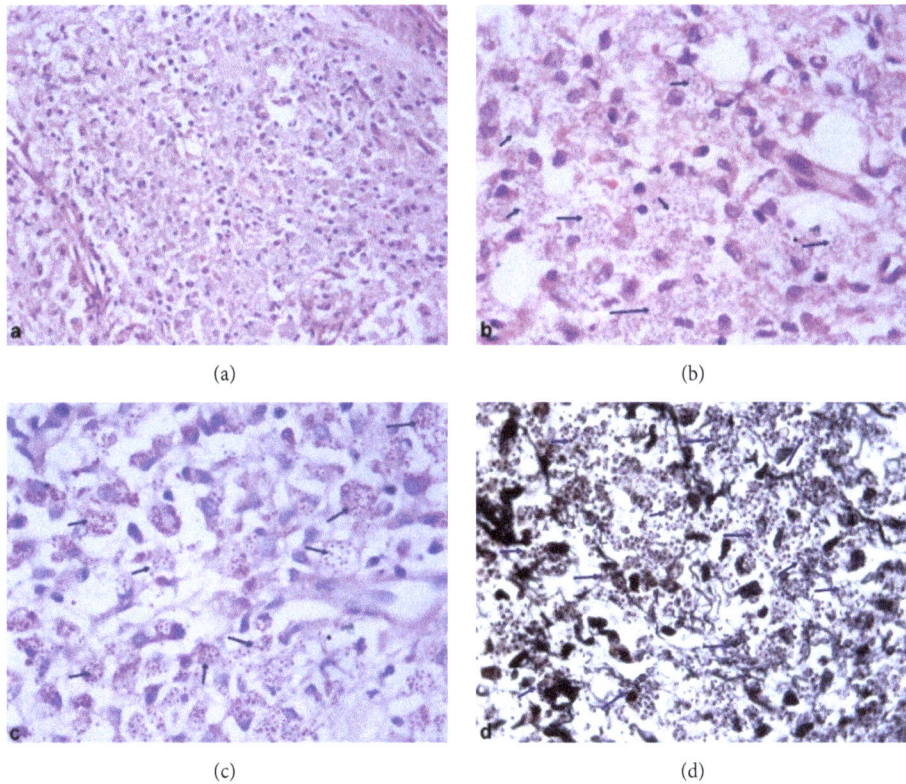

FIGURE 2: Skin biopsy shows a dense dermal histiocytic infiltrate with the presence of numerous intracellular spherical organisms surrounded by a halo in histiocytes, hematoxylin and eosin (H&E): (a) ×400 and (b) ×1000. These organisms stained positive with periodic acid Schiff (c) ×1000 and silver methenamine (d) ×1000 stains. All are morphologically compatible with *Histoplasma* as focused with arrows.

(1) Age (infants)

(2) AIDS

(3) Hematologic malignancies

(4) Solid organ transplant

(5) Hematopoietic stem cell transplant

(6) Immunosuppressive agents

   (a) Corticosteroids

   (b) Tumor necrosis factor antagonists

(7) Congenital T-cell deficiencies

(8) Gamma-interferon receptor deficiency

(9) Hyperimmunoglobulin M syndrome

(ii) Subacute, the most common type with a relentless course and focal lesions in various organs

(iii) Chronic, slowly progressive symptoms of organ involvement in old age and immunocompetent individuals with invariable death if not treated

Our case, in the absence of risk factors, belongs to the category of chronic PDH. The patient was a tea vendor by occupation. His shop was situated under a tree where a large number of birds nested. One possible source of infection could have been exposure to bird droppings. Further, his residence was close to Ganges belt from where cases of *Histoplasma* have been reported frequently [6]. There are not many studies to prove seasonal variation, but one French study showed a peak of infection during a long dry season [9]. Similar to our case that has been symptomatic in July 2014, there was another case presented in July 2012 as reported from Southern India [10].

No single organ is spared as dissemination proceeds but PDH should be considered as a possible differential diagnosis in all cases of fever of unknown origin (FUO), significant weight loss, adrenomegaly, hepatosplenomegaly, lymphadenopathy, or mucocutaneous lesions [11]. After self-limiting acute pulmonary histoplasmosis resolves due to adequate cellular immunity, calcified lung nodules and/or mediastinal lymph nodes remain which may persist for life [8]. Apical pleural thickening is common, but isolated pleural effusion (exudative, mostly hemorrhagic) is uncommon. Pleural effusion is common in a setting of acute pericarditis and is due to host immune response to fungi [12]. Our case had both calcified lymph nodes and exudative pleural effusion without features suggestive of pericarditis. Therefore, there is a high possibility of host immune response leading to the bilateral pleural effusion seen in our case. Lung biopsy depicted *Histoplasma* despite lack of any imaging evidence of acute/chronic pulmonary histoplasmosis, suggesting subtle involvement; however, acute pulmonary infections are not typically associated with a chest X-ray abnormality [7].

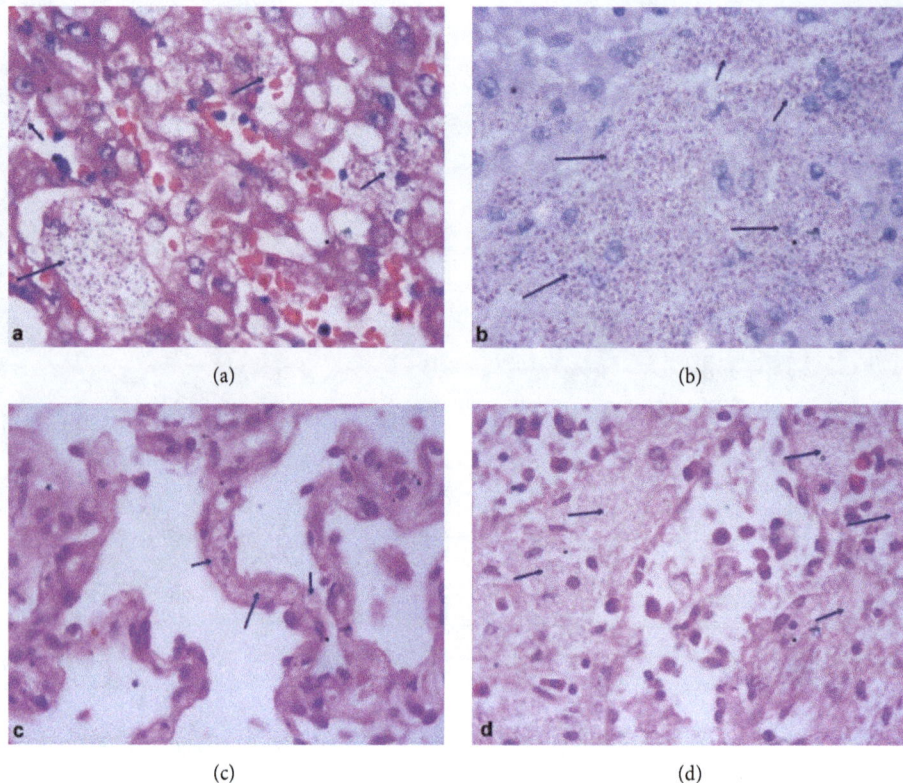

FIGURE 3: Liver biopsy shows numerous spherical organisms in the sinusoidal macrophages and Kupffer cells, (a) H&E ×1000, which stained positive with periodic acid Schiff stain (b) ×1000. Similar organisms are also seen in interstitial histiocytes in lung, (c) H&E ×1000, and splenic macrophages, (d) H&E ×1000. All are morphologically compatible with *Histoplasma* as focused with arrows.

Mucocutaneous histoplasmosis is very common in HIV patients and is rarely seen in immunocompetent individuals, but histoplasmosis in Asians has been shown to have higher mucocutaneous involvement in the latter group also. In one large case series having 61 immunocompetent patients, overall mucocutaneous involvement was found to be 36% [5]. Oral involvement in PDH, in the form of painful ulcers, nodules, or wart-like growths involving tongue, palate, gingiva, and oropharynx, (incidence 25–45%), needs to be differentiated from squamous cell carcinoma, hematological malignancies, tuberculosis, other deep fungal infections, or all manifestations of Crohn's disease or chronic traumatic ulcers [13]. In non-HIV patients, skin lesions were observed to be uncommon (9%) in one study [14]. The most common skin lesion is a papule, plaque, pustule, or nodule with or without central umbilication, resembling molluscum contagiosum, acneiform eruptions, or sebaceous hyperplasia [15]. Once detected, these classical mucocutaneous manifestations are hallmark of underlying PDH, especially in immunocompetent individuals like in our case, though localized skin involvement has also been rarely reported [13]. Biopsy of these lesions is a rapid way for diagnosis, preventing delay in administration of life-saving treatment. Our patient may have been diagnosed earlier if skin biopsy was done prior to the admission of the patient to the hospital.

Hematological manifestations like anemia, thrombocytopenia, pancytopenia, or increased ESR have been reported [6]. These are due to granulomatous involvement of bone marrow, secondary hemophagocytic lymphohistiocytosis, or immune mediated destruction of blood cells. Our patient had documented bone marrow involvement with possibly an element of immune thrombocytopenia since large platelets were seen in the peripheral smear. As Subbalaxmi et al. have reported, PDH should be considered in the differential diagnosis of thrombocytopenia with FUO irrespective of the patient's immune status and endemicity of the disease [10].

Gastrointestinal histoplasmosis (GIH) has been found in 70–90% of cases at autopsy but is rarely encountered during life because of minimal clinical symptoms and lack of suspicion [16]. Therefore, an active search through endoscopy should be made especially in patients with suspected PDH with apparently normal immune function, even in the absence of gastrointestinal symptoms. Endoscopy may show superficial mucosal ulceration, deep ulceration with or without perforation, or friable masses with or without obstruction [16]. Colon is the most common site involved in GIH followed by the small intestine [8]. Common symptoms are abdominal pain, diarrhea, nausea, vomiting, tenesmus, or constipation. Hepatomegaly and/or splenomegaly are reported in 30–100% of cases [16]. Our case had gastritis with submucosal hemorrhages and hepatosplenomegaly.

Culture is the gold standard for diagnosis, but histopathology/staining is the investigation of choice before starting treatment due to early reporting. The presence of tiny 2–$4\,\mu m$ spores with a clear zone around the nucleus, inside or outside macrophages or giant cells, visualized with hematoxylin & eosin, periodic acid Schiff, silver methenamine, Giemsa, lactophenol blue stains, or electron microscopy, is a distinguishing feature of *H. capsulatum* differentiating from *Leishmania*, *Penicillium marneffei*, *Cryptococcus neoformans*, and *Candida glabrata* [15]. Antigen detection and antibody serology are rapid diagnostic modalities; however, both have false positive and false negative results due to dependency on factors like quantity of antigen exposure, chronicity of disease, and immune status of patients [7]. One study showed culture positivity rates for lymph node, liver, and spleen biopsy samples, blood, and BAL to be 52.9%, with GI specimen showing a culture positivity rate of 90.9% [17]. Hence, all mucosal lesions identified at endoscopy should be cultured for fungi. This could not be done in our patient due to the high risk of bleeding.

Timely administration of antifungals decreases mortality to less than 25% in PDH, but, without treatment, the probablity of mortality is 80–100% [18]. For severe acute pulmonary histoplasmosis and severe PDH, Amphotericin-B, especially the liposomal formulation, is the drug of choice. For other types, azoles, mainly itraconazole, are sufficient. Relapse rate is high, up to 10–20% in PDH and up to 80% in AIDS associated cases [16].

4. Conclusions

(1) Mucocutaneous characteristics are pathognomonic of underlying PDH. Early local site biopsy can clinch the diagnosis and skin may be a window to diagnose deep fungal infections.

(2) GIH with diffuse gastritis and punctate submucosal bleeding spots is also an important finding. This may act as a window to diagnose PDH if biopsy is possible.

(3) One should consider histoplasmosis when symptoms are primarily respiratory (even with apparently normal chest imaging) with secondary dissemination of symptoms and signs. This is because the route of entry of this fungus is via the lungs.

(4) PDH is a highly underrecognized fungal infection in India even today. This case is again reminding us of the "Asian type of histoplasmosis."

(5) Lastly, this case reiterates the importance of doing biopsy on time before it is too late.

Competing Interests

The authors declare that they have no competing interests.

References

[1] S. T. Darling, "A Protozoön general infection producing pseudotubercles in the lungs and focal necroses in the liver, spleen and lymphnodes," *The Journal of the American Medical Association*, vol. 46, no. 17, pp. 1283–1285, 1906.

[2] R. P. Goswami, N. Pramanik, D. Banerjee, M. M. Raza, S. K. Guha, and P. K. Maiti, "Histoplasmosis in eastern India: the tip of the iceberg?" *Transactions of the Royal Society of Tropical Medicine and Hygiene*, vol. 93, no. 5, pp. 540–542, 1999.

[3] W. S. Symmers, "Histoplasmosis in southern and south-eastern Asia. A syndrome associated with a peculiar tissue form of histoplasma: a study of 48 cases," *Annales de la Société Belge de Médecine Tropicale*, vol. 52, no. 4, pp. 435–452, 1972.

[4] G. Panja and S. Sen, "A unique case of histoplasmosis," *Journal of the Indian Medical Association*, vol. 23, no. 6, pp. 257–258, 1954.

[5] S. Kathuria, M. R. Capoor, S. Yadav, A. Singh, and V. Ramesh, "Disseminated histoplasmosis in an apparently immunocompetent individual from north India: a case report and review," *Medical Mycology*, vol. 51, no. 7, pp. 774–778, 2013.

[6] D. De and U. K. Nath, "Disseminated histoplasmosis in immunocompetent individuals-not a so rare entity, in India," *Mediterranean Journal of Hematology and Infectious Diseases*, vol. 7, no. 1, Article ID e2015028, 2015.

[7] R. Kurowski and M. Ostapchuk, "Overview of histoplasmosis," *American Family Physician*, vol. 66, no. 12, pp. 2247–2252, 2002.

[8] C. A. Kauffman, "Histoplasmosis: a clinical and laboratory update," *Clinical Microbiology Reviews*, vol. 20, no. 1, pp. 115–132, 2007.

[9] M. Hanf, A. Adenis, B. Carme, P. Couppie, and M. Nacher, "Disseminated histoplasmosis seasonal incidence variations: a supplementary argument for recent infection?" *Journal of AIDS and Clinical Research*, vol. 3, no. 8, article 175, 2012.

[10] M. V. S. Subbalaxmi, P. Umabala, R. Paul, N. Chandra, Y. S. Raju, and S. M. Rudramurthy, "A rare presentation of progressive disseminated histoplasmosis in an immunocompetent patient from a non-endemic region," *Medical Mycology Case Reports*, vol. 2, no. 1, pp. 103–107, 2013.

[11] R. Gopalakrishnan, P. Senthur Nambi, V. Ramasubramanian, K. Abdul Ghafur, and A. Parameswaran, "Histoplasmosis in India: truly uncommon or uncommonly recognised?" *Journal of Association of Physicians of India*, vol. 60, no. 10, pp. 25–28, 2012.

[12] R. A. Goodwin Jr., J. E. Loyd, and R. M. des Prez, "Histoplasmosis in normal hosts," *Medicine*, vol. 60, no. 4, pp. 231–266, 1981.

[13] M. D. Mignogna, S. Fedele, L. Lo Russo, E. Ruoppo, and L. Lo Muzio, "A case of oral localized histoplasmosis in an immunocompetent patient," *European Journal of Clinical Microbiology and Infectious Diseases*, vol. 20, no. 10, pp. 753–755, 2001.

[14] M. Harnalikar, V. Kharkar, and U. Khopkar, "Disseminated cutaneous histoplasmosis in an immunocompetent adult," *Indian Journal of Dermatology*, vol. 57, no. 3, pp. 206–209, 2012.

[15] S. Vidyanath, P. M. Shameena, S. Sudha, and R. Nair, "Disseminated histoplasmosis with oral and cutaneous manifestations," *Journal of Oral and Maxillofacial Pathology*, vol. 17, no. 1, pp. 139–142, 2013.

[16] C. J. Kahi, L. J. Wheat, S. D. Allen, and G. A. Sarosi, "Gastrointestinal histoplasmosis," *The American Journal of Gastroenterology*, vol. 100, no. 1, pp. 220–231, 2005.

[17] L. Zhu, W. Zhang, L. Yang, T. Guo, C. Su, and J. Yang, "Disseminated histoplasmosis: intestinal multiple ulcers without gastrointestinal symptoms in an immune competent adult," *Journal of Cytology & Histology*, vol. 5, article 231, 2014.

[18] H. Rubin, M. L. Furcolow, J. L. Yates, and C. A. Brasher, "The course and prognosis of histoplasmosis," *The American Journal of Medicine*, vol. 27, no. 2, pp. 278–288, 1959.

Intra-Abdominal Actinomycosis Mimicking Malignant Abdominal Disease

Ali Ridha,[1] Njideka Oguejiofor,[2] Sarah Al-Abayechi,[1] and Emmanuel Njoku[2]

[1]University of Arkansas for Medical Science, 4301 West Markham Street, Little Rock, AR 72205, USA
[2]Chicago Medical School, Rosalind Franklin University of Medicine and Science, 3333 Green Bay Rd., North Chicago, IL 60064, USA

Correspondence should be addressed to Ali Ridha; alim.ridha@yahoo.com

Academic Editor: Gernot Walder

Abdominal actinomycosis is a rare infectious disease, caused by gram positive anaerobic bacteria, that may appear as an abdominal mass and/or abscess (Wagenlehner et al. 2003). This paper presents an unusual case of a hemodynamically stable 80-year-old man who presented to the emergency department with 4 weeks of worsening abdominal pain and swelling. He also complains of a 20-bound weight loss in 2 months. A large tender palpable mass in the right upper quadrant was noted on physical exam. Laboratory studies showed a normal white blood cell count, slightly decreased hemoglobin and hematocrit, and mildly elevated total bilirubin and alkaline phosphatase. A CT with contrast was done and showed a liver mass. Radiology and general surgery suspected malignancy and recommended CT guided biopsy. The sample revealed abundant neutrophils and gram positive rods. Cytology was negative for malignancy and cultures eventually grew actinomyces. High dose IV penicillin therapy was given for 4 weeks and with appropriate response transitioned to oral antibiotic for 9 months with complete resolution of symptoms.

1. Introduction

Actinomycosis is a rare chronic infectious disease caused by *Actinomyces israeli*, an aerobic or microaerophilic gram positive bacteria, present in the oral cavity, throughout the gastrointestinal tract, female genital tract, and the bronchus [1]. Actinomyces has low virulence; consequently disease occurs when the mucosal barrier has been compromised or in patients who are immune compromised [2]. Diagnosis preoperatively is rarely made due to variable clinical presentations. The majority of cases are diagnosed after the specimen in question has been resected and examined histologically [3].

Abdominal actinomycosis develops after a localized inflammatory process, prolonged IUD use, or recent abdominal surgery [4]. The appendix, cecum, and colon diverticulum are most affected. It is characterized by infiltrative and granulomatous inflammation similar in presentation to irritable bowel disease, tuberculosis, and malignancy macroscopically [4].

The direct extension of actinomyces, across the tissue, leads to formation of multiple abscesses, abundant granulation tissue, and sinuses [5]. The involvement of surrounding structures not only contributes to the insidious clinical course and delay of diagnosis, but also may mimic a tumor. This paper presents a case of intra-abdominal actinomycosis mimicking malignant abdominal disease.

2. Case Report

80-year-old man with a known past medical history of atrial fibrillation, hyperlipidemia, benign prostatic hyperplasia, osteoarthritis, and laparoscopic cholecystectomy in 2009 presented to the emergency department with a four-week history of abdominal pain and swelling localized to the right upper quadrant (RUQ). Patient reported that the abdominal pain was dull, aching, nonradiating, 7/10 in severity, aggravated by movement, alleviated by rest, and associated with loss of appetite and 20 pounds' weight loss in 2 months. He denied any associated fever.

Physical examination revealed an elderly male who appeared to be in mild painful distress. Vital signs were as follows: temperature 97.8°F, pulse 89/bpm, respirations 16/min, blood pressure 100/69 mm/Hg, and oxygen saturation 98% on room air. Abdominal exam revealed well healed old laparoscopic scars. There was a large palpable mass in the RUQ which was tender to palpation. There was no palpable hepatosplenomegaly, guarding or rebound with normal active bowel sounds. The rest of his exam was unremarkable.

Laboratory studies demonstrated a white blood cell count of 8.3 10^3/mcL, hemoglobin level 12.3 gm/dL, platelet count 315 10^3/mcL, and mean corpuscular volume 99.2 FL (82–99). Liver function tests were normal; alpha fetoprotein was normal at 1 ng/mL, and carcinoembryonic antigen was also unremarkable at 1.2 ng/mL.

Computerized tomography with contrast showed septated subpulmonic mass measuring 5.6 cm × 2.2 cm with internal high density anterior to the liver and adjacent to the diaphragm and 3.7 cm × 2.2 cm fluid collection posterior to the anterior abdominal wall musculature in the RUQ extending to the right rectus muscle (Figure 1). The radiologist suspected a malignancy with large hematoma knowing that he is chronically on Coumadin for atrial fibrillation. General surgery was called for evaluation and the surgeons recommended a CT guided biopsy of the mass and aspiration of the fluid collection. His Coumadin was held and a CT guided biopsy and aspiration were done with about 100 cc of thick viscus fluid drained. Fluid revealed abundant neutrophils and gram positive rods. Cultures eventually grew actinomyces and cytology was negative for any malignancy.

He was started on high dose intravenous penicillin G 3000000 units' every 4 hours for about 4 weeks with appropriate response. He was then transitioned to oral penicillin for about 9 months with complete resolution of symptoms.

3. Discussion

Actinomycosis is an infection caused by *Actinomyces* species. *Actinomyces* are gram positive, filamentous, nonsporing, and microaerophilic or obligate anaerobic bacteria. These bacteria normally colonize the flora of the oral cavity, genital tract, and upper gastrointestinal tract. They have a granulomatous inflammatory response causing pus production and abscess formation which is then followed by necrosis and extensive, reactive fibrosis [1]. The incidence of *Actinomyces* is 1 : 300000 [6]. Overall incidence of actinomycosis has been decreasing; however, abdominal and genital actinomycosis has been noted to be increasing in frequency due to increase of usage of intrauterine device [6].

Abdominal actinomycosis accounts for 20% of actinomycosis infection [7]. This particular type can occur due to a destruction of mucosal barriers, including perforated bowel, endoscopic procedures (like in our case), trauma, appendectomy, or due to an unknown cause [8]. One important challenge with actinomycosis infection is delayed diagnosis. It may present as a malignant disease, with symptoms of abdominal pain, asthenia, and weight loss.

Histopathologically, the organism produces the characteristic granulomatous inflammatory response. Confirmation is done by FNA or core biopsy by surgical exploration or radiological guided biopsy. Radiological techniques, including CT scan or magnetic resonance imaging (MRI), may show findings suggestive of the diagnosis of actinomycotic mass, in the right clinical setting. CT shows low-attenuation,

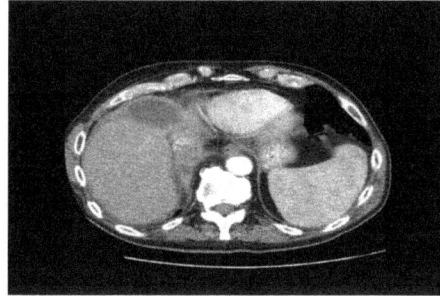

FIGURE 1: CT scan with contrast showing 5.6 cm × 2.2 cm liver mass and 3.7 cm × 2.2 cm fluid collection posterior to the anterior abdominal wall musculature.

focal areas of a solid mass and less frequently a thickened-wall cystic mass [9]. Actinomycosis treatment is centered on high dose antibiotics, including the standard treatment of 2–6 weeks IV penicillin G, followed by 6–12 months of oral penicillin [10].

4. Conclusion

Abdominal actinomycosis is an uncommon infectious disease that can mimic multiple disease processes. It may present as a malignant disease, with symptoms of abdominal pain, asthenia, and weight loss. High index of suspicion is needed to avoid delay in diagnosis. Confirmation is done by FNA or core biopsy by surgical exploration or radiological guided biopsy. In many patients prolonged treatment of high dose penicillin is required to be cured.

Competing Interests

The authors declare that there is no conflict of interests regarding the publication of this paper.

References

[1] F. M. E. Wagenlehner, B. Mohren, K. G. Naber, and H. F. K. Männl, "Abdominal actinomycosis," *Clinical Microbiology and Infection*, vol. 9, no. 8, pp. 881–885, 2003.

[2] Y. Sumer, B. Yilmaz, B. Emre, and C. Ugur, "Abdominal mass secondary to actinomyces infection: an unusual presentation and its treatment," *Journal of Postgraduate Medicine*, vol. 50, no. 2, pp. 115–117, 2004.

[3] T. Pusiol, D. Morichetti, C. Pedrazzani, and F. Ricci, "Abdominal-pelvic actinomycosis mimicking malignant neoplasm," *Infectious Diseases in Obstetrics and Gynecology*, vol. 2011, Article ID 747059, 4 pages, 2011.

[4] O. Sakrak, I. Muderrisoglu, A. Bedirl, O. Ince, and O. Canoz, "Acute abdomen secondary to colonic perforations: atypical presentation of actinomyces infection," *Journal of the American Society of Abdominal Surgeons*, pp. 18–21, 2015.

[5] H. Y. Sung, I. S. Lee, S. I. Kim et al., "Clinical features of abdominal actinomycosis: a 15-year experience of a single institute," *Journal of Korean Medical Science*, vol. 26, no. 7, pp. 932–937, 2011.

[6] G. Montori, A. Allegri, G. Merigo et al., "Intra-abdominal acti-
     nomycosis, the great mime: case report and literature review,"
     Emergency Medicine and Health Care, vol. 3, 2015.

[7] J. F. Yegüez, S. Martinez, L. R. Sands, and M. D. Hellinger, "Pelvic
     actinomycosis presenting as malignant large bowel obstruction:
     a case report and a review of the literature," *American Surgeon*,
     vol. 66, no. 1, pp. 85–90, 2000.

[8] S. H. Heo, S. S. Shin, J. W. Kim et al., "Imaging of actinomycosis
     in various organs: a comprehensive review," *Radiographics*, vol.
     34, no. 1, pp. 19–33, 2014.

[9] Ö. Şakrak, I. Müderrisoğlu, A. Bedirli, Ö. Ince, and Ö. Canöz,
     "Abdominal actinomycosis appearing as an intraabdominal
     tumoral mass," *Turkish Journal of Medical Sciences*, vol. 33, no.
     1, pp. 53–55, 2003.

[10] V. K. Wong, T. D. Turmezei, and V. C. Weston, "Actinomycosis,"
     BMJ (Online), vol. 343, no. 7827, article d6099, 2011.

A Rare Case of Mediterranean Spotted Fever and Encephalitis

Raquel Sousa Almeida, Petra M. Pego, Maria João Pinto, and João Matos Costa

3rd Department of Internal Medicine, Hospital Distrital de Santarém, Santarém, Portugal

Correspondence should be addressed to Raquel Sousa Almeida; almeida.raquelsousa@gmail.com

Academic Editor: Xavier Vallès

Mediterranean spotted fever is a tick-borne zoonotic disease caused by *Rickettsia conorii*. It is transmitted by the dog tick *Rhipicephalus sanguineus*. It usually presents as a benign self-limited disease characterized by a skin rash, high fever, and, sometimes, a characteristic ulcer at the tick bite site called *tache noir*. The course of this disease is usually benign, although severe manifestations have been previously described, mainly in adults. Neurological manifestations are very unusual. We present a case of Mediterranean spotted fever with encephalitis to highlight the importance of clinical suspicion, mainly in endemic areas, the potential severity of this disease, and the need of early initiation of therapy in order to prevent severe complications.

1. Introduction

Mediterranean spotted fever (MSF) is an emerging zoonosis caused by *Rickettsia conorii*, a member of the spotted fever group of rickettsiae [1]. *Rhipicephalus sanguineus* (dog tick) is the only recognized tick vector of rickettsiae identified in Portugal. Most of the cases occur during summer, during the period from July to September [2]. MSF is usually a benign and self-limited disease, characterized by skin rash, high fever, and a characteristic ulcer at the tick bite site called *tache noir*. Severe presentations are unusual but have been increasingly reported [3, 4]. Diagnosis is based on epidemiological, clinical, and laboratory criteria. The reference method is immunofluorescence which allows for the detection of IgM and IgG in the acute and convalescent sera [5]. Doxycycline (200 mg/day during 7–14 days, depending on the clinical course) is the drug of choice for the treatment of MSF [6].

2. Case Presentation

A 79-year-old male presented to the emergency department in August with high fever, headache, myalgia, nausea, and vomiting since the past six days and also with confusion and left hemiparesis since earlier that day. He had a previous history of arterial hypertension, diabetes mellitus, and chronic sinusitis. He lived in a rural area and had regular contact with dogs. On physical examination he was febrile (38,9°C), his blood pressure was 165/80 mmHg, and his pulse was regular, 120 beats per minute. He had a disseminated maculopapular rash, including the palms of the hands and the soles of the feet (Figures 1(a)–1(c)). A dark crusted lesion with a diameter of approximately 50 mm consistent with *tache noir* was noticed in the left inguinal region (Figure 1(d)). Neurological examination revealed decreased level of consciousness (Glasgow Coma Score of 10), left hemiparesis, and left hypoesthesia, including the face. Global aphasia and labial commissure deviation to the right side were also noted. The rest of the physical examination was normal, including absence of meningeal signs and normal flexor plantar reflexes. His haemoglobin level was 12.2 g/dL, his white blood cell count was 8700 cells/μL (88,5% neutrophils, 8% lymphocytes, and 3% monocytes), and his platelet count was 101 000 platelets/μL. His C-reactive protein level was 20,70 mg/dL. The remainder laboratory evaluation showed hyperglycaemia (167 g/dL), acute renal failure (2.2 mg/dL creatinine), and elevated liver enzymes (140 U/L aspartate aminotransferase, 136 alanine transferase U/L). Urinalysis and chest radiograph were unremarkable.

Cerebral computerized tomography (CT) scans were performed at admission and 48 hours later, both with no

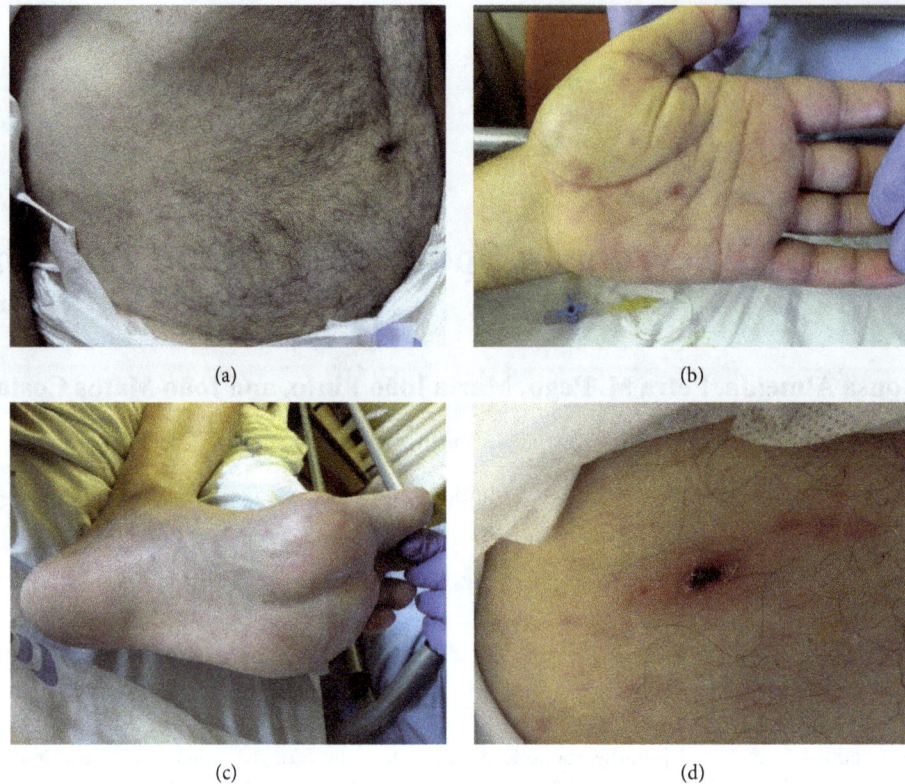

FIGURE 1: Maculopapular disseminated rash (a), including the palms of the hands (b) and the soles of the feet (c) and a dark brown inoculation eschar (*tache noir*) in the left inguinal region (d).

abnormalities. A lumbar puncture was performed on the first day of admission and cerebral spinal fluid (CSF) analysis revealed moderately elevated protein, normal glucose level, and pleocytosis (48 cells/μL) with polymorphonuclear predominance. Pending results of diagnostic studies, an empirical regimen of acyclovir, ceftriaxone, and doxycycline was started, with a slight neurological improvement in 24 hours. However, later that day, the patient presented with tonic-clonic seizures that ceased with intravenous diazepam and was transferred to the intensive care unit. The EEG examination was not performed as it was not available at the site and the patient was not clinically stable to be transferred. Microbiological cultures and PCR for herpes simplex virus in the CSF were negative. Serology by indirect immunofluorescence assay showed elevated IgM antibodies titer ($\geq$32; negative if < 32, positive if $\geq$ 32) for *Rickettsia conorii*, with nonelevated IgG (<64; negative result if < 64, suspicious if = 64, and positive if $\geq$ 128). After the third day in doxycycline therapy, there was a gradual clinical improvement, with progressive normalization of inflammatory markers, renal function, and liver enzymes. After eight days of doxycycline therapy, neurological examination was normal. He was discharged home with normal laboratory tests and with no neurological sequelae. In a new sample, taken 15 days after the initial presentation, the IgG antibodies for *Rickettsia conorii* were positive ($\geq$128). The patient has been followed in our clinic, with no episodes of seizures, neurological deficits, or other symptoms.

3. Discussion

In this patient, the first signs of were typical. The episode occurred during summer, with characteristic symptoms of fever, rash, and *tache noir* lesion and the acute and convalescent serological tests were confirmatory. However, it was complicated by neurological manifestations, acute renal failure, acute hepatic failure, and thrombocytopenia. The course of MSF is usually benign; however severe manifestations have been previously described. Advanced age, chronic alcoholism, immunocompromised status, glucose-6-phosphate dehydrogenase deficiency, prior prescription of inappropriate antimicrobial therapy, delay in treatment, and diabetes are risk factors for more severe presentations which can lead to a fatal outcome [2, 7]. The pathogenesis of MSF complications results from *Rickettsia* invasion and its multiplication in vascular endothelial cells, resulting in widespread vasculitis of capillaries, arterioles, and small arteries [7]. Renal impairment has been frequently described as a consequence of severe MSF [8]. In this patient, the delay in seeking medical attention and treatment, advanced age, and previous diabetes mellitus history probably accounted for the severity of the manifestations. Assuming the possible cross-reactions with other emerging *Rickettsia* of the spotted fever group, the use of standard serological tests for diagnosis is a limitation in our observation. Only five cases of adults with encephalitis related to *Rickettsia conorii* infection diagnosed by IFA and with CSF analysis description are described in the literature. The majority (three in five) of the cases reported pleocytosis in the CSF. Elevated protein levels were found in three cases. The glucose levels were normal in one case, slightly elevated in two, and decreased in one [1, 2, 9]. Of the four who survived, only one patient recovered without sequelae [1, 2, 9]. Although systematic pharmacokinetic studies are lacking for the concentration of doxycycline in CSF against *Rickettsia conorii*, a study on neuroborreliosis showed that daily doses of 200 mg of doxycycline produce a CSF concentration close to the MICs for susceptible bacteria, both in the absence and in the presence of meningeal inflammation [10]. Doxycycline is the most effective antibiotic against *Rickettsia conorii*, with a MIC of $0,06\,\mu\mathrm{g/mL}$ [11]. Fluoroquinolones may be considered a safe alternative to tetracyclines for the treatment of rickettsial diseases. However, the potential toxicity of doxycycline and fluoroquinolones contraindicates their use during pregnancy and childhood [12]. Clarithromycin is considered a valid alternative in patients with hypersensitivity to tetracyclines, in pregnant women and in children [13, 14].

4. Conclusion

Rickettsiosis is emerging infectious disease, which usually has a benign course. Nonetheless, clinical awareness is crucial, mainly in endemic areas, as they may present with severe life-threatening complications, such as encephalitis. This case report highlights the importance of early initiation of therapy in order to prevent these severe complications.

Competing Interests

The authors declare that they have no competing interests.

References

[1] C. Colomba, C. Imburgia, M. Trizzino, and L. Titone, "First case of Mediterranean spotted fever-associated rhabdomyolysis leading to fatal acute renal failure and encephalitis," *International Journal of Infectious Diseases*, vol. 26, pp. e12–e13, 2014.

[2] V. Duque, C. Ventura, D. Seixas et al., "Mediterranean spotted fever and encephalitis: a case report and review of the literature," *Journal of Infection and Chemotherapy*, vol. 18, no. 1, pp. 105–108, 2012.

[3] R. Demeester, M. Claus, M. Hildebrand, E. Vlieghe, and E. Bottieau, "Diversity of life-threatening complications due to Mediterranean spotted fever in returning travelers," *Journal of Travel Medicine*, vol. 17, no. 2, pp. 100–104, 2010.

[4] M. Amaro, F. Bacellar, and A. França, "Report of eight cases of fatal and severe Mediterranean spotted fever in Portugal," *Annals of the New York Academy of Sciences*, vol. 990, pp. 331–343, 2003.

[5] P. Brouqui, F. Bacellar, G. Baranton et al., "Guidelines for the diagnosis of tick-borne bacterial diseases in Europe," *Clinical Microbiology and Infection*, vol. 10, no. 12, pp. 1108–1132, 2004.

[6] M. Jensenius, P.-E. Fournier, and D. Raoult, "Rickettsioses and the international traveler," *Clinical Infectious Diseases*, vol. 39, no. 10, pp. 1493–1499, 2004.

[7] D. H. Walker and D. Raoult, "Rickettsia rickettsii and other spotted fever group rickettsiae (Rocky Mountain spotted fever and other spotted fevers)," in *Douglas and Bennett's Principles and Practice of Infectious Diseases*, Vo. G. L. Mandell, J. E. Bennett, and R. Dolin, Eds., pp. 2035–2042, Churchill Livingstone, New York, NY, USA, 5th edition, 2000.

[8] D. I. Montasser, Y. Zajjari, A. Alayoud et al., "Acute renal failure as a complication of Mediterranean spotted fever," *Nephrologie et Thérapeutique*, vol. 7, no. 4, pp. 245–247, 2011.

[9] L. Aliaga, P. Sánchez-Blázquez, J. Rodríguez-Granger, A. Sampedro, M. Orozco, and J. Pastor, "Mediterranean spotted fever with encephalitis," *Journal of Medical Microbiology*, vol. 58, no. 4, pp. 521–525, 2009.

[10] R. Nau, F. Sörgel, and H. Eiffert, "Penetration of drugs through the blood-cerebrospinal fluid/blood-brain barrier for treatment of central nervous system infections," *Clinical Microbiology Reviews*, vol. 23, no. 4, pp. 858–883, 2010.

[11] J.-M. Rolain, L. Stuhl, M. Maurin, and D. Raoult, "Evaluation of antibiotic susceptibilities of three rickettsial species including Rickettsia felis by a quantitative PCR DNA assay," *Antimicrobial Agents and Chemotherapy*, vol. 46, no. 9, pp. 2747–2751, 2002.

[12] J. M. Rolain, M. Maurin, G. Vestris, and D. Raoult, "In vitro susceptibilities of 27 rickettsiae to 13 antimicrobials," *Antimicrobial Agents and Chemotherapy*, vol. 42, no. 7, pp. 1537–1541, 1998.

[13] A. Cascio, C. Colomba, S. Antinori, D. L. Paterson, and L. Titone, "Clarithromycin versus azithromycin in the treatment of Mediterranean spotted fever in children: a randomized controlled trial," *Clinical Infectious Diseases*, vol. 34, no. 2, pp. 154–158, 2002.

[14] A. Cascio, C. Colomba, D. Di Rosa, L. Salsa, L. Di Martino, and L. Titone, "Efficacy and safety of clarithromycin as treatment for Mediterranean spotted fever in children: a randomized controlled trial," *Clinical Infectious Diseases*, vol. 33, no. 3, pp. 409–411, 2001.

Direct Acting Antivirals in Patients with Chronic Hepatitis C and Down Syndrome

Eric R. Yoo,[1] Ryan B. Perumpail,[2] George Cholankeril,[3] and Aijaz Ahmed[2]

[1]*Department of Medicine, University of Illinois College of Medicine, Chicago, IL, USA*
[2]*Division of Gastroenterology and Hepatology, Stanford University School of Medicine, Stanford, CA, USA*
[3]*Division of Gastroenterology and Hepatology, University of Tennessee Health Sciences Center, Memphis, TN, USA*

Correspondence should be addressed to Aijaz Ahmed; aijazahmed@stanford.edu

Academic Editor: Paola Di Carlo

Patients with Down syndrome who received blood transfusions, likely in conjunction with cardiothoracic surgery for congenital heart disease and prior to the implementation of blood-donor screening for hepatitis C virus infection, face a substantial risk of acquiring the infection. In the past, interferon-based therapy for chronic hepatitis C infection in patients with Down syndrome was noted to have lower efficacy and potentially higher risk of adverse effects. Recently, the treatment for chronic hepatitis C has been revolutionized with the introduction of interferon-free direct acting antivirals with favorable safety, tolerability, and efficacy profile. Based on our experiences, the newly approved sofosbuvir-based direct acting antiviral therapy is well tolerated and highly efficacious in this subpopulation of hepatitis C virus infected patients with Down syndrome.

1. Introduction

Prior to the implementation of blood-donor screening for hepatitis C virus infection, children who underwent cardiac surgery faced a substantial risk of acquiring the infection [1]. Chronic hepatitis C in patients with Down syndrome is usually a consequence of such childhood transfusions instituted in conjunction with cardiothoracic surgery for congenital heart disease [1–3]. To complicate matters further, an array of immunological disorders such as abnormal composition of peripheral blood lymphoid subsets, cellular dysfunction, and autoimmunity have been commonly noted in the setting of Down syndrome [4]. However, the majority of these patients do not manifest clear clinical features of immunological disorders. Despite these observations, limited experiences with interferon-based therapy in the setting of Down syndrome showed dismal results with none of the patients responding to treatment [5], raising the question whether immunological disturbances in patients with Down syndrome may result in poor performance of immune-dependent interferon therapy [4].

More recently, the treatment for chronic hepatitis C has been revolutionized with the introduction of interferon-free direct acting antivirals (DAA) with favorable safety, tolerability, and efficacy profile. Patients with chronic hepatitis C and Down syndrome form a unique group in which sofosbuvir- (SOF-) based DAA regimens may be promising and need further evaluation. We present our experience with the use of SOF-based regimens in this subpopulation of HCV-infected patients. Please note that the three patients presented below were monoinfected with chronic hepatitis C and with serologies negative for coinfection with hepatitis B virus or human immunodeficiency virus.

2. Case Presentations

2.1. Patient 1. Our first patient is a 27-year-old Caucasian man with trisomy 21, Down syndrome, and chronic hepatitis C virus, genotype 1b. He developed transfusion-related chronic hepatitis C, most likely following cardiothoracic surgery early in life for an endocardial cushion defect. Pretreatment laboratory data showed platelet count 98×10^3/microL, prothrombin time 14.2 seconds, INR 1.2, aspartate aminotransferase 74 units per liter (U/L), alanine aminotransferase 103 U/L, alkaline phosphatase 104 U/L, normal gamma-glutamyl transferase, total bilirubin 0.7 milligrams per deciliter (mg/dL), and hepatitis C virus RNA level 1.23 million International Units (IU)/mL. His liver biopsy in 2009 showed grade 3 inflammation and stage III fibrosis. A computerized tomography scan of the abdomen showed a nodular cirrhotic liver with mild splenomegaly. No hypervascular discrete hepatic lesions were noted to suggest hepatocellular carcinoma. He failed to respond to combination antiviral therapy using pegylated interferon plus ribavirin. He was retreated with telaprevir, pegylated interferon, and ribavirin. He did not respond to second course of antiviral therapy. He developed severe adverse effects during the two courses of interferon-based antiviral therapy requiring the use of growth factors and transfusions. He underwent retreatment with interferon and ribavirin free oral DAA regimen using SOF and simeprevir for 12 weeks in 2014 and developed a sustained virological response at 6 months following completion of antiviral therapy. He remained aviremic and without any liver related symptoms. His liver enzymes normalized during antiviral therapy and remained thrombocytopenic. He has been recommended to undergo surveillance for hepatocellular carcinoma every 6 months.

2.2. Patient 2. Our second patient is a 29-year-old Caucasian woman with Down syndrome. She underwent open heart surgery at age 6 months for an endocardial cushion defect in 1986. She required blood transfusions resulting in chronic hepatitis C virus RNA level 0.9 million IU/mL, genotype 2a. She has never undergone a liver biopsy. She did not demonstrate any stigmata of portal hypertension or advance liver disease. She underwent her first course of antiviral therapy for 12 weeks using SOF and ribavirin 400 mg twice a day in 2015. She tolerated the treatment well and developed minimal adverse effects during antiviral therapy. According to her caregiver, she was minimally fatigued during antiviral therapy; however, there were no major adverse effects. Her aminotransferases, alkaline phosphatase, gamma-glutamyl transferase, total bilirubin, platelets, and coagulation studies remained normal prior to and following completion of antiviral therapy. She was able to continue her daily chores and attend school. Our patient was noted to have undetectable levels of hepatitis C virus on completion of the antiviral, and 6 months later she developed a sustained virological response.

2.3. Patient 3. Our third patient is a 53-year-old Caucasian man with chronic hepatitis C, genotype 1b. He has been noted to have persistent thrombocytopenia consistent with portal hypertension and suggestive of advanced stage III to IV hepatic fibrosis. Pretreatment laboratory data showed platelet count 97×10^3/microL, coagulation studies normal, aspartate aminotransferase 54 U/L, alanine aminotransferase 49 U/L, alkaline phosphatase 189 U/L, gamma-glutamyl transferase normal, total bilirubin 0.5 mg/dL, and hepatitis C virus RNA level 27.8 million IU/mL. He did not undergo a liver biopsy. He underwent cardiothoracic surgery as a child and received transfusions leading to chronic hepatitis C. He was treated with SOF and ledipasvir combination therapy for 12 weeks in 2015. He developed a sustained virological response with undetectable levels of hepatitis C virus at 24 weeks following completion of antiviral therapy. The abnormalities in liver enzymes resolved within the first 8 weeks of antiviral therapy. He was asked to continue surveillance for hepatocellular carcinoma on a 6-monthly basis due to underlying advance liver disease (stage III to IV fibrosis).

3. Discussion

In our case series we report successful response rates to SOF-based DAA therapy in patients with Down syndrome. A detailed discussion was conducted with the court-appointed legal guardian—parents, family, and support staff members of the patients. In all three cases, treatment inquiry and request were initiated by the legal guardian of the patient. Efficacy data, side effect profile, treatment duration, black box warnings, and absolute contraindications noted in the package insert for SOF-based treatments were reviewed. Limitations of off-label therapy were also reviewed. Patients were very closely monitored during the therapy by the primary care provider with immediate access to the medical team. The three patients tolerated the therapy without any minor or major adverse effects and they did not experience any alterations in their quality of life, conducting their daily chores without interruption. They complained of antiviral therapy due to an already established firm support system provided by the primary care provider at home or nursing facility.

We did not experience any clinical evidence of immunological dysfunction in the three patients [4]. No new symptoms were reported during or after the SOF-based DAA therapy suspicious of immune-mediated disorder including skin rash, arthralgia, visual disturbances, infections, diarrhea, urinary complaints, and so forth. No new behavioral changes or psychiatric symptoms were reported. Two out of three patients demonstrated evidence of advance liver disease and were placed in a 6-monthly surveillance program for hepatocellular carcinoma. It is prudent to perform a comprehensive evaluation for advance fibrosis with patients with chronic hepatitis C and Down syndrome during their initial evaluation, as most of these patients were infected with hepatitis C virus prior to 1990 when screening protocols were not instituted by most blood banks in the United States. It may be challenging to perform liver biopsy in patients with Down syndrome due to pain associated with the procedure and the high level of cooperation needed from the patient. However, the recent availability of several noninvasive tests used to assess hepatic fibrosis may overcome these issues and be invaluable in this patient population.

4. Conclusion

Previously, interferon-based therapy for chronic hepatitis C infection in patients with Down syndrome was noted to have lower efficacy and potentially higher risk of adverse effects. However, based on our experience, the newly approved SOF-based antiviral therapy is well tolerated and highly efficacious in this patient population. We recommend that these patients with Down syndrome and chronic hepatitis C infection undergo close monitoring during their DAA therapy.

Competing Interests

There are no competing interests for Eric R. Yoo, Ryan B. Perumpail, and George Cholankeril. Aijaz Ahmed is a consultant and advisory board member for AbbVie Pharmaceuticals, Gilead Sciences, and Janssen Pharmaceutical. Aijaz Ahmed has research funding/grant from Gilead Sciences.

References

[1] M. Vogt, T. Lang, G. Frösner et al., "Prevalence and clinical outcome of hepatitis C infection in children who underwent cardiac surgery before the implementation of blood-donor screening," *New England Journal of Medicine*, vol. 341, no. 12, pp. 866–870, 1999.

[2] R. K. Chaudhary, E. Perry, F. Hicks, C. MacLean, and M. Morbey, "Hepatitis B and C infection in an institution for the developmentally handicapped," *The New England Journal of Medicine*, vol. 327, no. 27, p. 1953, 1992.

[3] M. Piccione, M. De Curtis, M. L. La Vecchia, A. Novissimo, and P. Vajro, "Hepatitis B and C infection in children with Down syndrome," *European Journal of Pediatrics*, vol. 156, no. 5, pp. 420–421, 1997.

[4] E. Cuadrado and M. J. Barrena, "Immune dysfunction in Down's syndrome: primary immune deficiency or early senescence of the immune system?" *Clinical Immunology and Immunopathology*, vol. 78, no. 3, pp. 209–214, 1996.

[5] Y. Miyoshi, H. Tajiri, M. Okaniwa et al., "Hepatitis C virus infection and interferon therapy in patients with Down syndrome," *Pediatrics International*, vol. 50, no. 1, pp. 7–11, 2008.

Treatment of Polymicrobial Osteomyelitis with Ceftolozane-Tazobactam: Case Report and Sensitivity Testing of Isolates

Jeffrey C. Jolliff,[1,2] **Jackie Ho,**[1] **Jeremiah Joson,**[1,2] **Arash Heidari,**[1] **and Royce Johnson**[1]

[1]*Kern Medical, 1700 Mount Vernon Avenue, Bakersfield, CA 93306-4018, USA*
[2]*University of the Pacific School of Pharmacy & Health Sciences, 3601 Pacific Avenue, Stockton, CA 95211-0109, USA*

Correspondence should be addressed to Jackie Ho; jackie.ho@tu.edu

Academic Editor: Arlene C. Sena

Stenotrophomonas maltophilia is an inherently multidrug resistant (MDR) opportunistic pathogen with many mechanisms of resistance. SENTRY studies reveal decreasing sensitivities of *S. maltophilia* to trimethoprim-sulfamethoxazole and fluoroquinolones. Ceftolozane-tazobactam (Zerbaxa, Merck & Co., Inc.) a novel intravenous combination agent of a third-generation cephalosporin and β-lactamase inhibitor was demonstrated to have *in vitro* activity against many Gram-positive, Gram-negative, and MDR organisms. Data for ceftolozane-tazobactam's use outside of Food and Drug Administration (FDA) approved indications has been limited thus far to two case reports which demonstrated its efficacy in pan-resistant *Pseudomonas aeruginosa* pneumonia. Herein, we describe the first published case of treatment of MDR *S. maltophilia* in polymicrobial osteomyelitis with long-term (>14 days) ceftolozane-tazobactam and metronidazole. Ceftolozane-tazobactam may offer a possible alternative for clinicians faced with limited options in the treatment of resistant pathogens including MDR *S. maltophilia*.

1. Introduction

Stenotrophomonas maltophilia is an inherently multidrug resistant (MDR) opportunistic pathogen with many mechanisms of resistance which may challenge clinicians to find safe and effective treatment regimens. Antimicrobial resistance mechanisms include β-lactamase production, the presence of class 1 integrons and ISCR elements (resistance to trimethoprim-sulfamethoxazole, TMP-SMX), expression of quinolone resistance (*Qnr*) genes, and multidrug efflux pumps [1].

Although TMP-SMX is often regarded as the drug of choice with fluoroquinolones (FQs) as reasonable alternatives, SENTRY studies reveal decreasing sensitivities of *S. maltophilia* to TMP-SMX (96.0% to 94.5%) and levofloxacin (83.4% to 77.3%) [2–4]. Other options with historically good susceptibility profiles but rising resistance rates include ceftazidime, ticarcillin-clavulanate, and tetracyclines [1]. Therefore, knowledge of the activity of other compounds, including

new agents, which might be effective in treating *S. maltophilia* is desirable.

Ceftolozane-tazobactam (Zerbaxa, Merck & Co., Inc.) is a novel intravenous combination agent of a third-generation cephalosporin and β-lactamase inhibitor Food and Drug Administration (FDA) approved in 2014 for the treatment of complicated intra-abdominal (cIAI) (when combined with metronidazole) and complicated urinary tract infection (cUTI) (Figure 1) [5]. Ceftolozane-tazobactam has demonstrated *in vitro* activity against many Gram-positive, Gram-negative, and MDR organisms. It retains activity against ESBL-producing Enterobacteriaceae (TEM-SHV, CTX-M, and OXA) and MDR *Pseudomonas aeruginosa* with resistance mechanisms including chromosomal AmpC, loss of outer membrane porin (OprD), and upregulation of efflux pumps (MexY and MexAB). Its activity against MDR *P. aeruginosa* is surpassed only by colistin [6].

Data for ceftolozane-tazobactam's use outside of the FDA approved indications (cIAI and cUTI) has been limited thus

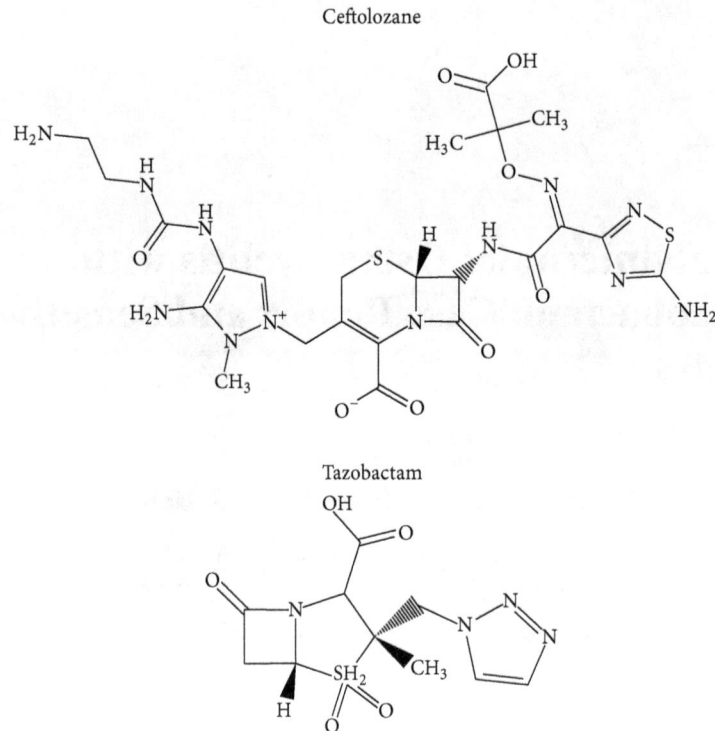

FIGURE 1: Chemical structure of ceftolozane-tazobactam.

far to two case reports which demonstrated its efficacy in pan-resistant *P. aeruginosa* pneumonia [7, 8].

Herein, we describe the first published case of treatment of MDR *S. maltophilia* in polymicrobial osteomyelitis with long-term (>14 days) ceftolozane-tazobactam and metronidazole.

2. Case Presentation

A 20-year-old male with no significant past medical history presented to the emergency department after suffering a crush injury to his right foot. After incision and drainage (I&D) of the wound and open reduction internal fixation of the navicular, tarsal, and metatarsals, he was discharged on cephalexin 500 mg orally (PO) every 6 hours.

Subsequent clinic visits revealed delayed wound healing and moderate-to-severe edema. By postoperative week six, the wound had dehisced with signs of necrosis and abscess formation. He underwent surgical intervention the following day where the wound was incised and drained, hardware was removed, and cultures were obtained. He was sent home on levofloxacin 750 mg PO daily and told to follow up in one week. Upon return, inspection of his foot showed exposed metatarsal bone which was dark and foul smelling. He was admitted for further management.

Wound cultures taken at surgery the week prior resulted in *Klebsiella pneumoniae, Enterobacter cloacae, Streptococcus anginosus*, and *Bacteroides ovatus*. Piperacillin-tazobactam

3.375 g IV every 6 hours was started. Another I&D was performed with cultures taken from necrotic bone. A PICC line was placed to initiate a prolonged course of antimicrobials.

On day 4, bone cultures returned *S. anginosus, Granulicatella adiacens*, and MDR *S. maltophilia*, resistant to TMP-SMX and levofloxacin. Etests were ordered to explore alternative antimicrobial options: ceftolozane-tazobactam, minimum inhibitory concentration (MIC) 0.5 mg/L; tigecycline MIC 2 mg/L; ceftazidime MIC 2 mg/L; and colistin MIC 0.5 mg/L. Due to concerns that monotherapy would not suffice and the need for simplified outpatient parenteral antimicrobial therapy to facilitate patient discharge, ceftolozane-tazobactam was favored [9–11].

The antibiotic regimen was therefore changed to ceftolozane-tazobactam 1.5 g IV every 8 hours plus metronidazole 500 mg PO every 8 hours (for coverage against *Bacteroides ovatus*) for six weeks with wound VAC to be changed every other day. At six- and ten-week follow-up, his wound was noted to be healing nicely with no purulence or serous drainage; inflammatory symptoms were also absent. At week 14, granulation tissue had failed to completely cover exposed bone, so patient underwent reconstruction of right foot defect with a fasciocutaneous flap. Cultures were obtained from the excised subcutaneous tissue which resulted in pan-sensitive coagulase positive *Staphylococcus, Staphylococcus lugdunensis*, and *Gemella morbillorum*; however, antimicrobial therapy was forgone as no overt signs of infection were present. Also of note, this culture was negative for the previously cultured organisms (*S. anginosus*,

TABLE 1: Ratio of ceftolozane concentrations between bone tissue and plasma.

	Dose	Time after last dose (hours)	Bone: serum concentration ratio
Rabbit model	1 g q 8 h	1.5	*Marrow*: 14.1%–17.5% *Bone*: 6.2%–9.0%
Rat model	20 mg/kg	2	27%
		8	40%

Source: unpublished manufacturer data.

TABLE 2: Bone penetration of cephalosporins and β-lactamase inhibitors [12].

	Time after last dose (hours)	Bone (mg/kg): serum concentration (mg/L) ratio[a]	Method
Cephalosporins			
Ceftriaxone	0.2–8	0.07–0.17	HPLC
Cefotaxime	0.75–4	0.02–0.28	Bioassay
Cefuroxime (osteomyelitis)	1	0.04–0.08	HPLC
Cefazolin	0.9	0.179	HPLC
Cefepime	1-2	0.46–0.76	HPLC
Ceftazidime (ischemic bone)	1-2	0.04–0.08	HPLC
Ceftazidime	2	0.54	Bioassay
β-Lactamase inhibitors			
Clavulanic acid	1	1.14–1.76	Bioassay
Sulbactam	0.25–4	0.17–0.71	Gas chromatography
Tazobactam	*1.5*	*0.22–0.26*	*HPLC*

[a]Assumed bone density of 1 kg/L was assumed if not reported.
HPLC: high-performance liquid chromatography.

Granulicatella adiacens, and *S. maltophilia*). At 30-week follow-up, fasciocutaneous graft had taken well and no signs of infection were present.

3. Discussion

Ceftolozane-tazobactam's many unique properties including the presence of a 7-aminothiadiazole (activity against Gram-negative organisms), alkoximino group (stability against β-lactamases), dimethylacetic acid moiety (activity against *P. aeruginosa*), and a bulky pyrazole ring (stability in the presence of AmpC β-lactamase) allow for increased activity against broad-spectrum Gram-negative organisms including some ESBL-producing Enterobacteriaceae and MDR *P. aeruginosa* [5, 6].

Ceftolozane-tazobactam's activity against these MDR Gram-negative pathogens in cIAI and cUTI is promising to clinicians. However, further information regarding its utility for off-label indications is speculative at best and based mostly upon unpublished manufacturer data from Phase I and II trials. In the case of osteomyelitis, variable bone to plasma ratio has been seen in animal data ranging from 5.2% to 9.0% in rabbit model and up to 40.0% in rat model femur concentration (Table 1). Nonetheless these ranges of results are comparable to cephalosporins that are widely used in osteomyelitis such as cefazolin and cefepime which have bone concentrations at 17.9% and 46%–76%, respectively (Table 2) [12]. While there are no Clinical & Laboratory Standards Institute (CLSI) approved MIC to predict sensitivity to *S. maltophilia*, one may speculate that a breakpoint of 0.5 mg/L may offer a reasonable chance of treatment success.

In this patient case, ceftolozane-tazobactam was demonstrated *in vitro* to be active against the offending pathogens including MDR *S. maltophilia*. The wound evidenced healing during and after completing antibiotic therapy and at posttreatment follow-up visits. Tolerability to ceftolozane-tazobactam beyond 14 days of treatment has previously not been demonstrated but was well tolerated in this case with no adverse drug reactions.

While further investigations are needed to examine ceftolozane-tazobactam's utility in off-label indication, the authors felt that it was important to share this experience with ceftolozane-tazobactam in this case of polymicrobial osteomyelitis. Ceftolozane-tazobactam may offer a possible alternative for clinicians faced with limited options in the treatment of resistant pathogens including MDR *S. maltophilia*.

Competing Interests

The authors declare that they have no competing interests.

References

[1] Y.-T. Chang, C.-Y. Lin, Y.-H. Chen, and P.-R. Hsueh, "Update on infections caused by Stenotrophomonas maltophilia with particular attention to resistance mechanisms and therapeutic options," *Frontiers in Microbiology*, vol. 6, article 893, 2015.

[2] M. E. Falagas, P.-E. Valkimadi, Y.-T. Huang, D. K. Matthaiou, and P.-R. Hsueh, "Therapeutic options for *Stenotrophomonas maltophilia* infections beyond co-trimoxazole: a systematic review," *Journal of Antimicrobial Chemotherapy*, vol. 62, no. 5, pp. 889–894, 2008.

[3] D. J. Farrell, H. S. Sader, and R. N. Jones, "Antimicrobial susceptibilities of a worldwide collection of *Stenotrophomonas maltophilia* isolates tested against tigecycline and agents commonly used for *S. maltophilia* infections," *Antimicrobial Agents and Chemotherapy*, vol. 54, no. 6, pp. 2735–2737, 2010.

[4] H. S. Sader, R. K. Flamm, and R. N. Jones, "Tigecycline activity tested against antimicrobial resistant surveillance subsets of clinical bacteria collected worldwide (2011)," *Diagnostic Microbiology and Infectious Disease*, vol. 76, no. 2, pp. 217–221, 2013.

[5] J. C. Cho, M. A. Fiorenza, and S. J. Estrada, "Ceftolozane/tazobactam: a novel cephalosporin/β-lactamase inhibitor combination," *Pharmacotherapy*, vol. 35, no. 7, pp. 701–715, 2015.

[6] D. Cluck, P. Lewis, B. Stayer, J. Spivey, and J. Moorman, "Ceftolozane-tazobactam: a new-generation cephalosporin," *American Journal of Health-System Pharmacy*, vol. 72, no. 24, pp. 2135–2146, 2015.

[7] R. Soliman, S. Lynch, E. Meader et al., "Successful ceftolozane/tazobactam treatment of chronic pulmonary infection with pan–resistant *Pseudomonas aeruginosa*," *JMM Case Reports*, 2015.

[8] A. Alqaid, C. K. Dougherty, and S. Ahmad, "Triple antibiotic therapy with ceftolozane/tazobactam, colistin and rifampin for pan-resistant Pseudomonas aeruginosa ventilator-associated pneumonia," *SWRCCC*, vol. 3, no. 11, pp. 35–39, 2015.

[9] J. E. Garcia Sanchez, M. L. Vazquez Lopez, A. M. Blazquez De Castro et al., "Aztreonam/clavulanic acid in the treatment of serious infections caused by *Stenotrophomonas maltophilia* in neutropenic patients: case reports," *Journal of Chemotherapy*, vol. 9, no. 3, pp. 238–240, 1997.

[10] C. Leung, P. Drew, and E. A. Azzopardi, "Extended multidrug-resistant *Stenotrophomonas maltophilia* septicemia in a severely burnt patient," *Journal of Burn Care and Research*, vol. 31, no. 6, p. 966, 2010.

[11] P. N. Pérez, M. A. Ramírez, J. A. Fernández, and L. L. de Guevara, "A patient presenting with cholangitis due to *Stenotrophomonas maltophilia* and *Pseudomonas aeruginosa* successfully treated with intrabiliary colistine," *Infectious Disease Reports*, vol. 6, no. 2, pp. 17–19, 2014.

[12] C. B. Landersdorfer, J. B. Bulitta, M. Kinzig, U. Holzgrabe, and F. Sörgel, "Penetration of antibacterials into bone: pharmacokinetic, pharmacodynamic and bioanalytical considerations," *Clinical Pharmacokinetics*, vol. 48, no. 2, pp. 89–124, 2009.

A Rare Case of Glossitis due to *Pasteurella multocida* after a Cat Scratch

Negin Niknam, Thien Doan, and Elizabeth Revere

Hofstra Northwell School of Medicine, Hempstead, NY, USA

Correspondence should be addressed to Negin Niknam; negin.niknam93@gmail.com

Academic Editor: Larry M. Bush

Pasteurella is one of the zoonotic pathogens that can cause variety of serious infections in animals and humans such as bacteremia, septic shock, endocarditis, meningitis, prosthetic and native valve infections, osteomyelitis, skin and soft tissue infections, abscesses, and even pneumonia with empyema. However, there have been few reports of upper respiratory involvements like tonsillitis and epiglottitis in humans. We present a case of recurrent *Pasteurella* glossitis after a cat scratch which has not been reported in humans.

1. Introduction

Pasteurella are small Gram-negative coccobacilli that are primarily animal pathogens. *Pasteurella multocida* is a component of the normal upper respiratory tract flora of fowl and mammals, especially felines. Other *Pasteurella* species can be found in the oral cavity of a variety of animals including dogs, cats, pigs, hamsters, and horses.

Pasteurella can cause a variety of diseases in animals, such as fowl cholera in domestic fowl, shipping fever in cattle, hemorrhagic septicemia in cattle and lambs, fibrinous pneumonia in cattle, snuffles in rabbits, and other focal infections [1]. However these organisms can cause several infections in humans, usually as a result of cat scratches or cat or dog bites or licks. There have been multiple cases of septic shock [2, 3], bacteremia [4], prosthetic valve endocarditis [5, 6], aortic endograft infection [7], primary shoulder involvement [8], total knee replacement infection [9], meningitis [10, 11], and even pneumonia [12, 13] or empyema [14]. It was also reported in deep sternal wound infection [15], peritonitis due to peritoneal dialysis [16, 17], endophthalmitis [18], chorioamnionitis from vaginal transmission [19], frontal osteomyelitis Pott's puffy tumor [20], infection in solid organ transplantation [21], lung and liver abscess [22], and even failed renal transplant [23]. However, there were rare cases of tonsillitis [24] or epiglottitis [25, 26] in humans. There has been one report of Ludwig's angina after a dog bite [27] but glossitis was mostly seen in animals [28].

2. Case Presentation

A 56-year-old male with a past medical history of hypertension, hyperlipidemia, gastroesophageal reflux disease, recurrent otitis media leading to hearing impairment, and tonsillectomy, presented to the Emergency Department with tongue swelling, dysphagia, drooling, and shortness of breath. He stated that about 5 days prior to presentation he experienced throat pain and went to his Ear, Nose, Throat (ENT) specialist, who felt his symptoms could be due to lymphadenitis. He was prescribed Clindamycin, which the patient had tolerated in the past. He continued to have worsening throat pain and difficulty swallowing and presented to the Emergency Department. In the Emergency Department a CT scan of his neck was performed and was unremarkable as well as direct laryngoscopy. He was discharged with Dexamethasone and Ketorolac. The next day he started to develop severe tongue pain and swelling to the point that he could not speak or move his tongue. He was evaluated by ENT specialist who noticed tongue edema tenderness and enlargement suggestive of glossitis with no posterior pharyngeal edema.

His laboratory work shown was remarkable for a white blood cell count: 14.1 K/uL, neutrophil count: 11.73 K/uL, hemoglobin: 15.2 g/dL, and platelets count: 177 K/uL.

A repeat CT scan of the neck with contrast showed asymmetric fatty reticulation along the left sublingual space without focal mass or rim-enhancing fluid collection and no evidence of odontogenic abscess. Blood cultures were sent and the patient was admitted to the ICU for glossitis or possible Ludwig's angina. He was initially started on Dexamethasone and Clindamycin in view of his penicillin allergy which was remote and reported as a rash.

On the second day, blood cultures revealed Gram-negative rods. The antibiotics were switched from Clindamycin to Aztreonam and Metronidazole. The next day the Gram-negative organism was identified as *Pasteurella multocida*. On further investigation, the patient stated that he was scratched by his new cat two weeks prior on his right wrist, which resolved without complications. Aztreonam and Metronidazole were discontinued and the patient was started on Imipenem.

Further laboratory work showed improving leukocytosis and repeat blood cultures were negative the next day. Echocardiogram was performed and showed normal valves and normal right ventricular size and function, but moderate to severe global left ventricular dysfunction. The patient was diagnosed with systolic heart failure. The patient's symptoms gradually resolved and he was discharged home with Ertapenem via PICC line for a total of 14 days. However, 10 days after discharge the patient presented again with a milder swelling of his tongue with no signs of sepsis or airway compromise. He was admitted again and blood cultures were sent which were negative. The white blood cell count and neck and chest X-rays were within normal limits. The course of Ertapenem was completed and he was discharged home. The patient did not report any further episodes of tongue or throat swelling.

3. Discussion

P. multocida can cause a range of infections in wild and domesticated animals as well as humans from a mild wound infection to severe sepsis and death. The diseases are usually different in animals, such as the glossitis that was reported only in animals.

Infections with *P. multocida* can be divided into three categories in humans:

(i) Skin and soft tissue infections: following animal bites or scratches; bites and scratches can also result in abscesses, necrotizing soft tissue infections, septic arthritis, and osteomyelitis.

(ii) Serious invasive infection often unrelated to animal bites, such as meningitis, intraabdominal infection, endocarditis, or ocular infection.

(iii) Oral and respiratory infections, usually in the setting of chronic pulmonary disease.

Pasteurella respiratory infections are rare and have no distinctive characteristics. *P. multocida* may not be suspected as the infecting pathogen but should be considered as a serious pathogen in patients with cat exposure including bites, licks, and scratches.

Glossitis has been never reported in humans and is not well described in the literature. In our case diagnosis was made clinically.

4. Conclusion

Glossitis could be a rare presentation of *Pasteurella multocida*, which can be diagnosed clinically and treated the same as other *Pasteurella* infections.

Competing Interests

The authors declare that there is no conflict of interests regarding the publication of this paper.

References

[1] P. N. Acha and B. Szyfres, *Zoonoses and Communicable Diseases Common to Man and Animals*, Pan American Health Organization, Washington, DC, USA, 2001.

[2] A. C. Adler, C. Cestero, and R. B. Brown, "Septic shock from *Pasturella multocida* following a cat bite: case report and review of literature," *Connecticut Medicine*, vol. 75, no. 10, pp. 603–605, 2011.

[3] J. Orsini, R. Perez, A. Llosa, and N. Araguez, "Non-zoonotic *Pasteurella multocida* infection as a cause of septic shock in a patient with liver cirrhosis: a case report and review of the literature," *Journal of Global Infectious Diseases*, vol. 5, no. 4, pp. 176–178, 2013.

[4] P. Courtin, E. Brugière, D. Torro, D. Magnin, P. Guinot, and J. L. Lemaître, "Pasteurella multocida septicemia. Apropos of a case," *Cahiers d'Anesthesiologie*, vol. 42, no. 5, pp. 609–611, 1994.

[5] R. E. Nettles and D. J. Sexton, "*Pasteurella multocida* prosthetic valve endocarditis: case report and review," *Clinical Infectious Diseases*, vol. 25, no. 4, pp. 920–921, 1997.

[6] F. Camou, O. Guisset, S. Pereyre et al., "Endocarditis due to *Pasteurella* sp. Two cases," *Médecine et Maladies Infectieuses*, vol. 35, no. 11, pp. 556–559, 2005.

[7] E. J. Silberfein, P. H. Lin, R. L. Bush, W. Zhou, and A. B. Lumsden, "Aortic endograft infection due to *Pasteurella multocida* following a rabbit bite," *Journal of Vascular Surgery*, vol. 43, no. 2, pp. 393–395, 2006.

[8] D. Y. Ding, A. Orengo, M. J. Alaia, and J. D. Zuckerman, "*Pasteurella multocida* infection in a primary shoulder arthroplasty after cat scratch: case report and review of literature," *Journal of Shoulder and Elbow Surgery*, vol. 24, no. 6, pp. e159–e163, 2015.

[9] K. B. Ferguson, R. Bharadwaj, A. MacDonald, B. Syme, and A. M. Bal, "*Pasteurella multocida* infected total knee arthroplasty: a case report and review of the literature," *Annals of the Royal College of Surgeons of England*, vol. 96, no. 2, pp. e1–e4, 2014.

[10] S. Kawashima, N. Matsukawa, Y. Ueki, M. Hattori, and K. Ojika, "*Pasteurella multocida* meningitis caused by kissing animals: a case report and review of the literature," *Journal of Neurology*, vol. 257, no. 4, pp. 653–654, 2010.

[11] A. Kumar, H. R. Devlin, and H. Vellend, "*Pasteurella multocida* meningitis in an adult: case report and review," *Reviews of Infectious Diseases*, vol. 12, no. 3, pp. 440–448, 1990.

[12] J. Ferreira, K. Treger, and K. Busey, "Pneumonia and disseminated bacteremia with *Pasteurella multocida* in the immune competent host: a case report and a review of the literature," *Respiratory Medicine Case Reports*, vol. 15, pp. 54–56, 2015.

[13] Y. Oyama, K. Naoki, H. Kunikane et al., "Severe *Pasteurella multocida* pneumonia by close contact with a pet in chronic respiratory failure," *Nihon Naika Gakkai Zasshi*, vol. 96, no. 7, pp. 1467–1469, 2007.

[14] T. Unoki, I. Nakamura, T. Mori, T. Kamei, M. Kunihiro, and N. Ueda, "An autopsied case of *Pasteurella multocida* empyema with review of the literature," *Kansenshogaku Zasshi*, vol. 58, no. 7, pp. 703–708, 1984.

[15] R. Baillot, P. Voisine, L. M. Côté, and Y. Longtin, "Deep sternal wound infection due to *Pasteurella multocida*: the first case report and review of literature," *Infection*, vol. 39, no. 6, pp. 575–578, 2011.

[16] P. G. Poliquin, P. Lagacé-Wiens, M. Verrelli, D. W. Allen, and J. M. Embil, "*Pasteurella* species peritoneal dialysis-associated peritonitis: household pets as a risk factor," *Canadian Journal of Infectious Diseases and Medical Microbiology*, vol. 26, no. 1, pp. 52–55, 2015.

[17] P. M. Sol, N. C. van de Kar, and M. F. Schreuder, "Cat induced Pasteurella multocida peritonitis in peritoneal dialysis: a case report and review of the literature," *International Journal of Hygiene and Environmental Health*, vol. 216, no. 2, pp. 211–213, 2013.

[18] N. P. L. D. Burgener, E. Baglivo, S. Harbarth, C. Sahabo, D. Pittet, and A. B. Safran, "Pasteurella multocida endophthalmitis: case report and review of the literature," *Klinische Monatsblatter fur Augenheilkunde*, vol. 222, no. 3, pp. 231–233, 2005.

[19] G. P. Wong, N. Cimolai, J. E. Dimmick, and T. R. Martin, "*Pasteurella multocida* chorioamnionitis from vaginal transmission," *Acta Obstetricia et Gynecologica Scandinavica*, vol. 71, no. 5, pp. 384–387, 1992.

[20] R. Skomro and K. L. McClean, "Frontal osteomyelitis (Pott's puffy tumour) associated with *Pasteurella multocida*—a case report and review of the literature," *Canadian Journal of Infectious Diseases*, vol. 9, no. 2, pp. 115–121, 1998.

[21] E. S. Christenson, H. M. Ahmed, and C. M. Durand, "Pasteurella multocida infection in solid organ transplantation," *The Lancet Infectious Diseases*, vol. 15, no. 2, pp. 235–240, 2015.

[22] P. Goussard, R. P. Gie, F. Steyn, G. J. Rossouw, and S. Kling, "Pasteurella multocida lung and liver abscess in an immune-competent child," *Pediatric Pulmonology*, vol. 41, no. 3, pp. 275–278, 2006.

[23] R. R. Mayo and D. Lipschutz, "An interesting case of failed renal transplant complicated by a lymphocele infected with *Pasteurella multocida* and a review of the literature," *American Journal of Nephrology*, vol. 16, no. 4, pp. 361–366, 1996.

[24] G. D. Ramdeen, R. J. Smith, E. A. Smith, and L. M. Baddour, "*Pasteurella multocida* tonsillitis: case report and review," *Clinical Infectious Diseases*, vol. 20, no. 4, pp. 1055–1057, 1995.

[25] N. Wine, Y. Lim, and J. Fierer, "*Pasteurella multocida* epiglottitis," *Archives of Otolaryngology—Head and Neck Surgery*, vol. 123, no. 7, pp. 759–761, 1997.

[26] P. J. Harris and M. B. Osswald, "*Pasteurella multocida* epiglottitis: a review and report of a new case with associated chronic lymphocytic leukemia," *Ear, Nose and Throat Journal*, vol. 89, no. 12, article E4, 2010.

[27] M. S. Dryden and D. Dalgliesh, "Pasteurella multocida from a dog causing Ludwig's angina," *The Lancet*, vol. 347, no. 8994, p. 123, 1996.

[28] J. Arnbjerg, "*Pasteurella multocida* from canine and feline teeth, with a case report of glossitis calcinosa in a dog caused by *P. multocida*," *Nordisk Veterinaermedicin*, vol. 30, no. 7-8, pp. 324–332, 1978.

Refractory Toxic Shock-Like Syndrome from *Streptococcus dysgalactiae* ssp. *equisimilis* and Intravenous Immunoglobulin as Salvage Therapy

Marjan Islam,[1] Dennis Karter,[1] Jerry Altshuler,[2] Diana Altshuler,[3] David Schwartz,[4,5] and Gianluca Torregrossa[6]

[1]*Department of Medicine, Mount Sinai Beth Israel, New York, NY 10003, USA*
[2]*Department of Pharmacy, Mount Sinai Beth Israel, New York, NY 10003, USA*
[3]*Department of Pharmacy, NYU Langone Medical Center, New York, NY 10016, USA*
[4]*Department of Medicine, NYU Langone Medical Center, New York, NY 10016, USA*
[5]*NYU School of Medicine, New York, NY 10016, USA*
[6]*Department of Cardiac Surgery, Mount Sinai Beth Israel, New York, NY 10003, USA*

Correspondence should be addressed to Marjan Islam; mislam@chpnet.org

Academic Editor: Antonella Marangoni

Infections from *Streptococcus dysgalactiae* ssp. *equisimilis* (SDSE) can cause a wide variety of infections, ranging from mild cellulitis to invasive disease, such as endocarditis and streptococcal toxic shock-like syndrome (TSLS). Despite prompt and appropriate antibiotics, mortality rates associated with shock have remained exceedingly high, prompting the need for adjunctive therapy. IVIG has been proposed as a possible adjunct, given its ability to neutralize a wide variety of superantigens and modulate a dysregulated inflammatory response. We present the first reported cases of successful IVIG therapy for reversing shock in the treatment of SDSE TSLS.

1. Introduction

Streptococcus dysgalactiae ssp. *equisimilis* (SDSE) are gram-positive β-hemolytic group C and G streptococci that commonly colonize the human respiratory, gastrointestinal, and female genital tracts. Epidemiologically and pathologically, this species is very similar to Group A streptococcus, capable of causing infections ranging from mild cellulitis or pharyngitis, to life-threatening invasive disease such as necrotizing fasciitis, meningitis, endocarditis, and septic shock. It has rarely been reported to cause streptococcal toxic shock-like syndrome (TSLS), with some strains found to produce streptococcal exotoxins [1]. We present what we believe to be the first 2 reported cases of successful intravenous immunoglobulin (IVIG) therapy for adult refractory SDSE TSLS.

2. Case Report 1

An 82-year-old male with history of heart failure, atrial fibrillation, diabetes, and multiple prior admissions for cellulitis presented to the ED with right lower-extremity erythema with associated altered mental status, fever of 101.8°F, hypotension (72/40 mmHg), and tachycardia (146 bpm). He was admitted to the MICU for septic shock from presumed cellulitis, with initial labs significant for a lactate of 4.5 mmol/L, acute kidney injury (SCr 1.9 mg/dL), leukocytosis (white blood cell count 17 k/μL, 88% neutrophils), and a procalcitonin of 38.64 ng/mL. He was requiring 26 mcg/min of norepinephrine for refractory hypotension, and vancomycin with piperacillin/tazobactam for cellulitis was initiated.

On day 2, his blood cultures grew SDSE, and vasopressin (0.04 U/min) and dobutamine were added to maintain cardiac output due to a presumed sepsis-induced myocardial depression. Despite hemodynamic support, the patient remained in shock, raising concern for development of a refractory TSLS. Surgery was consulted for potential necrotizing fasciitis and IVIG (Gamunex®-C) (1 g/kg day 1, 0.5 g/kg days 2-3) and clindamycin were initiated.

The following evening, the patient's vasopressor requirements had lessened, eventually titrated off completely over the following 24 hours. His lactate had cleared, and he did not require any surgical intervention. He was narrowed to penicillin on day 3 and transferred out of the MICU the following day. Workup for a source was inconclusive, with an abdominal CT scan showing no fluid collections or abscess. He was deemed stable for discharge on day 8.

3. Case Report 2

A 37-year-old male with history of coarctation of the aorta presented to the ED with fevers and diaphoresis for 2 weeks. He was initially treated for flu-like symptoms but developed rigors, abdominal pain, and jaundice, prompting him to return to our institution. On admission, he was febrile to 101°F, thrombocytopenic (platelet count 15 k/μL), with leukocytosis (white blood cell count 17.5 k/μL, 96% neutrophils), and with acute renal failure (SCr 1.79 mg/dL). He was started on broad spectrum antibiotics, which were subsequently narrowed to ceftriaxone (a rash developed with penicillin) and clindamycin after sensitivities revealed penicillin-susceptible SDSE (penicillin MIC < 0.06). Gentamicin was later added in the setting of persistent fevers and tachycardia. A transesophageal echocardiogram (TEE) revealed a 1.6 cm mobile tricuspid valve vegetation and a possible abscess at the aortic root after initial transthoracic echocardiogram (TTE) was inconclusive. His admission EKG showed a new 1st degree AV block.

By day 9, his heart block progressed to type II second-degree AV block, with periods of complete heart block. With concern for infectious spread to the conduction system and a perivalvular abscess, he was taken emergently to the OR for radical debridement of the aortic roots, aortomitral curtain, and interatrial septum. He underwent an extensive bovine patch repair of the aortomitral curtain, interatrial septum, and pericardium. He also underwent enlargement of the aortic annulus and roots and placement of a mechanical aortic valve and permanent pacemaker. Pathology from the aortic valve revealed acute inflammatory cells with gram-positive cocci. Postoperatively, the patient remained febrile, and antimicrobials were transiently broadened. On day 14, a TTE revealed a new mitral valve vegetation, with a perforated anterior leaflet and severe mitral regurgitation.

On day 26, repeat TEE revealed progression of mitral valve endocarditis, with a flail anterior leaflet with a second perforation, mandating surgical intervention. On day 28, the patient underwent repeat sternotomy with debridement of the mitral valve endocarditis and extensive reconstruction of the cardiac skeleton, requiring a repeat aortic and mitral valve replacement. Postoperatively, he became hypotensive and progressed into a refractory vasoplegic shock. He was given 2 doses of methylene blue and started on epinephrine

(5 mcg/min), norepinephrine (19 mcg/min), and vasopressin (0.1 U/min). Despite adequate vasopressors, he remained vasoplegic, and IVIG was attempted as salvage therapy. He underwent 2 days of 100 g (1 g/kg adjust body weight) IVIG (Gamunex-C), which allowed for titration off vasopressor support over the following 2 days.

An extensive infectious workup followed to identify other potential causes for a possible culture-negative endocarditis, including serology for *B. henselae, B. quintana, Brucella, Coccidioides, Q Fever,* and *Rocky Mountain Spotted Fever,* and PCR for *Tropheryma whipplei,* all of which returned negative. On day 46, the patient underwent a final TTE, which showed no valvular vegetation. He was deemed stable for discharge, with follow-up in the cardiac surgery clinic.

4. Discussion

SDSE belong to a group of pyogenic streptococci, often referred to as β-hemolytic streptococci. While they were considered nonpathogenic for years, recent population-based studies have revealed invasive SDSE to have a similar disease profile as invasive *Streptococcus pyogenes* [1]. SDSE primarily present as skin and soft tissue infections, though invasive forms may present as osteomyelitis, pulmonary or intra-abdominal abscesses, meningitis, endocarditis, or necrotizing fasciitis. Septic shock and multisystem organ failure may result from TSLS. While injection drug users and immunosuppression pose increased risk, previously healthy individuals can develop severe infections as well [2].

Molecular studies have shown SDSE to display nearly identical virulence factors as *S. pyogenes,* though the etiology behind the emergence of more human-invasive strains remains undetermined. The principal mechanism appears to be translocation of mobile DNA elements into bacterial genomes by bacteriophages [1]. Indeed certain superantigen genes such as *speA, speC,* and *speM* have been found in SDSE strains nearly identical to those in *S. pyogenes.* Further, SDSE have consistently displayed the M protein common to *S. pyogenes,* conferring resistance to phagocytosis. In addition, *S. pyogenes* and SDSE share adhesion virulence factors such as fibronectin and plasminogen binding proteins, allowing for colonization of epithelium and invasion into the bloodstream [1].

Streptococcal TSLS is the most severe manifestation of invasive disease from streptococci, with case-mortality rates reported as high as 81% [3]. The pathogenesis behind SDSE-mediated shock likely involves the release of superantigens known as streptococcal pyrogenic exotoxins (SPEs). SPEs activate T-cell receptor molecules that directly interact with the MHC class II on antigen-presenting cells, leading to massive T-cell proliferation and a cytokine storm [2]. The effects of such a large influx of cytokines can precipitate severe vasoplegia and hemodynamic collapse, conferring the mortality seen in streptococcal TSLS [4].

SDSE remains nearly universally susceptible to penicillin and other β-lactam agents [1]. Clinical investigations have identified the need for an adjunctive therapy however, as high mortality rates persist despite prompt antimicrobial therapy. Since many streptococcal superantigens contribute to the pathogenesis of invasive streptococcal infections, IVIG has been suggested as the plausible adjunct, given its ability to modulate the inflammatory response elicited by virulence factors and counteract a wide variety of superantigens simultaneously [5]. It is postulated that only individuals who lack neutralizing antibodies to the putative virulence factors, such as the SPEs or M-protein, develop invasive streptococcal infections and TSLS [6]. Indeed studies have demonstrated patients with bacteremia and TSLS lacked antibodies directed against *speB*, suggesting passive immunization of patients lacking neutralizing antibodies may modify the course of this toxin-mediated disease [7].

Prior reports demonstrated IVIG's capability to block in vitro T-cell activation of staphylococcal and streptococcal superantigens. Emerging evidence has also suggested IVIG may contain superantigen-neutralizing antibodies [8]. Multiple case reports have demonstrated improved clinical outcomes in patients with TSLS who have received IVIG [9–11], while larger clinical series have supported its use. Kaul et al. demonstrated a higher 30-day survival in patients with TSLS who received IVIG compared to controls (67% versus 34%, $p = 0.02$), demonstrating an odds ratio for survival of 8.1 (CI 1.6–45, $p = < 0.01$) [8]. Further, they demonstrated reduction in bacterial mitogenicity and T-cell production of IL-6 and TNF-α in patients who received IVIG [8]. Darenberg et al. compared IVIG therapy to placebo in patients with streptococcal TSLS and demonstrated a 3.6-fold lower mortality rate in the IVIG group, though the study was underpowered ($p = 0.3$) [12]. The IVIG group also had significantly lower sepsis-related organ failure assessment scores on days 2 ($p = 0.02$) and 3 ($p = 0.04$) compared to placebo, while also demonstrating increased plasma neutralizing activity against superantigens expressed by autologous isolates ($p = 0.03$) [12].

Upon revisiting the cases presented, it is plausible that our patients lacked the appropriate antibodies necessary to eradicate a putative virulence factor, leading to an invasive SDSE infection and ultimately succumbing into a refractory TSLS. Administration of IVIG likely helped modulate their profoundly dysregulated inflammatory responses, neutralizing the virulent super-antigens expressed by SDSE and allowing for hemodynamics to normalize. The successful use of IVIG for refractory TSLS demonstrates the utility of this novel adjunctive therapy, while highlighting the changing epidemiology and pathogenicity of SDSE.

Additional Points

The information in this paper was not presented in any meetings at the time of submission.

Competing Interests

None of the authors have a financial relationship with a commercial entity that has an interest in the subject of this paper.

References

[1] C. M. Brandt and B. Spellerberg, "Human infections due to *Streptococcus dysgalactiae* Subspedes *equisimilis*," *Clinical Infectious Diseases*, vol. 49, no. 5, pp. 766–772, 2009.

[2] T. M. Korman, A. Boers, T. M. Gooding, N. Curtis, and K. Visvanathan, "Fatal case of toxic shock-like syndrome due to group C streptococcus associated with superantigen exotoxin," *Journal of Clinical Microbiology*, vol. 42, no. 6, pp. 2866–2869, 2004.

[3] S. Natoli, C. Fimiani, N. Faglieri et al., "Toxic shock syndrome due to group C Streptococci. A case report," *Intensive Care Medicine*, vol. 22, no. 9, pp. 985–989, 1996.

[4] I. C. Ojukwu, D. W. Newton, A. E. Luque, M. Y. S. Kotb, and M. Menegus, "Invasive Group C Streptococcus infection associated with rhabdomyolysis and disseminated intravascular coagulation in a previously healthy adult," *Scandinavian Journal of Infectious Diseases*, vol. 33, no. 3, pp. 227–229, 2001.

[5] A. Norrby-Teglund, H. Basma, J. Andersson, A. McGeer, D. E. Low, and M. Kotb, "Varying titers of neutralizing antibodies to streptococcal superantigens in different preparations of normal polyspecific immunoglobulin G: implications for therapeutic efficacy," *Clinical Infectious Diseases*, vol. 26, no. 3, pp. 631–638, 1998.

[6] S. E. Holm, A. Norrby, A.-M. Bergholm, and M. Norgren, "Aspects of pathogenesis of serious group A streptococcal infections in Sweden, 1988-1989," *Journal of Infectious Diseases*, vol. 166, no. 1, pp. 31–37, 1992.

[7] W. Barry, L. Hudgins, S. T. Donta, and E. L. Pesanti, "Intravenous immunoglobulin therapy for toxic shock syndrome," *The Journal of the American Medical Association*, vol. 267, no. 24, pp. 3315–3316, 1992.

[8] R. Kaul, A. McGeer, A. Norrby–Teglund et al., "Intravenous immunoglobulin therapy for streptococcal toxic shock syndrome—a comparative observational study," *Clinical Infectious Diseases*, vol. 28, no. 4, pp. 800–807, 1999.

[9] D. Nadal, R. P. Lauener, C. P. Braegger et al., "T cell activation and cytokine release in streptococcal toxic shock-like syndrome," *The Journal of Pediatrics*, vol. 122, no. 5, pp. 727–729, 1993.

[10] J. M. Yong, R. J. Holdsworth, and D. Parratt, "Necrotising fasciitis," *The Lancet*, vol. 343, no. 8910, pp. 1427–1428, 1994.

[11] F. Lamothe, P. D'Amico, P. Ghosn, C. Tremblay, J. Braidy, and J.-V. Patenaude, "Clinical usefulness of intravenous human immunoglobulins in invasive group A streptococcal infections: case report and review," *Clinical Infectious Diseases*, vol. 21, no. 6, pp. 1469–1470, 1995.

[12] J. Darenberg, N. Ihendyane, J. Sjölin et al., "Intravenous immunoglobulin G therapy in streptococcal toxic shock syndrome: a European randomized, double-blind, placebo-controlled trial," *Clinical Infectious Diseases*, vol. 37, no. 3, pp. 333–340, 2003.

9

Strongyloides Hyperinfection in a Renal Transplant Patient: Always Be on the Lookout

Murtaza Mazhar,[1] Ijlal Akbar Ali,[1] and Nelson Iván Agudelo Higuita[2]

[1]Department of Internal Medicine, Suite 6300, 800 Stanton L Young Boulevard, Oklahoma University Health Sciences Center, Oklahoma City, OK 73104, USA
[2]Department of Infectious Diseases, Suite 7300, 800 Stanton L Young Boulevard, Oklahoma University Health Sciences Center, Oklahoma City, OK 73104, USA

Correspondence should be addressed to Ijlal Akbar Ali; ijlalakbar-ali@ouhsc.edu

Academic Editor: Fariborz Mansour-ghanaei

We present a case of a 71-year-old Vietnamese man with chronic kidney disease secondary to adult polycystic kidney disease. He had been a prisoner of war before undergoing a successful cadaveric renal transplant in the United States. He presented to clinic one year after the transplant with gross hematuria, productive cough, intermittent chills, and weight loss. Long standing peripheral eosinophilia of 600–1200/μL triggered further evaluation. A wet mount of stool revealed *Strongyloides stercoralis* larvae. A computed tomography (CT) of chest showed findings suggestive of extension of the infection to the lungs. The patient was treated with a three-week course of ivermectin with complete resolution of signs, symptoms, peripheral eosinophilia, and the positive IgG serology. Strongyloides infection in renal transplant patient is very rare and often presents with hyperinfection, associated with high mortality rates. The American Transplant Society recommends pretransplant screening with stool examination and *Strongyloides stercoralis* antibody in recipients and donors from endemic areas or with eosinophilia. It is imperative that healthcare professionals involved in the care of these individuals be cognizant of these recommendations as it is a very preventable and treatable entity.

1. Introduction

Strongyloides stercoralis is an intestinal nematode that is unique in its ability to complete its entire life cycle in the human host. The infection can be therefore present for decades without causing symptoms. In immunocompromised hosts, progression of the chronic intestinal infection can lead to a potentially fatal hyperinfection syndrome. We describe an interesting case of an immunocompromised Vietnamese man with likely hyperinfection two decades after initial exposure to the parasite.

2. Case Presentation

A 71-year-old Vietnamese man was diagnosed with chronic kidney disease secondary to adult polycystic kidney disease two years after immigrating to the United States. He had been a prisoner of war for 14 years in the jungles of Vietnam 5

years before arriving to the US. He underwent a successful cadaveric renal transplant 19 years after immigration from a US-born donor. No other details from the donor were available. The patient's immunosuppressive regimen consisted of prednisone, mycophenolate mofetil, and tacrolimus. One year after the transplant, he presented to his nephrologist for the evaluation of gross hematuria. He also reported cough productive of yellow sputum, shortness of breath, intermittent chills, weight loss, and fatigue of several weeks duration. The physical exam was notable for the presence of rales on both lung bases, left more than right. The abdomen was soft with no hepatosplenomegaly or masses. No rash was noted.

A urine analysis showed hematuria, pyuria, and proteinuria. The urine culture failed to isolate an organism. A cystoscopy showed no abnormalities and a cytology of a bladder wash showed atypical inflammatory cells. He was empirically treated with a ten-day course of cephalexin for a presumed urinary tract infection with resolution of the

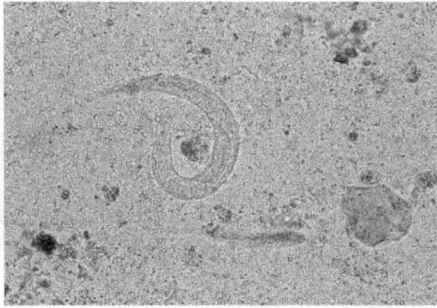

FIGURE 1: Wet mount of stool showing Strongyloides larvae.

hematuria. Peripheral eosinophilia of $1200/\mu$L (normal range $0–500/\mu$L) [1] was noted on the complete blood count (CBC) and further evaluation of the records showed that he had had intermittent mild peripheral blood eosinophilia ($600–800/\mu$L range) for at least 7 years before transplantation. No screening for *S. stercoralis* had been done and screening for HTLV-1 was negative. A *Strongyloides stercoralis* IgG was therefore obtained which yielded a positive result of 1.96 IU (<1 IU is considered negative). Numerous Strongyloides larvae were easily identified on a wet mount of a stool specimen by their morphological characteristics of a large genital primordium and short buccal capsule (Figure 1). Larvae were not detected in the urine or sputum despite repeated testing. Blood cultures were negative. A computed tomography (CT) of the chest showed mild peribronchial thickening with a mosaic pattern within the bilateral lobes and ill-defined patchy nodular opacity within the posterior segment of the right upper lobe suggestive of infectious etiology. The patient was treated with a three-week course of ivermectin at a dose of 200 μg/kg/day with resolution of his symptoms before the end of therapy and therefore a bronchoalveolar lavage was not pursued. Larvae were no longer visualized in 3 consecutive stool specimens using an agar culture method at the end of treatment and 2 weeks after completion of therapy. The peripheral eosinophilia resolved 4 weeks after therapy, and the IgG reverted to negative after 3 months of completion of treatment. The patient continues to be monitored clinically for recurrence and is currently free of symptoms.

3. Case Discussion

The global burden caused by *Strongyloides stercoralis* is not known, with estimates of 370 million infected people worldwide [2]. The parasite is present in tropical, subtropical, and temperate areas [3]. Humans become infected when filariform (L3) larvae penetrate the skin or the oral mucosa. The larvae migrate through the blood stream to the lungs, and then they enter the airway, are swallowed, and eventually reach the small intestine where they mature into adult females capable of laying eggs without the aid of males (parthenogenetic females). The eggs are embryonated upon release and hatch internally. The resultant rhabditiform (L1) larvae are released in the stool to the external environment where they mature into filariform larvae. The rhabditiform

larvae can also develop into free-living adult worms capable of producing infective filariform larvae. The crucial characteristic that sets *S. stercoralis* aside from other helminthic infections is the capability of the rhabditiform larvae to molt into infective filariform larvae in the intestine. These tissue-penetrating larvae can enter the circulation through the colonic wall or perianal skin and complete an internal cycle. This process, known as autoinfection, is the mechanism by which the infection is established for the life of the infected individual [4, 5].

Approximately 50% of patients with chronic infection have no symptoms. Nonspecific gastrointestinal complaints, pulmonary, and cutaneous symptoms are the most commonly reported manifestations in those that are symptomatic [4]. Hyperinfection usually develops in immunocompromised states when reduced immune surveillance leads to an unrestricted proliferation of worms through accelerated autoinfection. The distinction between autoinfection and hyperinfection is therefore quantitative rather than specifically defined. In our case, the respiratory complaints, abnormal imaging findings, and resolution of symptoms with treatment are highly suggestive of an accelerated autoinfection involving the lungs despite the failure to isolate larvae from a sputum sample. The nematode, larvae, and on occasions eggs can be detected in extra-intestinal regions like the lungs [6]. Pulmonary manifestations are the rule and patchy fleeting pulmonary infiltrates are usually seen. Diffuse bronchopneumonia and severe alveolar hemorrhage can lead to death [4, 6]. Disseminated strongyloidiasis is typically referred to the condition when worms are found in ectopic sites other than the lungs (e.g., brain). In hyperinfection and dissemination, enteric bacteria or fungi can be carried by larvae leading to potentially deadly metastatic infection elsewhere (e.g., pneumonia, meningitis) or septicemia [4, 6].

The incidence of *Strongyloides* hyperinfection after renal transplantation is unknown and believed to be uncommon. Hyperinfection typically occurs during the first 3 months after transplantation with mortality rates reaching up to 50% [6]. Although transmission of Strongyloides can occur from an infected renal allograft [7], most are the result of the uncontrolled proliferation of the nematode in an immunocompromised recipient with potential exposure before transplantation. In our case, the patient had eosinophilia for several years before transplantation making acquisition of the infection in the jungles of Vietnam likely.

Strongyloidiasis is known to be endemic in Vietnam [3]. For example, the prevalence of infection among Vietnam veterans ranges from 1.6 to 11.6% [8, 9]. For this reason and for the potentially deadly complications of untreated disease, refugees from South East Asia should receive preemptive treatment before arrival to the US. The Division of Global Migration and Quarantine of the Center for Disease Control and Prevention (since 2005) recommends prearrival ivermectin at a dose of 200 μg/kg/day orally once a day for 2 days for those without contraindications [10]. Our patient arrived to the US before this recommendation was enacted.

The American Society of Transplantation recommends pretransplant screening with stool examination and *Strongyloides stercoralis* immunoglobulin G enzyme-linked immunosorbent assay (ELISA) antibody in recipients and donors from endemic areas or with eosinophilia [11, 12]. The tests have diagnostic limitations. Different serological assays have been evaluated with estimated sensitivities between 84% and 95% in chronically infected patients [13] with specificity being 100% with an acceptable cut-off for sensitivity [14]. Interpretation of positive results needs to be done with caution as cross-reactivity exists with *Ascaris lumbricoides* and *Schistosoma* spp. [5]. In addition, seropositivity can persist for years despite appropriate treatment and a negative result does not exclude the diagnosis. Molecular methods in diagnosing the infection are still limited owing to results from different studies showing these tests to be less sensitive than serological tests although it is still unclear if molecular tests are more sensitive compared to traditional fecal testing due to variability in different studies conducted so far [15]. Our patient was not screened or presumptively treated for this parasitic infection for unclear reasons.

Coprological examination alone has poor sensitivity (15–30% for a single specimen) due to the fact that larvae are excreted intermittently and in small quantities [5]. The sensitivity of a stool exam can increase by performing more laborious and expensive testing. For example, the sensitivity increases to almost 100% if 7 consecutive daily stool specimens are examined by experienced personnel [15]. Study by Sato et al. reported the agar culture plate method to have a sensitivity of 96% when multiple stool samples were tested, the detection rate being less than 60% if only single sample was tested [5, 16]. The goal of treatment is complete eradication of Strongyloides to prevent serious disease. Due to these limitations, presumptive treatment is recommended by some for patients with risk factors and negative serology and stool examination [6].

A definite test of cure does not exist since a negative stool agar culture plate does not guarantee cure and serology may remain positive for years despite a curative treatment course. It is important to remember that treatment failure or relapse is more common in immunocompromised patients and therefore treatment should be preferentially administered before transplantation [4, 6].

Ivermectin results in more people cured than albendazole and is at least as well tolerated. In trials of ivermectin with thiabendazole, both have similar cure rates but ivermectin is better tolerated [17]. The duration of therapy in immunocompromised patients is unclear. For chronic intestinal strongyloidiasis, ivermectin should be administered for a minimum of two weeks of daily therapy to extend over the full life cycle of the parasite, followed by posttreatment monitoring of stool samples and antibody titers to document clearance. Hyperinfection requires a longer course of treatment and current guidance dictates for ivermectin to be given until microscopic clearance of larvae from infected sites is documented [6].

4. Conclusion

Despite the high mortality rate and being a preventable and treatable entity, hyperinfection due to *Strongyloides* continues to be reported in renal transplant recipients. Comprehensive guidance regarding the prevention and treatment of parasitic diseases in the setting of solid organ transplantation has been published. It is imperative that healthcare professionals involved in the care of these individuals be cognizant of the importance to follow such recommendations.

Competing Interests

The authors declare that there is no conflict of interests regarding the publication of this paper.

Acknowledgments

The authors would like to thank Dr. Rina Girard de Kaminsky for her valuable comments.

References

[1] F. Roufosse and P. F. Weller, "Practical approach to the patient with hypereosinophilia," *Journal of Allergy and Clinical Immunology*, vol. 126, no. 1, pp. 39–44, 2010.

[2] Z. Bisoffi, D. Buonfrate, A. Montresor et al., "Strongyloides stercoralis: a plea for action," *PLoS Neglected Tropical Diseases*, vol. 7, no. 5, article e2214, 2013.

[3] S. Puthiyakunnon, S. Boddu, Y. Li et al., "Strongyloidiasis—an insight into its global prevalence and management," *PLoS Neglected Tropical Diseases*, vol. 8, no. 8, Article ID e3018, 2014.

[4] P. B. Keiser and T. B. Nutman, "Strongyloides stercoralis in the immunocompromised population," *Clinical Microbiology Reviews*, vol. 17, no. 1, pp. 208–217, 2004.

[5] A. A. Siddiqui and S. L. Berk, "Diagnosis of Strongyloides stercoralis infection," *Clinical Infectious Diseases*, vol. 33, no. 7, pp. 1040–1047, 2001.

[6] A. C. Roxby, G. S. Gottlieb, and A. P. Limaye, "Strongyloidiasis in transplant patients," *Clinical Infectious Diseases*, vol. 49, no. 9, pp. 1411–1423, 2009.

[7] D. A. Roseman, D. Kabbani, J. Kwah et al., "Strongyloides stercoralis transmission by kidney transplantation in two recipients from a common donor," *American Journal of Transplantation*, vol. 13, no. 9, pp. 2483–2486, 2013.

[8] R. M. Genta, R. Weesner, R. W. Douce, T. Huitger O'connor, and P. D. Walzer, "Strongyloidiasis in US veterans of the vietnam and other wars," *JAMA*, vol. 258, no. 1, pp. 49–52, 1987.

[9] H. Rahmanian, A. C. Macfarlane, K. E. Rowland, L. J. Einsiedel, and S. J. Neuhaus, "Seroprevalence of Strongyloides stercoralis in a South Australian Vietnam veteran cohort," *Australian and New Zealand Journal of Public Health*, vol. 39, no. 4, pp. 331–335, 2015.

[10] W. M. Stauffer, P. T. Cantey, S. Montgomery et al., "Presumptive treatment and medical screening for parasites in refugees resettling to the United States," *Current Infectious Disease Reports*, vol. 15, no. 3, pp. 222–231, 2013.

[11] S. A. Fischer and K. Lu, "Screening of donor and recipient in solid organ transplantation," *American Journal of Transplantation*, vol. 13, supplement 4, pp. 9–21, 2013.

[12] B. S. Schwartz, S. D. Mawhorter, and AST Infectious Diseases Community of Practice, "Parasitic infections in solid organ transplantation," *American Journal of Transplantation*, vol. 2, pp. 280–303, 2013.

[13] D. Buonfrate, F. Formenti, F. Perandin, and Z. Bisoffi, "Novel
      approaches to the diagnosis of Strongyloides stercoralis infec-
      tion," *Clinical Microbiology and Infection*, vol. 21, no. 6, pp. 543–
      552, 2015.

[14] Z. Bisoffi, D. Buonfrate, M. Sequi et al., "Diagnostic accuracy of
      five serologic tests for Strongyloides stercoralis infection," *PLoS
      Neglected Tropical Diseases*, vol. 8, no. 1, Article ID e2640, 2014.

[15] A. Requena-Méndez, P. Chiodini, Z. Bisoffi, D. Buonfrate, E.
      Gotuzzo, and J. Muñoz, "The laboratory diagnosis and follow up
      of strongyloidiasis: a systematic review," *PLoS Neglected Tropical
      Diseases*, vol. 7, no. 1, article e2002, 2013.

[16] Y. Sato, J. Kobayashi, H. Toma, and Y. Shiroma, "Efficacy of stool
      examination for detection of Strongyloides infection," *American
      Journal of Tropical Medicine and Hygiene*, vol. 53, no. 3, pp. 248–
      250, 1995.

[17] C. Henriquez-Camacho, E. Gotuzzo, J. Echevarria, A. C. White
      Jr., A. Terashima, F. Samalvides et al., "Ivermectin versus alben-
      dazole or thiabendazole for *Strongyloides stercoralis* infection,"
      The Cochrane Database of Systematic Reviews, no. 1, Article ID
      CD007745, 2016.

10

Neurobrucellosis: A Case Report from Himachal Pradesh, India, and Review of the Literature

Sujeet Raina,[1] Ashish Sharma,[2] Rajesh Sharma,[1] and Amit Bhardwaj[2]

[1]*Department of Medicine, Dr. RPGMC, Tanda, Kangra 176001, India*
[2]*Department of Neurology, Dr. RPGMC, Tanda, Kangra 176001, India*

Correspondence should be addressed to Sujeet Raina; sujeetrashmishera@yahoo.co.in

Academic Editor: Antonella Marangoni

Human brucellosis is a multisystem disease that commonly presents as a febrile illness along with variable spectrum of clinical manifestations. Neurological complications include encephalitis, meningoencephalitis, radiculitis, myelitis, peripheral and cranial neuropathies, subarachnoid hemorrhage, and psychiatric manifestations. We report a case diagnosed as neurobrucellosis who presented with fever and bilateral upper motor neuron symptoms and signs along with bilateral sensorineural deafness. Diagnosis was confirmed by Rose Bengal Test (RBT) and standard tube agglutination test (SAT).

1. Introduction

Brucellosis is the commonest bacterial zoonosis and causes more than 500 000 human infections per year worldwide [1]. The disease has a widespread geographic distribution and is labelled as regionally emerging zoonotic disease [2]. It also comes under the WHO list of neglected tropical zoonotic infection. Brucellosis has a variable clinical manifestation due to extensive involvement of organ systems during infection. Neurobrucellosis is a complication of systemic brucellosis infection. The frequency of neurobrucellosis has been reported as 5–7% in the literature [3]. Neurological complications include encephalitis, meningoencephalitis, radiculitis, myelitis, peripheral and cranial neuropathies, subarachnoid hemorrhage, psychiatric manifestations, brain abscess, and demyelinating syndrome [3, 4]. Human brucellosis has been reported from different states of India. The seroprevalence of brucellosis among occupationally exposed human beings was observed to be 6.66% in Himachal Pradesh, India [5]. Rural population is predominantly agrarian society linked with animal husbandry and shepherding in the state. Migratory pastoralism is very common in the Himalaya and a number of nomadic communities practise this migratory system of goat and sheep rearing in Himachal Pradesh, India. Despite well documented seroprevalence, human brucellosis is less commonly reported from the state [6]. Disease is usually not considered as a cause of meningitis in this region which leads to missed or delayed diagnosis. This could be because of the lack of awareness, suspicion, and diagnostic facilties at the health provider's end. We report a case of neurobrucellosis who presented with fever and bilateral upper motor neuron symptoms and signs along with bilateral sensorineural deafness. Diagnosis was based on consistent clinical features, radiological imaging, positive serum Rose Bengal Test (RBT) and serum standard tube agglutination test (SAT) and a favourable response to therapy.

2. Case Report

A 24-year-old male was admitted in March 2014, with history of fever for 3 months. The fever was documented up to 103°F and was associated with sweating. There was history of insidious onset, progressive weakness of both lower limbs proximal more than distal in the form of not being able to stand from squatting, climbing up, and getting down stairs for the last 2 months. Simultaneously, he noticed proximal weakness in both upper limbs in the form of inability to lift heavy objects as he used to previously. Patient also gave history of difficulty in walking for the same duration. History of increased frequency of micturition accompanied with urgency and precipitancy was present for the last month. In addition patient had developed impairment in hearing for the

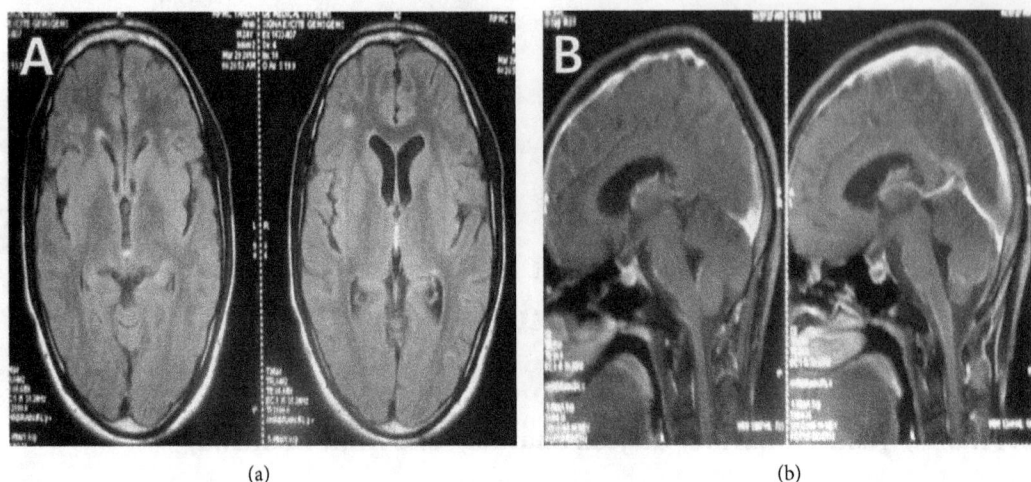

(a)   (b)

FIGURE 1: (a) Axial FLAIR images showing white matter periventricular and subcortical hyperintensities bilaterally. (b) After contrast brainstem meningeal enhancement is seen.

last month. No history of headache, vomiting, ear discharge, altered sensorium, or seizures was reported. Review of other systems was normal. No significant past history was present. The patient belonged to a rural area and was associated with livestock rearing. He used to consume raw milk of goat. (This history was disclosed retrospectively.) On examination patient was febrile. Rest of the general physical examination was normal. On nervous system examination, our patient was conscious with the mini-mental state examination score of 28/30. Examination of cranial nerves revealed bilateral sensory neural deafness. Motor examination revealed normal muscle bulk, spasticity in upper and lower limbs, grade IV power in proximal muscles of both upper and lower limbs, symmetrically brisk deep tendon reflexes, and bilaterally extensor plantar response. Sensory examination was normal. Gait was spastic. No meningeal signs were present. Rest of the neurological examination was normal. Review of other systemic examinations was normal. On investigations hemoglobin was 11.6 gm% and total leukocyte count was 7200/cmm. Peripheral smear revealed a microcytic hypochromic picture. Biochemistry showed normal blood glucose and renal and liver functions. Cerebrospinal fluid (CSF) analysis had proteins: 273 mg/dL; glucose: 29 mg/dL (concomitant blood glucose: 101 mg/dL); adenosine deaminase: 19.5 U/L. On microscopic examination of CSF total WBCs count was 288/cmm; neutrophils were 12%; lymphocytes were 88%; total RBCs count was 16/cmm. CSF was VDRL nonreactive, negative for cryptococcal infection and negative for acid fast bacilli by ZN stain. Chest X-ray and ultrasonography of abdomen were normal. As a part of fever workup his blood sample was sent to Department of Veterinary Microbiology, College of Veterinary and Animal Sciences, CSK HPKV Palampur, Himachal Pradesh, for diagnosis of brucellosis. Blood sample was positive for RBT. SAT was positive in 1 : 640 titers. Subsequently brain magnetic resonance imaging (MRI) was done. On T2W and FLAIR images white matter hyperintensities bilaterally involving periventricular white matter and centrum semiovale (mainly

involving frontal lobes) with involvement of subcortical U fibres at places were observed. After contrast brainstem meningeal enhancement was seen (Figures 1(a) and 1(b)). On pure tone audiometry bilateral moderate sensorineural hearing loss was documented. Patient was prescribed doxycycline 100 mg twice a day, rifampicin 600 mg once a day, and cotrimoxazole (160 mg trimethoprim and 800 mg sulfamethoxazole) twice a day. Patient became afebrile on fourth day of treatment. All three drugs were continued for three months. At the end of three months patient remained afebrile, deafness recovered, and bladder dysfunction and spastic gait improved. He had resumed his routine work. He faced difficulty only in running around. His upper motor neuron signs persisted on clinical examination. Repeat SAT titer was 1 : 160. So drugs were continued for another three months (total 6 months). Follow-up MRI at 6 months of treatment showed partial resolution of subcortical and periventricular white matter lesions in bilateral inferior frontal regions. Resolution of brainstem meningeal enhancement was also seen (Figures 2(a) and 2(b)). Patient had a sequelae in the form of brisk deep tendon reflexes and bilaterally extensor plantar response after 6 months of therapy which was subsequently stopped. The functional status had a score of 1 on modified Rankin scale.

3. Discussion

Brucellosis is considered a deceptive infectious disease in India [7]. Human brucellosis is well reported in India; however there are only few reports on neurobrucellosis [8–10]. Neurological complications of brucellosis are infrequent but an important clinical entity. Clinical presentation of central nervous involvement is variable. Nervous system involvement is generally in meningoencephalitis form. Development of basal meningitis may lead to lymphocytic pleocytosis, cranial nerve involvement, or intracranial hypertension [11]. Guven et al. [4] observed that headache, blurred vision, loss of vision, hearing loss, and confusion were significantly

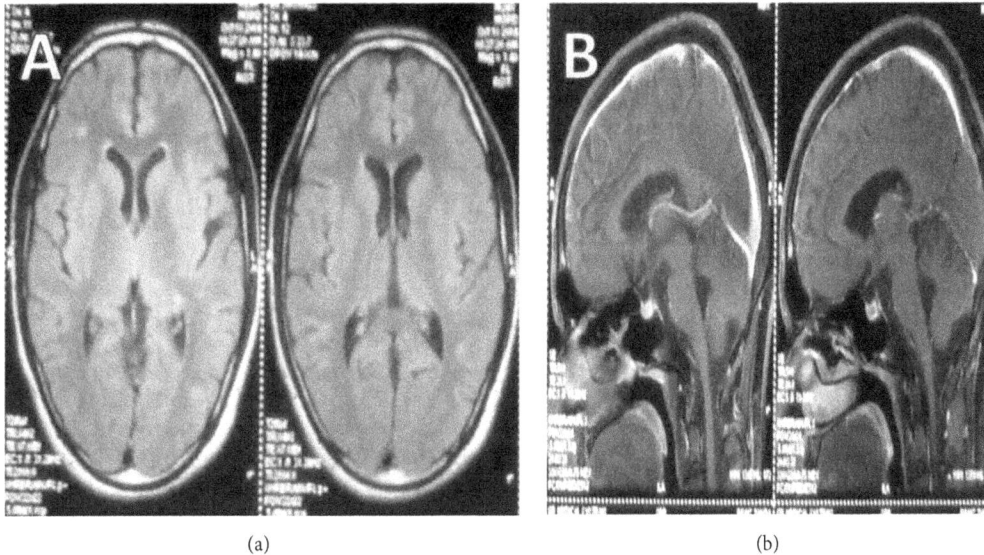

FIGURE 2: Follow-up MRI 6 months later showing (a) axial FLAIR images showing partially resolved white matter periventricular and subcortical hyperintensities. (b) After contrast, no brainstem meningeal enhancement is seen.

associated with neurobrucellosis. Muscular weakness, disorientation, neck rigidity, changes in deep tendon reflexes, and paresthesias were also more common amid the patients. Among cranial nerves abducens, facial and vestibulocochlear were affected more than other cranial nerves in neurobrucellosis. Peripheral nerve involvement was observed as radiculopathy or polyradiculopathy. Signs and symptoms of meningeal involvement are nonspecific in neurobrucellosis and meningeal signs are infrequently present [11].

Brucella bacteria may affect the nervous system directly or indirectly, as a result of cytokine or endotoxin on the neural tissue. Cytotoxic T lymphocytes and microglia activation play an immunopathologic role in this disease. Infection triggers the immune mechanism leading to a demyelinating state of cerebral and spinal cord [11].

In neurobrucellosis imaging findings may be found in four types: normal, meningeal contrast enhancement, white matter changes, and vascular changes [11]. In addition to nonenhancing bilateral white matter lesions deep grey matter involvement has also been documented [10].

Most important differential diagnosis of brucellosis is tuberculosis in our country. Both chronic granulomatous infectious diseases are endemic in our country. There is a clear overlap between neurobrucellosis and tuberculosis both in terms of clinical presentation, laboratory parameters, and neuroimaging. Hearing loss due to vestibulocochlear nerve involvement, deep grey matter involvement, and extensive white matter lesions on neuroimaging mimicking demyelinating disorders seems to be unique for brucellosis [10, 12].

Neurobrucellosis is a diagnostic puzzle as there is a lack of consensus in diagnostic criteria. According to Kochlar et al. [8], the criteria necessary for definite diagnosis of neurobrucellosis are (i) neurological dysfunction not explained by other neurologic diseases, (ii) abnormal CSF indicating lymphocytic pleocytosis and increased protein, (iii) positive CSF culture for Brucella organisms or positive Brucella IgG

agglutination titer in the blood and CSF, and (iv) response to specific chemotherapy with a significant drop in the CSF lymphocyte count and protein concentration. Recently Guven et al. [4] diagnosed neurobrucellosis by the presence of any one of the following criteria: (1) symptoms and signs suspect of neurobrucellosis, (2) isolation of Brucella species from cerebrospinal fluid (CSF) and/or presence of anti-Brucella antibodies in CSF, (3) the presence of lymphocytosis, increased protein, and decreased glucose levels in the CSF, or (4) findings in cranial MRI or computed tomography (CT). Erdem et al. [13] defined chronic Brucella meningitis on the basis of following criteria:

(1) The manifestation of clinical neurological symptoms for over 4 weeks

(2) The presence of typical CSF evidence with meningitis (protein concentrations >50 mg/dL, pleocytosis over $10/mm^3$, and CSF glucose to serum glucose ratios <0.5)

(3) Positive bacterial culture or serological test results for brucellosis in CSF (positive Rose Bengal Test or serum tube agglutination) or in blood (positive Rose Bengal Test and serum tube agglutination with a titer ≥1/160) or positive bone marrow culture

(4) Nonappearance of any alternative neurological diagnosis

These criteria were applied in the case definition of 177 patients with chronic brucellar meningitis or meningoencephalitis in a multicenter, retrospective Istanbul 2 study. Based on the results of the study, the sensitivities of the principal serological tests like serum SAT, RBT, and ELISA as well as CSF RBT and SAT were analyzed. The sensitivities of the tests were 94% for serum SAT, 96% for serum RBT, 78% for CSF SAT, and 71% for CSF RBT. The data supported the view that blood serological tests were significantly more sensitive than CSF tests [13]. CSF culture, when positive, is considered the gold standard in the laboratory diagnosis of neurobrucellosis [14]. However, serological approaches are the mainstays in the diagnosis of neurobrucellosis due to the relatively lower efficacy of bacterial culture. Our patient fulfilled all the four criteria of neurobrucellosis as laid in the case definition by Erdem et al. [13].

In patients with consistent clinical features, overemphasis on determination of CSF *Brucella* agglutination titers and isolation of *Brucella* from CSF can be done away in diagnostic criteria with in resource limited settings like our country [12].

There is no consensus for choice of antibiotic, dose, and duration of the treatment for neurobrucellosis. Dual- or triple-combination therapy with doxycycline, rifampicin, trimethoprim-sulfamethoxazole, streptomycin, or ceftriaxone for >2 months (3–6 months) has been recommended [4].

Short-course steroid therapy has been found to be effective in minimizing the residual deficits in those with arachnoiditis, optic neuritis, and multiple-sclerosis-like presentation [15]. Sequelae among survivors despite appropriate antibiotic therapy are well known [4, 9, 16]. They are significant if patient has diffuse CNS, encephalitis, or spinal cord involvement compared to meningitis as a presentation. They have been reported as aphasia, hearing loss, hemiparesis, and visual impairment. Mortality is uncommon [4, 11, 17].

Most of the laboratories lack facilities for diagnosis of human brucellosis in India. In presence of appropriate history and clinical findings, RBT is a very useful test for the diagnosis of human brucellosis. Being simple and affordable it should be an ideal test for diagnosis of brucellosis in patients with clinical setting in our rural hospitals [18].

Competing Interests

The authors declare that there are no competing interests regarding the publication of this paper.

Acknowledgments

The authors thank Department of Veterinary Microbiology, College of Veterinary and Animal Sciences, CSK HPKV Palampur, Himachal Pradesh, for providing resources for the reported study.

References

[1] G. Pappas, P. Papadimitriou, N. Akritidis, L. Christou, and E. V. Tsianos, "The new global map of human brucellosis," *The Lancet Infectious Diseases*, vol. 6, no. 2, pp. 91–99, 2006.

[2] B. G. Mantur and S. K. Amarnath, "Brucellosis in India—a review," *Journal of Biosciences*, vol. 33, no. 4, pp. 539–547, 2008.

[3] G. Pappas, N. Akritidis, M. Bosilkovski, and E. Tsianos, "Medical progress Brucellosis," *New England Journal of Medicine*, vol. 352, no. 22, pp. 2325–2367, 2005.

[4] T. Guven, K. Ugurlu, O. Ergonul et al., "Neurobrucellosis: clinical and diagnostic features," *Clinical Infectious Diseases*, vol. 56, no. 10, pp. 1407–1412, 2013.

[5] Shalmali, A. K. Panda, and R. Chahota, "Sero-prevalence of brucellosis in occupationally exposed human beings of Himachal Pradesh (India)," *Journal of Communicable Diseases*, vol. 44, no. 2, pp. 91–95, 2012.

[6] R. Chahota, A. Dattal, S. D. Thakur, and M. Sharma, "Isolation of *Brucella melitensis* from a human case of chronic additive polyarthritis," *Indian Journal of Medical Microbiology*, vol. 33, no. 3, pp. 429–432, 2015.

[7] H. L. Smits and S. M. Kadri, "Brucellosis in India: a deceptive infectious disease," *Indian Journal of Medical Research*, vol. 122, no. 5, pp. 375–384, 2005.

[8] D. K. Kochlar, B. L. Kumawat, N. Agarwal et al., "Meningoencephalitis in brucellosis," *Neurology India*, vol. 48, no. 2, pp. 170–173, 2000.

[9] D. K. Kochar, B. K. Gupta, A. Gupta et al., "Hospital based case series of 175 cases of serologically confirmed Brucellosis in Bikaner," *Journal of Association of Physician of India*, vol. 48, no. 4, pp. 170–173, 2007.

[10] R. Rajan, D. Khurana, and P. Kesav, "Teaching neuroimages: deep gray matter involvement in neurobrucellosis," *Neurology*, vol. 80, no. 3, pp. E28–E29, 2013.

[11] N. Ceran, R. Turkoglu, I. Erdem et al., "Neurobrucellosis: clinical, diagnostic, therapeutic features and outcome. Unusual clinical presentations in an endemic region," *Brazilian Journal of Infectious Diseases*, vol. 15, no. 1, pp. 52–59, 2011.

[12] P. Kesav, V. Y. Vishnu, and D. Khurana, "Is neurobrucellosis the Pandora's box of modern medicine?" *Clinical Infectious Diseases*, vol. 57, no. 7, pp. 1056–1057, 2013.

[13] H. Erdem, S. Kilic, B. Sener et al., "Diagnosis of chronic brucellar meningitis and meningoencephalitis: the results of the Istanbul-2 study," *Clinical Microbiology and Infection*, vol. 19, no. 2, pp. E80–E86, 2013.

[14] G. F. Araj, "Update on laboratory diagnosis of human brucellosis," *International Journal of Antimicrobial Agents*, vol. 36, supplement 1, pp. S12–S17, 2010.

[15] A. R. Lulu, G. F. Araj, M. I. Khateeb, M. Y. Mustafa, A. R. Yusuf, and F. F. Fenech, "Human brucellosis in Kuwait: a prospective study of 400 cases," *Quarterly Journal of Medicine*, vol. 66, no. 1, pp. 39–54, 1988.

[16] R. A. Shakir, A. S. N. Al-Din, G. F. Araj, A. R. Lulu, A. R. Mousa, and M. A. Saadah, "Clinical categories of neurobrucellosis: a report on 19 cases," *Brain*, vol. 110, no. 1, pp. 213–223, 1987.

[17] H. Karsen, S. T. Koruk, F. Duygu, K. Yapici, and M. Kati, "Review of 17 cases of neurobrucellosis: clinical manifestations, diagnosis, and management," *Archives of Iranian Medicine*, vol. 15, no. 8, pp. 491–494, 2012.

[18] R. Díaz, A. Casanova, J. Ariza, and I. Moriyón, "The Rose Bengal Test in human brucellosis: a neglected test for the diagnosis of a neglected disease," *PLoS Neglected Tropical Diseases*, vol. 5, no. 4, article e950, 2011.

11

Persistent Bacteremia from *Pseudomonas aeruginosa* with *In Vitro* Resistance to the Novel Antibiotics Ceftolozane-Tazobactam and Ceftazidime-Avibactam

Louie Mar Gangcuangco,[1] **Patricia Clark,**[2] **Cynthia Stewart,**[2]
Goran Miljkovic,[1,3] **and Zane K. Saul**[1,3]

[1]*Department of Internal Medicine, Yale New Haven Health-Bridgeport Hospital, Bridgeport, CT, USA*
[2]*Department of Microbiology, Yale New Haven Health-Bridgeport Hospital, Bridgeport, CT, USA*
[3]*Internal Medicine and Infectious Disease Associates P.C., Stratford, CT, USA*

Correspondence should be addressed to Louie Mar Gangcuangco; louiemarmd@gmail.com

Academic Editor: Tomoyuki Shibata

Ceftazidime-avibactam and ceftolozane-tazobactam are new antimicrobials with activity against multidrug-resistant *Pseudomonas aeruginosa*. We present the first case of persistent *P. aeruginosa* bacteremia with *in vitro* resistance to these novel antimicrobials. A 68-year-old man with newly diagnosed follicular lymphoma was admitted to the medical intensive care unit for sepsis and right lower extremity cellulitis. The patient was placed empirically on vancomycin and piperacillin-tazobactam. Blood cultures from Day 1 of hospitalization grew *P. aeruginosa* susceptible to piperacillin-tazobactam and cefepime identified using VITEK 2 (Biomerieux, Lenexa, KS). Repeat blood cultures from Day 5 grew *P. aeruginosa* resistant to all cephalosporins, as well as to meropenem by Day 10. Susceptibility testing performed by measuring minimum inhibitory concentration by *E*-test (Biomerieux, Lenexa, KS) revealed that blood cultures from Day 10 were resistant to ceftazidime-avibactam and ceftolozane-tazobactam. The Verigene Blood Culture-Gram-Negative (BC-GN) microarray-based assay (Nanosphere, Inc., Northbrook, IL) was used to investigate underlying resistance mechanism in the *P. aeruginosa* isolate but CTX-M, KPC, NDM, VIM, IMP, and OXA gene were not detected. This case report highlights the well-documented phenomenon of antimicrobial resistance development in *P. aeruginosa* even during the course of appropriate antibiotic therapy. In the era of increasing multidrug-resistant organisms, routine susceptibility testing of *P. aeruginosa* to ceftazidime-avibactam and ceftolozane-tazobactam is warranted. Emerging resistance mechanisms to these novel antibiotics need to be further investigated.

1. Introduction

Sepsis from *Pseudomonas aeruginosa* bacteremia may be fatal and necessitates prompt antimicrobial therapy. Newer antimicrobials have been developed to address the rise of multidrug-resistant *P. aeruginosa* [1]. Among these are ceftolozane-tazobactam, a combination of a fifth-generation cephalosporin and a β-lactamase inhibitor, and ceftazidime-avibactam, a combination of a third-generation cephalosporin and a non-β-lactam β-lactamase inhibitor [2]. We present the first case report of persistent *P. aeruginosa* bacteremia resistant to these novel antibiotics.

2. Case Presentation

A 68-year-old man presents to the Emergency Department for a 6-month history of worsening fatigue, anorexia, and weight loss. CT scan of the abdomen showed enlarged lymph nodes. Axillary lymph node biopsy showed follicular lymphoma with bone marrow involvement. The patient was started on chemotherapy with rituximab, etoposide, prednisolone, oncovin, cyclophosphamide, and hydroxyl-daunorubicin (R-EPOCH). Second cycle consisted of rituximab, cyclophosphamide, hydroxyl-daunorubicin, oncovin, and prednisone (R-CHOP). The patient had a prolonged hospital course (3 months) complicated by tumor lysis syndrome, febrile neutropenia (treated with aztreonam, cefepime, and anidulafungin), acute renal failure requiring hemodialysis, right lower extremity cellulitis treated with a 7-day course of intravenous vancomycin, and *Clostridium difficile* colitis treated with oral metronidazole.

On hospital discharge, outpatient chemotherapy consisted of bendamustine and rituximab. Two weeks later, the patient presented to the clinic for recurrence of right lower extremity cellulitis. Physical exam revealed erythema and induration of the right upper leg with extension to the groin and left medial thigh. One dose of intravenous ceftriaxone was administered and amoxicillin-clavulanate 500 mg three times a day was started. The patient presented 1 day later to the Emergency Department with increased shortness of breath, loose bowel movement, hypotension (80/40), tachycardia (129 beats/minute), temperature of 99.6°F, and oxygen saturation of 75% in room air. Empiric vancomycin and piperacillin-tazobactam were started and 6 liters of normal saline bolus led to improvement in blood pressure. Hospital course is summarized in Table 1.

Blood cultures from the day of admission grew *P. aeruginosa* (Table 2), identified using VITEK 2 (Biomerieux, Lenexa, KS). Blood cultures persistently grew *P. aeruginosa* initially susceptible to piperacillin-tazobactam and cefepime, with subsequent resistance to all cephalosporins and penicillins by Day 5 and resistance to meropenem by Day 10. Antimicrobial susceptibility testing to ceftolozane-tazobactam and ceftazidime-avibactam was performed for the *P. aeruginosa* isolate from Day 10 by measuring minimum inhibitory concentration using *E*-test (Biomerieux, Lenexa, KS). *E*-test showed 0 mm zone of inhibition for ceftazidime-avibactam (resistant) and 16 mm for ceftolozane-tazobactam (resistant).

The patient had an extensive work-up to find the source of *P. aeruginosa* bacteremia. Transesophageal echocardiogram did not show vegetation or endocarditis. Noncontrast CT scan of the chest, abdomen, and pelvis revealed bilateral pleural effusions but no abscess. Low platelet counts precluded thoracentesis. Urine cultures (Day 1, Day 10, and Day 15), as well as catheter tip culture of peripherally inserted central catheter line (PICC line), did not grow bacteria.

Antimicrobial coverage was adjusted appropriately based on blood culture susceptibility reports. Despite medical treatment, the patient developed progressive acidosis, respiratory distress, and hypotension. By Day 15, he required three vasopressors. A decision was made to shift the patient from full interventions to comfort measures only. He was extubated and expired on Day 16 of hospitalization.

To determine possible underlying resistance mechanisms in the *P. aeruginosa* isolate, the Verigene Blood Culture-Gram-Negative (BC-GN) microarray-based assay (Nanosphere, Inc., Northbrook, IL) was utilized following previously published methods [3]. In brief, we seeded a known negative blood culture bottle with the *P. aeruginosa* isolate using 100 mL of a 0.5 McFarland standard in normal saline. Blood culture bottles were placed on the BACTEC automated blood culture monitoring system (BD Diagnostics, Franklin Lakes, NJ, USA). Once they were flagged positive, we took four 1 mL aliquots and placed them in sterile tubes. The tubes were immediately placed in −70°F freezer before shipping on dry ice to Nanosphere, Inc. (Illinois, USA). The Verigene BC-GN detected *P. aeruginosa*. However, all resistance markers tested were negative (CTX-M, KPC, NDM, VIM, IMP, or OXA gene).

3. Discussion

We present the first documented case of persistent *P. aeruginosa* bacteremia resistant to the novel antimicrobials ceftazidime-avibactam and ceftolozane-tazobactam. A recent publication on a multidrug-resistant *P. aeruginosa* bacteremia was reported by Bremmer and colleagues, but the isolate was susceptible to ceftolozane-tazobactam [4]. In our current report, a rapid development of antibiotic resistance was observed despite appropriate antimicrobial therapy and, intriguingly, with resistance to ceftazidime-avibactam and ceftolozane-tazobactam, agents that have been only recently approved by the US Food and Drug Administration. This case raises the following important questions: (1) Must patients remain on double antimicrobial coverage for *P. aeruginosa* pending *repeat* blood cultures? (2) Should screening for resistance determinants be routinely performed for *P. aeruginosa*?

The rationale for double antibiotic coverage/combination therapy against suspected *P. aeruginosa* infection is to increase the chance that the patient receives an active agent awaiting final susceptibility results. Combination therapy also has a theoretical benefit in decreasing the emergence of resistance and may confer synergistic effect. Although the routine use of combination antimicrobials for *P. aeruginosa* remains controversial, there is evidence that a subset of patients who are at high risk for resistant strains (i.e., patients with neutropenia, burn, severe sepsis, or shock) may benefit from combination therapy [5]. Measuring peak and minimum inhibitory concentrations for ciprofloxacin and aminoglycosides was also shown to be associated with increased success/clinical cure in *P. aeruginosa* bacteremia [6].

In our current report, despite appropriate antimicrobial therapy and initial isolate susceptible to piperacillin-tazobactam, the patient continued to have bacteremia. There are two possible reasons for this: (1) the patient has multiple *P. aeruginosa* strains and the predominant phenotype from Day 1 was eradicated by piperacillin-tazobactam, with the carbapenem-resistant strains subsequently becoming the predominant phenotype in the repeat blood cultures or (2) the initial *P. aeruginosa* isolate developed resistance from mutation/acquisition of exogenous resistance determinants.

The ability of *P. aeruginosa* to develop resistance during antimicrobial therapy has been well-documented in literature and involves complex mechanisms, including chromosomally encoded AmpC cephalosporinase, outer membrane porin (OprD), and multidrug efflux pumps [7]. AmpC β-lactamases are chromosomally encoded cephalosporinases. AmpC enzymes may be induced and expressed at high levels by mutation. Overexpression of AmpC confers resistance to broad-spectrum cephalosporins, including ceftazidime [8]. Furthermore, structural modifications in AmpC may impact the ability of avibactam to protect ceftazidime from hydrolysis [9]. A study comparing wild-type and mutator

TABLE 1: Significant events in the patient's hospital course.

Hospital day	Significant event	Tmax (°F)	WBC (cells/mm³)	Antibiotics
1	Admission to the medical ICU, being started on norepinephrine for hypotension Blood cultures drawn Right radial A-line and left femoral central line inserted	103.0	4.61	Piperacillin-tazobactam 4.5 g IV every 8 hours Vancomycin IV*
2	Noncontrast CT scan of abdomen and pelvis showed bilateral pleural effusion, moderate ascites, generalized anasarca, no abscess Day 1 blood cultures grew P. aeruginosa	100.7	11.16	
3	Stool C. difficile enzyme immune-assay positive** Rising creatinine (1.8 mg/dL)	99.8	15.60	Cefepime 2 gm IV daily
4	Urinary catheter removed Femoral line removed PICC line inserted Hemoglobin decreased from 7.2 to 6.8 g/dL	98.3	17.07	
5	Platelets decreased from 27 to 16 × 10³/microliter 1 unit of packed RBC transfused Repeat blood cultures drawn Blood pressure stable off vasopressor, arterial line removed	97.7	14.29	
6	Repeat blood culture negative to date Transferred to general medical floor	97.8	6.38	
7	Repeat blood culture × 1, no growth Minimal bleeding from nares, platelets transfused	97.8	12.4	
8	Blood culture from Day 5 resistant to cefepime 1 unit of packed RBC transfused	98.2	11.93	Meropenem 1 g IV every 8 hours
9	Transthoracic 2D ECHO showed possible valvular vegetations HIDA scan, negative	99.0	9.68	
10	Intubated for decreased respiratory rate and apnea, hypotension (75/50), altered mental status Repeat blood cultures were drawn Transferred back to the medical ICU	98.4	5.96	Meropenem 1 g IV every 8 hours + tobramycin*
11	Hypotension despite fluid resuscitation Phenylephrine started	98.0	6.29	
12	Transesophageal echocardiogram did not reveal vegetations PICC line removed and sent for culture Stable respiratory status; patient extubated Worsening renal function and oliguria	98.3	4.35	
13	Blood culture from Day 10 grew P. aeruginosa resistant to meropenem; E-test performed for P. aeruginosa isolate from Day 10 showed resistance to ceftazidime-avibactam and ceftolozane-tazobactam	99.3	3.84	Tobramycin 1.7 mg/kg every 12 hours
14	Increasing tachypnea, tachycardia, lethargy Absolute neutrophil count dropped to 590 cells/mm³	98.5	1.54	
15	Reintubated for respiratory distress Hypotension despite fluids; patient on three vasopressors (norepinephrine, phenylephrine, vasopressin) Repeat blood cultures drawn	98.5	2.53	Tobramycin 1.7 mg/kg every 12 hours Anidulafungin 200 mg IV Cefepime 2 gm IV daily Vancomycin IV
16	Family decided to change the patient's code status from full interventions to comfort measures only He was extubated and expired			

*Tobramycin and vancomycin doses were adjusted by pharmacy based on peak and trough blood levels.
*Patient was on oral vancomycin empirically for C. difficile since Day 1 of hospitalization.
HIDA scan: hepatobiliary iminodiacetic acid scan; IV, intravenous; PICC: peripherally-inserted central catheter; and Tmax, maximum temperature.

TABLE 2: Antimicrobial susceptibility of *Pseudomonas aeruginosa* isolated from the blood.

Antimicrobial	Day 1		Day 5		Day 10[*]		Day 15	
	MIC	Int	MIC	Int	MIC	Int	MIC	Int
Piperacillin-tazobactam	32	S	≥128	R	≥128	R	≥128	R
Cefepime	8	S	32	R	≥64	R	≥64	R
Aztreonam	16	I	16	I	≥64	R	≥64	R
Meropenem	4	S	4	S	≥16	R	≥16	R
Amikacin	16	S	16	S	16	S	16	S
Gentamicin	8	I	8	I	≥16	R	≥16	R
Tobramycin	≤1	S	≤1	S	≤1	S	≤1	S
Ciprofloxacin	≥4	R	≤4	R	≥4	R	≥4	R
Tigecycline	≥8	R	≤8	R	≥8	R	≥8	R

Int, interpretation; MIC, minimum inhibitory concentration; R, resistant; S, susceptible; and I, intermediate.
[*]Antimicrobial susceptibility testing of *P. aeruginosa* against ceftolozane-tazobactam (C/T) and ceftazidime-avibactam (CZA) by *E*-test was performed for the *Pseudomonas* isolate from Day 10. *E*-test showed 0 mm zone of inhibition for CZA (resistant) and 16 mm for C/T (resistant). Cefepime was used as a surrogate for ceftazidime susceptibility.

P. aeruginosa strains showed that the development of high-level resistance to ceftolozane-tazobactam occurs in the presence of *P. aeruginosa* mutator strains and that multiple mutations result in overexpression and structural modifications of AmpC [10]. Resistance to carbapenems, on the other hand, can arise from a simple mutation in *P. aeruginosa* and one mechanism is through the loss of OprD, a carbapenem-specific porin [11].

We initially thought that the *P. aeruginosa* isolate from our current patient produces metallo-β-lactamase, which confers resistance to both cephalosporins and carbapenems [12]. However, it was surprising that the Verigene BC-GN did not detect any of the carbapenemases tested (KPC, NDM, VIM, IMP, or OXA gene). The resistance that we observed may be due to a mechanism not in the BC-GN panel, or the *P. aeruginosa* strain may have acquired resistance through other novel mechanisms. Unfortunately, our limited resources precluded us from testing the isolate for possible chromosomal resistance mechanisms at a reference laboratory.

Another limitation of our case report is the lack of testing of the initial isolate's susceptibility to ceftolozane-tazobactam and ceftazidime-avibactam from Day 1. Per our Microbiology lab protocol, positive blood culture samples are discarded 1 week after the Microbiology report has been finalized. When the patient's blood culture sample from Day 10 showed resistance to meropenem and the decision was made to test for ceftolozane-tazobactam and ceftazidime-avibactam, blood sample from Day 1 was no longer available. Hence, susceptibility testing was performed only on the most recent blood culture (Day 10).

Unlike the presence of extended-spectrum β-lactamase production in *Enterobacteriaceae*, the presence of resistance determinants in *P. aeruginosa* is not routinely tested in most hospitals. Whether testing for carbapenemases and other resistance determinants prior to initiation of antimicrobial treatment would impact mortality among patients with *P. aeruginosa* bacteremia remains to be elucidated. Continued antimicrobial susceptibility surveillance, development of cost-effective screening tests for antimicrobial resistance, and further studies on appropriate treatment strategies in persistent *P. aeruginosa* bacteremia are warranted.

Competing Interests

Investigators requested Nanosphere (Northbrook, IL) to test the *P. aeruginosa* isolate for resistance determinants using the Verigene Blood Culture-Gram-Negative assay. The authors have no conflict of interests to disclose.

Acknowledgments

The authors would like to thank the staff of the Bridgeport Hospital Department of Microbiology for their assistance in antimicrobial culture and susceptibility testing. Financial support for publication was subsidized by the Office of Graduate Medical Education of Yale New Haven Health-Bridgeport Hospital. No other funding sources were obtained for this report.

References

[1] D. van Duin and R. A. Bonomo, "Ceftazidime/avibactam and ceftolozane/tazobactam: second-generation β-lactam/β-lactamase inhibitor combinations," *Clinical Infectious Diseases*, vol. 63, no. 2, pp. 234–241, 2016.

[2] R. Draenert, U. Seybold, E. Grützner, and J. R. Bogner, "Novel antibiotics: are we still in the pre-post-antibiotic era?" *Infection*, vol. 43, no. 2, pp. 145–151, 2015.

[3] M. Dodemont, R. De Mendonça, C. Nonhoff, S. Roisin, and O. Denis, "Performance of the verigene gram-negative blood culture assay for rapid detection of bacteria and resistance determinants," *Journal of Clinical Microbiology*, vol. 52, no. 8, pp. 3085–3087, 2014.

[4] D. N. Bremmer, D. P. Nicolau, P. Burcham, A. Chunduri, G. Shidham, and K. A. Bauer, "Ceftolozane/tazobactam pharmacokinetics in a critically ill adult receiving continuous renal replacement therapy," *Pharmacotherapy*, vol. 36, no. 5, pp. e30–e33, 2016.

[5] N. Safdar, J. Handelsman, and D. G. Maki, "Does combination antimicrobial therapy reduce mortality in Gram-negative bacteraemia? A meta-analysis," *Lancet Infectious Diseases*, vol. 4, no. 8, pp. 519–527, 2004.

[6] S. Zelenitsky, L. Barns, I. Findlay et al., "Analysis of microbiological trends in peritoneal dialysis-related peritonitis from 1991 to 1998," *American Journal of Kidney Diseases*, vol. 36, no. 5, pp. 1009–1013, 2000.

[7] P. D. Lister, D. J. Wolter, and N. D. Hanson, "Antibacterial-resistant *Pseudomonas aeruginosa*: clinical impact and complex regulation of chromosomally encoded resistance mechanisms," *Clinical Microbiology Reviews*, vol. 22, no. 4, pp. 582–610, 2009.

[8] G. A. Jacoby, "AmpC β-lactamases," *Clinical Microbiology Reviews*, vol. 22, no. 1, pp. 161–182, 2009.

[9] S. D. Lahiri, G. K. Walkup, J. D. Whiteaker et al., "Selection and molecular characterization of ceftazidime/avibactamresistant mutants in Pseudomonas aeruginosa strains containing derepressed AmpC," *Journal of Antimicrobial Chemotherapy*, vol. 70, no. 6, pp. 1650–1658, 2015.

[10] G. Cabot, S. Bruchmann, X. Mulet et al., "*Pseudomonas aeruginosa* ceftolozane-tazobactam resistance development requires multiple mutations leading to overexpression and structural modification of AmpC," *Antimicrobial Agents and Chemotherapy*, vol. 58, no. 6, pp. 3091–3099, 2014.

[11] D. M. Livermore, "Has the era of untreatable infections arrived?" *Journal of Antimicrobial Chemotherapy*, vol. 64, supplement 1, pp. i29–i36, 2009.

[12] E. B. Hirsch and V. H. Tam, "Impact of multidrug-resistant *Pseudomonas aeruginosa* infection on patient outcomes," *Expert Review of Pharmacoeconomics and Outcomes Research*, vol. 10, no. 4, pp. 441–451, 2010.

12

First Case of Lung Abscess due to *Salmonella enterica* Serovar Abony in an Immunocompetent Adult Patient

Vassiliki Pitiriga,[1] **John Dendrinos,**[2] **Emanuel Nikitiadis,**[2]
Georgia Vrioni,[1] **and Athanassios Tsakris**[1]

[1]*Department of Microbiology, Medical School, National and Kapodistrian University of Athens, M. Asias 75, Goudi, 11527 Athens, Greece*
[2]*Metropolitan Hospital, Ethnarchou Makariou 9 & El. Venizelou 1, N. Faliro, 18547 Athens, Greece*

Correspondence should be addressed to Vassiliki Pitiriga; siliapit@hotmail.com

Academic Editor: Lawrence Yamuah

In healthy individuals, nontyphoidal *Salmonella* species predominantly cause a self-limited form of gastroenteritis, while they infrequently invade or cause fatal disease. Extraintestinal manifestations of nontyphoidal *Salmonella* infections are not common and mainly occur among individuals with specific risk factors; among them, focal lung infection is a rare complication caused by nontyphoidal *Salmonella* strains typically occurring in immunocompromised patients with prior lung disease. We describe the first case of a localized lung abscess formation in an immunocompetent healthy female adult due to *Salmonella enterica* serovar Abony. The patient underwent lobectomy and was discharged after full clinical recovery. This case report highlights nontyphoidal *Salmonellae* infections as a potential causative agent of pleuropulmonary infections even in immunocompetent healthy adults.

1. Introduction

In developed countries, nontyphoidal *Salmonellae* (NTS) strains are a leading cause of self-limiting enterocolitis in healthy population; they are estimated to cause 94 million cases of gastroenteritis and 115,000 deaths globally each year [1]. Up to 5% of patients will develop secondary bacteremia [2], with low attributable mortality (1–5%). Localized extraintestinal infections develop as secondary complications in approximately 5–10% of cases with NTS bacteremia [3] and occur predominately in a wide variety of immunocompromised individuals [4], including patients with severe underlying diseases [5], immunocompromised elderly patients [6, 7], or children [8]. Mainly they involve the gastrointestinal tract, endothelial surfaces [9], pericardium [10], meninges [11], lungs, joints, and bones [12], or soft tissues. Among them, pleuropulmonary NTS infection is an infrequent manifestation [13, 14] mostly occurring in immunocompromised patients with prior lung or pleural pathology [15].

In healthy immunocompetent individuals, extraintestinal complications caused by NTS remain uncommon [16–19]. We present the first case of a lung abscess caused by *Salmonella* serovar Abony in an immunocompetent healthy young adult with no prior history of pulmonary disease or presence of any underlying disease.

2. Case Presentation

A 26-year-old female of Hellenic ethnicity was admitted to our outpatient clinic, reporting a 10-day history of low grade fever, chills, nausea, headache, urge to vomiting, and a dull pain over the right kidney area. Her past medical history was free of any chronic or acute infection or systemic disease, except for a prior admission to our hospital 1 year ago due to diarrhea not associated with any specific microorganism.

Her physical examination revealed temperature of 38°C, normal blood pressure (110/70 mmHg), and tachycardia (HR = 160 bpm). During palpation, a slight pain in right upper abdominal area was revealed with no other specific signs and symptoms. The respiratory examination was remarkable for dullness to percussion with decreased breath sounds over the lower right lung base. The remainder of the physical

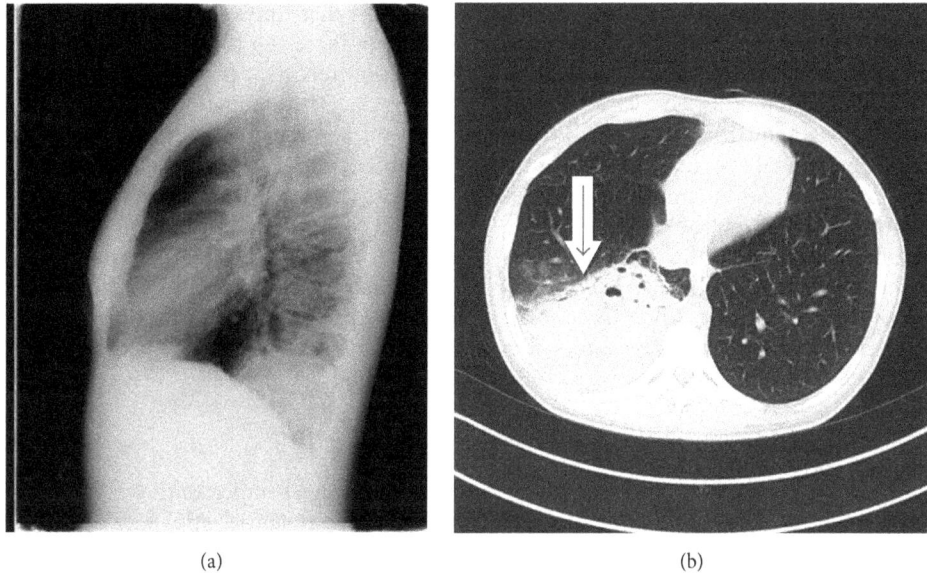

(a)   (b)

FIGURE 1: (a) Chest radiograph on presentation; (b) chest CT scanning on day 3 of admission, showing a large abscess in the right lower lobe.

examination was unremarkable. Initial laboratory findings revealed a polymorphonuclear leucocytosis of 13.700/mm^3 with 72% neutrophils and 18% lymphocytes, ESR of 29 mm/hr, and C-reactive protein of 5.31 mg/dL. No other pathological findings were indicated from the biochemical testing. Detailed investigations did not reveal any predisposing factors or evidence of an underlying immunodeficiency. More specifically, there was no evidence of malnutrition, no history of therapy with glucocorticoids or other immunosuppressive drugs, and no indication of immunoglobulin excess or deficiency through quantitative serum immunoglobulin tests, and blood tests were negative for chronic infections (HIV, viral hepatitis, etc.) or autoimmune disorders (antinuclear antibodies and other autoantibodies). Chest X-ray examination showed pneumonic infiltration in the lower one-third of the right hemithorax and laterally located dense appearance resembling left pleural effusion. Based on this evidence, the patient was diagnosed as having community-acquired pneumonia and after blood cultures were taken, antimicrobial treatment was initiated with intravenous ceftriaxone 1 gr/day + azithromycin 500 mg/day. Sputum, protected specimen brush (PSB) material of bronchial secretions, and three sets of blood specimens were also taken on admission for cultures which did not yield any pathogens.

Within the following two days, the patient's fever rose to 40°C despite the administration of antimicrobial therapy, and her condition deteriorated by developing dry cough, chest pain, total absence of breath sound during auscultation in right hemithorax, and dyspnea. Additionally, a strong right lumbar pain appeared. Three additional sets of blood cultures, taken while the patient was febrile, were negative.

On the third day, computed tomography (CT) scanning of the chest was performed and revealed a lung thick-walled abscess formation in the right lower lobe, with a surrounding inflammatory infiltrate, extended atelectasis, and pleural

effusion to the right lower lobe. Figures 1(a) and 1(b) exhibit the size and morphology of the lung abscess. A subsequent ultrasound examination of the patient's liver, carried out in order to examine whether there was any subdiaphragmatic extension or origin of the infection, did not reveal any relevant evidence.

The combination of ceftriaxone + azithromycin was consequently discontinued and replaced by moxifloxacin 400 mg/day + tazobactam plus piperacillin (0.5 + 4.0) gr × 3/day + clindamycin 600 mg × 3/day. PCR for tuberculosis was performed and anti-*Echinococcus* IgG and IgM antibody titers were measured; however all the results were negative.

The next days, her fever did not subside, CRP levels rose gradually to 16.85 mg/dL, and the pleural effusion continued to rise. Blood cultures remained all negative for any bacterial growth.

On the sixth day of admission, the patient underwent lobectomy, owing to the lack of response to antibiotic therapy, the deterioration of symptoms, and the difficulty in approaching the specific lobe area by thoracentesis. Approximately 700 mL of pleural fluid was collected and sent to laboratory for biochemical analysis, Gram stain, cultures, and antimicrobial profile. Biochemical analysis of the pleural fluid showed the following: glucose of 74 mg/dL, lactate dehydrogenase of 730 U/L, total protein of 3.9 g/dL, and white blood cell count of 15.400/mm^3 with 80% polymorphs. Gram staining and cultures of the pleural fluid were negative. In addition, the aspiration of the abscess revealed yellowish pus (about 45 mL) that was also sent for laboratory analysis the same day. Cultures of the pus sample collected from the abscess yielded a Gram-negative aerobic rod identified as *Salmonella enterica* subsp. *enterica* serovar Abony. *Salmonella* isolate was identified to the genus level by both the automated Vitek-2 System (bioMerieux, Inc., Hazelwood, MO) and the API 20E (bioMerieux, Inc., Hazelwood, MO).

Serotyping of the isolate was performed using the somatic O and flagellar H antisera according to the Kauffman-White classification scheme (Difco Laboratories, Detroit, MI, USA). Molecular confirmation of *Salmonella* serotyping was carried out using the DNA microarray system Premi-Test® Salmonella (DSM Nutritional Products, Check-Points, Wageningen, Netherlands) [20]. Antimicrobial susceptibility testing was initially performed by the Vitek-2 System, according to the recommendations of the National Committee for Clinical Laboratory Standards [21] and confirmed by E-test (bioMerieux, Inc., Hazelwood, MO). The isolate was susceptible to commonly used antibiotics (ampicillin MIC of 0.75 μg/mL, ceftriaxone MIC of 0.085 μg/mL, cefotaxime MIC of 0.082 μg/mL, ceftazidime MIC of 0.115 μg/mL, ciprofloxacin MIC of 0.032 μg/mL, moxifloxacin MIC of 0.016 μg/mL, and trimethoprim-sulfamethoxazole MIC of 0.064 μg/mL). Based on the laboratory report, the antimicrobial therapy was changed on the eighth day after admission, to sulfamethoxazole/trimethoprim (800 + 160) mg × 2/day, moxifloxacin 400 mg/day, and clindamycin 600 mg × 3/day, along with supportive therapy.

The postoperative clinical condition of the patient improved noticeably. Six days after surgery, the patient's symptoms resolved and she was discharged on sulfamethoxazole/trimethoprim (800 + 160) mg × 2/day and ciprofloxacin 500 mg × 2/day, for 20 days.

3. Discussion

Even though the prevalence of invasive NTS in humans by means of bacteremia and extraintestinal infections is increasing worldwide among immunocompromised patients, particularly in developing countries, likely secondary to the high prevalence of coexisting malnutrition, malaria, and HIV infection, it remains uncommon in immunocompetent subjects [22]. Especially for NTS pleuropulmonary infection as a secondary manifestation in healthy individuals, only two reports exist in the literature documenting *Salmonella* Group B spp. as the primary cause of lung abscess in two immunocompetent female children [23, 24]. In another report of Genzen et al. [25], even though the 55-year-old man diagnosed with pulmonary *Salmonella* serovar Typhimurium infection was considered as immunocompetent, his medical history of chronic alcoholism and bronchitis should be taken into account as a significant predisposing factor for the invasive development of the infection. To our knowledge, this is the first report of lung abscess caused by NTS presenting in an immunocompetent healthy individual of the adult age group. Moreover, only one case report has been described in the literature documenting *Salmonella* serovar Abony to cause severe invasive disease, by means of disseminated intravascular coagulation, in an immunocompromised elderly patient [26]. We report for the first time an extraintestinal complication of lung abscess caused by *Salmonella* serovar Abony.

Lung infections by NTS may occur via several routes such as direct extension from a nearby infection, aspiration of gastric secretions, or hematogenous dissemination from the gastrointestinal tract. In the present case, our patient reported a history of diarrhea one year before the onset of

illness. At that time, she was admitted to our clinic with a history of loose stools for a period of the prior ten days. She was given treatment with ciprofloxacin for three days before admission. On examination, she was not febrile and the stools were not accompanied by mucus or blood, while vomiting was absent. Stool and blood cultures were negative, possibly due to the antibiotic treatment and she was discharged 4 days after without identification of the infectious causative agent. This incident might be connected with the existing pulmonary complication, as it provides an indication of a potential gastrointestinal infection by *Salmonella* Abony with a subsequent seeding of the pathogen to the lungs through bacteremia.

4. Conclusion

This case report indicates that NTS strains should be considered as a potential etiological agent of infection in the differential diagnosis of pleuropulmonary infection causes, even among immunocompetent healthy adults.

Competing Interests

The authors declare that they have no conflict of interests relevant to this paper.

References

[1] S. E. Majowicz, J. Musto, E. Scallan et al., "The global burden of nontyphoidal *Salmonella* gastroenteritis," *Clinical Infectious Diseases*, vol. 50, no. 6, pp. 882–889, 2010.

[2] E. L. Hohmann, "Nontyphoidal salmonellosis," *Clinical Infectious Diseases*, vol. 32, no. 2, pp. 263–269, 2001.

[3] D. A. Pegues, M. E. Ohl, and S. I. Miller, "*Salmonella* species, including *Salmonella typhi*," in *Principles and Practice of Infectious Diseases*, G. L. Mandell, J. E. Bennett, and R. Dolin, Eds., pp. 2636–2654, Churchill Livingstone, Philadelphia, Pa, USA, 6th edition, 2005.

[4] M. A. Gordon, "*Salmonella* infections in immunocompromised adults," *Journal of Infection*, vol. 56, no. 6, pp. 413–422, 2008.

[5] B. Cabaret, M.-L. Couëc, M. Lorrot, E. Launay, and C. Gras-Le Guen, "Multifocal osteoarticular infection caused by *Salmonella* non typhi in a child with sickle cell disease," *Archives de Pediatrie*, vol. 20, no. 4, pp. 398–402, 2013.

[6] P.-L. Chen, C.-M. Chang, C.-J. Wu et al., "Extraintestinal focal infections in adults with nontyphoid *Salmonella* bacteraemia: predisposing factors and clinical outcome," *Journal of Internal Medicine*, vol. 261, no. 1, pp. 91–100, 2007.

[7] R.-B. Hsu, Y.-G. Tsay, R. J. Chen, and S.-H. Chu, "Risk factors for primary bacteremia and endovascular infection in patients without acquired immunodeficiency syndrome who have nontyphoid salmonellosis," *Clinical Infectious Diseases*, vol. 36, no. 7, pp. 829–834, 2003.

[8] E. Çiftçi, H. Güriz, A. D. Aysev, E. Ince, B. Erdem, and U. Doğru, "*Salmonella* bacteraemia in Turkish children: 37 cases seen in a university hospital between 1993 and 2002," *Annals of Tropical Paediatrics*, vol. 24, no. 1, pp. 75–80, 2004.

[9] R.-B. Hsu and F.-Y. Lin, "Risk factors for bacteraemia and endovascular infection due to non-typhoid *Salmonella*: a reappraisal," *Quarterly Journal of Medicine*, vol. 98, no. 11, pp. 821–827, 2005.

[10] D. Ortiz, E. M. Siegal, C. Kramer, B. K. Khandheria, and E. Brauer, "Nontyphoidal cardiac salmonellosis: two case reports and a review of the literature," *Texas Heart Institute Journal*, vol. 41, no. 4, pp. 401–406, 2014.

[11] E. M. Molyneux, L. A. Mankhambo, P. Ajib et al., "The outcome of non-typhoidal *Salmonella* meningitis in Malawian children, 1997–2006," *Annals of Tropical Paediatrics*, vol. 29, no. 1, pp. 13–22, 2009.

[12] A. Dutta and C. H. Allen, "Non-typhoidal *Salmonella* osteomyelitis in the midfoot of a healthy child and review of the literature," *Journal of Infectious Diseases and Therapy*, vol. 1, no. 2, article 107, 2013.

[13] P.-L. Chen, C.-J. Wu, C.-M. Chang et al., "Extraintestinal focal infections in adults with *Salmonella enterica* serotype Choleraesuis bacteremia," *Journal of Microbiology, Immunology and Infection*, vol. 40, no. 3, pp. 240–247, 2007.

[14] E. Moraitou, I. Karydis, D. Nikita, and M. E. Falagas, "Case report: parotid abscess due to *Salmonella enterica* serovar Enteritidis in an immunocompetent adult," *International Journal of Medical Microbiology*, vol. 297, no. 2, pp. 123–126, 2007.

[15] C. Saturveithan, "*Salmonella* osteomyelitis in a one year old child without sickle cell disease: a case report," *Malaysian Orthopaedic Journal*, vol. 8, pp. 52–54, 2014.

[16] J. C. Kam, S. Abdul-Jawad, C. Modi et al., "Pleural Empyema due to Group D Salmonella," *Case Reports in Gastrointestinal Medicine*, vol. 2012, Article ID 524561, 4 pages, 2012.

[17] N. F. Crum, "Non-typhi *Salmonella* empyema: case report and review of the literature," *Scandinavian Journal of Infectious Diseases*, vol. 37, no. 11-12, pp. 852–857, 2005.

[18] R. L. Hall, R. Partridge, N. Venkatraman, and M. Wiselka, "Invasive non-typhoidal *Salmonella* infection with multifocal seeding in an immunocompetent host: an emerging disease in the developed world," *BMJ Case Reports*, vol. 2013, 2013.

[19] W.-J. Lin, C.-C. Wang, S.-N. Cheng, W.-T. Lo, and C.-H. Hung, "Hand abscess, phlebitis, and bacteremia due to *Salmonella enterica* serotype Augustenborg," *Journal of Microbiology, Immunology and Infection*, vol. 39, no. 6, pp. 519–522, 2006.

[20] P. Andreoli, J. Thijssen, R. Anthony, P. Vos, and W. De Levita, "Fast method for detecting micro-organisms in food samples 2004," Patent WO2004106547 A3.

[21] National Committee for Clinical Laboratory Standards, "Performance standards for antimicrobial susceptibility testing; 24th informational supplement," Tech. Rep. M100-S11, National Committee for Clinical Laboratory Standards, Wayne, Pa, USA, 2014.

[22] E. Galanakis, M. Bitsori, S. Maraki, C. Giannakopoulou, G. Samonis, and Y. Tselentis, "Invasive non-typhoidal salmonellosis in immunocompetent infants and children," *International Journal of Infectious Diseases*, vol. 11, no. 1, pp. 36–39, 2007.

[23] R. Thapa, A. Ghosh, D. Mallick, and B. Biswas, "Lung abscess secondary to non-typhoidal salmonellosis in an immunocompetent girl," *Singapore Medical Journal*, vol. 50, no. 10, pp. 1033–1035, 2009.

[24] B. Adhisivam, S. Mahadevan, and C. Udaykumar, "Lung abscess caused by *Salmonella*," *Indian Journal of Pediatrics*, vol. 73, no. 5, pp. 450–451, 2006.

[25] J. R. Genzen, D. M. Towle, J. D. Kravetz, and S. M. Campbell, "*Salmonella typhimurium* pulmonary infection in an immunocompetent patient," *Connecticut Medicine*, vol. 72, no. 3, pp. 139–142, 2008.

[26] S. C. Glover, C. C. Smith, and I. A. Porter, "Fatal *Salmonella* septicaemia with disseminated intravascular coagulation and renal failure," *Journal of Medical Microbiology*, vol. 15, no. 1, pp. 117–121, 1982.

13

Autoantibodies in a Three-Year-Old Girl with Visceral Leishmaniasis: A Potential Diagnostic Pitfall

Gholamreza Pouladfar,[1] Zahra Jafarpour,[1] Amir Hossein Babaei,[1,2] Bahman Pourabbas,[1] Bita Geramizadeh,[3] and Anahita Sanaei Dashti[1]

[1]*Professor Alborzi Clinical Microbiology Research Center, Namazi Hospital, Shiraz University of Medical Sciences, Shiraz, Iran*
[2]*Student Research Committee, Shiraz University of Medical Sciences, Neshat Street, Shiraz 71348 43638, Iran*
[3]*Transplant Research Center, Pathology Department, Shiraz University of Medical Sciences, Shiraz, Iran*

Correspondence should be addressed to Amir Hossein Babaei; babaei93@yahoo.com

Academic Editor: Sinésio Talhari

Visceral leishmaniasis (VL), a life-threatening parasitic infection, is endemic in the Mediterranean region. Diagnosis of VL is based on epidemiologic, clinical, and laboratory findings. However, sometimes, clinical features and laboratory findings overlap with those of autoimmune diseases. In some cases, autoantibodies are detected in patients with VL and this could be a potential diagnostic pitfall. In this study, we have reported on a three-year-old girl from a VL-endemic area in Iran, who presented with prolonged fever and splenomegaly. Bone marrow examination, serologic tests, and the molecular PCR assay were performed; however, results were inconclusive. The levels of anti-double stranded DNA, cytoplasmic antineutrophil cytoplasmic autoantibody, and perinuclear antineutrophil cytoplasmic autoantibody were elevated and, at the end, splenic biopsy was performed. The splenic tissue PCR test detected the DNA of *Leishmania infantum*. The patient's condition improved with anti-*Leishmania* therapy, and the autoantibodies disappeared within the following four months. Clinical presentations and laboratory findings of VL and autoimmune diseases may overlap in some patients.

1. Introduction

Visceral leishmaniasis (VL) is an endemic parasitic infection, occurring in India, Africa, South America, the Middle East region, and the eastern Mediterranean region. VL is an endemic disease in northwest (Ardebil and East Azerbaijan provinces) and southwest (Fars and Bushehr provinces) of Iran [1]. It could be life-threatening if diagnosis is delayed and treatment is inappropriate [2]. In the eastern Mediterranean region, *Leishmania infantum* (*L. infantum*) is the main cause of VL. In Iran, *L. infantum* is the leading cause of VL, while *L. tropica* has been recognized as the second most common cause [3, 4].

Suspicion of VL is usually based on demographic, clinical, and laboratory findings. A patient with VL shows a number of clinical features such as fever, malaise, weight loss, and hepatosplenomegaly, as well as some nonspecific laboratory findings like pancytopenia, hypergammaglobulinemia, elevated C-reactive protein (CRP) level, and high erythrocyte sedimentation rate (ESR). These clinical features and laboratory findings could mimic those of autoimmune diseases [5, 6]. Sometimes, autoantibodies such as antinuclear antibody (ANA), anti-double stranded DNA (anti-dsDNA), cytoplasmic antineutrophil cytoplasmic autoantibody (C-ANCA), perinuclear antineutrophil cytoplasmic autoantibody (P-ANCA), rheumatoid factor (RF), and anti-smooth muscle antibodies (ASMA) are detected in patients with VL. These may lead to a potential diagnostic pitfall [5, 7]. Indeed, several reports have described the misdiagnosis of VL as an autoimmune disease which has led to fatal outcomes [7, 8].

In this work, we report the case study of a three-year-old girl with the final diagnosis of visceral leishmaniasis, where autoimmune antibodies in the serum were elevated, resulting in an initial misleading diagnosis.

2. The Case

A three-year-old girl was referred to the Namazi Teaching Hospital, affiliated to Shiraz University of Medical Sciences, with a history of fever for seven days, as well as splenomegaly. She was referred from an endemic area of VL in Fars province, southeastern Iran. The notable findings in the general physical examination were an axillary temperature of 40°C and a palpable spleen just below the costal margin. Based on the history and physical examination there were no other explanations for other sources of infection.

On admission, a complete blood count revealed pancytopenia. The hemoglobin level was 9.3 g/dL, and there were a mean corpuscular volume of 77 femtoliters, white blood cell (WBC) count of 4400/mm^3 with 35% neutrophils, 62% lymphocytes, and a platelet count of 119000/mm^3. The reticulocyte count was 1.2% and the direct and indirect Coombs tests were negative. Liver function test results were as follows: albumin 3.8 mg/dL, globulin 2.8 mg/dL, alanine aminotransferase (ALT) 16 U/L, aspartate aminotransferase (AST) 51 U/L, alkaline phosphatase 267 U/L, serum lactate dehydrogenase 1474 U/L (normal level below 480 U/L), total bilirubin 0.5 mg/dL, and direct bilirubin 0.1. Prothrombin time and partial thromboplastin time were within the normal range. The systemic inflammation indices were abnormal, including an ESR of 75 mm/h and a CRP level of 11 mg/dL. The ferritin level was 690 ng/mL (normal: 10–124 ng/mL). The renal function was normal.

Urine, blood, and stool cultures were also negative. In thick and thin smears for malaria, no parasites were detected. The DNA quantitative PCR for cytomegalovirus and EBV, the Wright and Widal tests, and HIV antibody were all negative. The Epstein-Barr virus, viral-capsid antigen (EBV-VCA) IgM was within the normal range. The Venereal Disease Research Laboratory (VDRL) test for syphilis and the cold agglutinin tests were also negative. The serum immunofluorescence assay (IFA) for determining *Leishmania* antibodies and quantitative PCR for detecting *L. infantum* kinetoplast DNA were performed by methods described previously and results were negative [4, 9].

Some autoimmune lab findings, including RF, ANA, anti-cardiolipin antibodies (ACLA), anti-Smith (anti-Sm), anti-Sjögren's syndrome related antigen A (anti-SSA/Ro), anti-Sjögren's syndrome related antigen B (anti-SSB/La), and anti-topoisomerase I (anti-Scl-70) antibodies, were negative. On the other hand, others were positive including anti-dsDNA, 42.2 U/mL (positive above 24), C-ANCA, 27.3 U/mL (positive above 18), and P-ANCA, 26.3 U/mL (positive above 18). The serums C3 and C4 were within normal range.

Abdominal ultrasonography and CT scan both confirmed splenomegaly. Bone marrow smears and biopsy indicated mild hypocellular marrow; however the myeloid and erythroid maturation was normal. The PCR test for detection of *L. infantum* in bone marrow was negative. There was no evidence of malignancy or an infiltrative disease and no Leishman bodies were seen.

For evaluating the competency of the immune system, quantitative serum immunoglobulin tests, the CH50 assay, the dihydrorhodamine (DHR) flow cytometric test, and the

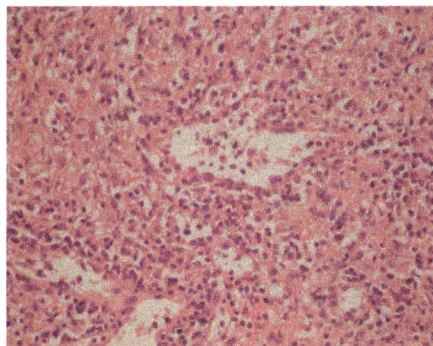

FIGURE 1: Splenic section H&E; red pulps expanded by heavy infiltration of plasma cells and histiocytes. No Leishman body is present.

T-cell and B-cell counts by flow cytometry were performed, and their results were normal.

One week after admission, the patient's condition started to deteriorate and pancytopenia worsened (hemoglobin 6.1 mg/dL, WBC 2.8/mm^3, and platelet 29000/mm^3). Despite the negative results in our initial investigations for VL diagnosis, we made the decision to start VL treatment with amphotericin B deoxycholate (AmB-d, 1 mg/kg per day by infusion, daily). This decision was made based on demographic data, clinical and laboratory findings, and exclusion of other probable causes.

One week after AmB-d administration, the patient's condition started to improve dramatically. Ultimately, VL was diagnosed when an open spleen biopsy was performed. A histological examination of the spleen biopsy showed red pulp expansion with heavy infiltration of plasma cells and histiocytes. This was highly suggestive of VL. No Leishman bodies were detected (Figure 1). The qualitative PCR in the spleen tissue revealed *L. infantum* kinetoplast DNA. On the tenth day of treatment with AmB-d, the platelet count started to increase; therefore, we changed AmB-d to intramuscular Glucantime at 20 mg/kg per day for a period of 20 days.

Four months after her therapy, the patient was in good clinical condition and free of any complaints. She had normal blood counts, inflammatory indices, and biochemical analyses. Anti-dsDNA, C-ANCA, and P-ANCA levels had become normal (3.24 U/mL, 2.14 U/mL, and 1.42 U/mL, resp., normal below 5 U/mL).

3. Discussion

Clinical presentations and laboratory findings of VL and autoimmune diseases may overlap in some cases. The similarity in clinical presentations (fever, pallor, anorexia, malaise, weight loss, and hepatosplenomegaly) and laboratory findings (anemia, leucopenia, thrombocytopenia, hypergammaglobulinemia, hypoalbuminemia, low serum complement levels, high levels of inflammatory markers like ESR and CRP, and the presence of anti-dsDNA, C-ANCA, and P-ANCA) could therefore be misleading in differentiating VL from autoimmune diseases [10, 11].

It was previously reported that some patients with VL had been misdiagnosed with autoimmune hepatitis [12, 13], primary biliary cirrhosis, and systemic lupus erythematosus [7, 14]. These misdiagnoses sometimes led to fatal outcomes [7, 8]. In addition, VL could develop in patients with autoimmune diseases who were treated with immunosuppressive medications. Overlapping clinical manifestations could lead to delayed diagnosis of VL and fatal consequences [15, 16].

Sometimes autoantibodies like ANA, P-ANCA, C-ANCA, RF, anti-dsDNA, anti-Sm, anti-SSA/Ro, anti-SSB/La, and ASMA are detected in patients with VL [5, 7]. There are three major theories for the formation of autoantibodies in VL patients. The first theory claims that the destruction of tissues by the protozoa causes the release of self-antigens and their exposure to the immune system. The second theory claims that polyclonal B-cell activation and the altered function of regulatory and suppressor T-cells lead to the formation of autoantibodies. The last theory claims that molecular mimicry of the host antigens by antigens of *Leishmania* can cause a cross-reactivity [5, 7, 13].

The gold standard of VL diagnosis still remains the detection of parasites in the bone marrow aspiration or splenic tissue by smear or culture [17]. Indeed, splenic smears have the highest sensitivity for detecting VL (93.1–98.7%), compared to bone marrow and lymph node smears (52–85% and 52–58%, resp.). Serological tests such as IFA, which are frequently performed in areas where VL is endemic, serve as a highly sensitive diagnostic method in immunocompetent patients. The sensitivity and specificity of IFA for VL are shown to be 96% and 98%, respectively [18]. Molecular tests such as PCR have been proposed as highly sensitive methods in VL diagnosis. In a recent meta-analysis, the pooled sensitivity of PCR in whole blood was 93.1% (95% confidence interval (CI), 90.0 to 95.2), and the specificity was 95.6% (95% CI, 87.0 to 98.6) [17]. The sensitivity of the PCR assay in bone marrow aspirate samples is 95.7% [19]. There have not been many studies investigating the sensitivity and specificity of PCR in human spleen tissues. In a study carried out in southern Iran, PCR revealed the existence of parasite DNA in all 22 splenic aspirate specimens of confirmed VL patients [9]. In the patient of this study, splenic tissue PCR was the only diagnostic test that confirmed VL.

In conclusion, the presence of autoantibodies can be a potential pitfall which can lead to the diagnosis of autoimmune diseases instead of VL. Maintaining high clinical indexes for suspicion of VL in patients who are referred from endemic areas plays a crucial role in efficiently managing and treating patients, unless clinical findings and lab tests rule out VL suspicion.

Competing Interests

The authors declare that they have no competing interests.

References

[1] A. Heidari, M. Mohebali, K. Kabir et al., "Visceral leishmaniasis in rural areas of Alborz province of Iran and implication to health policy," *Korean Journal of Parasitology*, vol. 53, no. 4, pp. 379–383, 2015.

[2] J. Alvar, I. D. Vélez, C. Bern et al., "Leishmaniasis worldwide and global estimates of its incidence," *PLoS ONE*, vol. 7, no. 5, Article ID e35671, 2012.

[3] M. Mohebali, "Visceral leishmaniasis in Iran: review of the epidemiological and clinical features," *Iranian Journal of Parasitology*, vol. 8, no. 3, pp. 348–358, 2013.

[4] B. Pourabbas, A. Ghadimi Moghadam, G. Pouladfar, Z. Rezaee, and A. Alborzi, "Quantification of *Leishmania infantum* kinetoplast DNA for monitoring the response to meglumine antimoniate therapy in visceral leishmaniasis," *The American Journal of Tropical Medicine and Hygiene*, vol. 88, no. 5, pp. 868–871, 2013.

[5] M. Nozzi, M. Del Torto, F. Chiarelli, and L. Breda, "Leishmaniasis and autoimmune diseases in pediatric age," *Cellular Immunology*, vol. 292, no. 1, pp. 9–13, 2014.

[6] I. U. Santana, B. Dias, E. A. S. Nunes, F. A. C. D. Rocha, F. S. Silva, and M. B. Santiago, "Visceral leishmaniasis mimicking systemic lupus erythematosus: case series and a systematic literature review," *Seminars in Arthritis and Rheumatism*, vol. 44, pp. 658–665, 2015.

[7] E. Liberopoulos, A. Kei, F. Apostolou, and M. Elisaf, "Autoimmune manifestations in patients with visceral leishmaniasis," *Journal of Microbiology, Immunology and Infection*, vol. 46, no. 4, pp. 302–305, 2013.

[8] I. D. Xynos, M. G. Tektonidou, D. Pikazis, and N. V. Sipsas, "Leishmaniasis, autoimmune rheumatic disease, and antitumor necrosis factor therapy, Europe," *Emerging Infectious Diseases*, vol. 15, no. 6, pp. 956–959, 2009.

[9] A. Alborzi, M. Rasouli, Z. Nademi, M. R. Kadivar, and B. Pourabbas, "Evaluation of rK39 strip test for the diagnosis of visceral leishmaniasis in infants," *Eastern Mediterranean Health Journal*, vol. 12, no. 3-4, pp. 294–299, 2006.

[10] S. Lakhal, M. Benabid, I. B. Sghaier et al., "The sera from adult patients with suggestive signs of autoimmune diseases present antinuclear autoantibodies that cross-react with *Leishmania infantum* conserved proteins: crude *Leishmania* histone and Soluble *Leishmania* antigens," *Immunologic Research*, vol. 61, no. 1-2, pp. 154–159, 2015.

[11] N. Pasyar, A. Alborzi, and G. R. Pouladfar, "Short report: evaluation of serum procalcitonin levels for diagnosis of secondary bacterial infections in visceral leishmaniasis patients," *American Journal of Tropical Medicine and Hygiene*, vol. 86, no. 1, pp. 119–121, 2012.

[12] S. Sotirakou and G. Wozniak, "Clinical expression of autoimmune hepatitis in a nine-year-old girl with visceral leishmaniasis," *Polish Journal of Pathology*, vol. 62, no. 2, pp. 118–119, 2011.

[13] O. G. Tunccan, A. Tufan, G. Telli et al., "Visceral leishmaniasis mimicking autoimmune hepatitis, primary biliary cirrhosis, and systemic lupus erythematosus overlap," *Korean Journal of Parasitology*, vol. 50, no. 2, pp. 133–136, 2012.

[14] A. I. Elshafie, M. Mullazehi, and J. Rönnelid, "General false positive ELISA reactions in visceral leishmaniasis. Implications for the use of enzyme immunoassay analyses in tropical Africa," *Journal of Immunological Methods*, vol. 431, pp. 66–71, 2016.

[15] G. S. Karagiannidis, M. Mantzourani, J. Meletis, A. N. Anastasopoulou, and G. A. Vaiopoulos, "Visceral leishmaniasis in a rheumatoid arthritis patient treated with methotrexate," *Journal of Clinical Rheumatology*, vol. 18, article 59, 2012.

[16] K. Kritikos, E. Haritatos, S. Tsigkos et al., "An atypical presentation of visceral leishmaniasis infection in a patient with rheumatoid arthritis treated with infliximab," *Journal of Clinical Rheumatology*, vol. 16, no. 1, pp. 38–39, 2010.

[17] C. M. de Ruiter, C. van der Veer, M. M. G. Leeflang, S. Deborggraeve, C. Lucas, and E. R. Adams, "Molecular tools for diagnosis of visceral leishmaniasis: systematic review and meta-analysis of diagnostic test accuracy," *Journal of Clinical Microbiology*, vol. 52, no. 9, pp. 3147–3155, 2014.

[18] P. Srivastava, A. Dayama, S. Mehrotra, and S. Sundar, "Diagnosis of visceral leishmaniasis," *Transactions of the Royal Society of Tropical Medicine and Hygiene*, vol. 105, no. 1, pp. 1–6, 2011.

[19] R. Reithinger and J.-C. Dujardin, "Molecular diagnosis of leishmaniasis: current status and future applications," *Journal of Clinical Microbiology*, vol. 45, no. 1, pp. 21–25, 2007.

14

A Rare Case of Coexistence of Borderline Lepromatous Leprosy with Tuberculosis Verrucosa Cutis

Biswajit Dey,[1] Debasis Gochhait,[1] Nagendran Prabhakaran,[2]
Laxmisha Chandrashekar,[2] and Biswanath Behera[2]

[1]Department of Pathology, Jawaharlal Institute of Postgraduate Medical Education and Research (JIPMER), Pondicherry, India
[2]Department of Dermatology, Jawaharlal Institute of Postgraduate Medical Education and Research (JIPMER), Pondicherry, India

Correspondence should be addressed to Debasis Gochhait; publicationmail@rediffmail.com

Academic Editor: Sinésio Talhari

Occurrence of pulmonary tuberculosis with leprosy is known but association of cutaneous tuberculosis with leprosy is rare. We report a case of borderline lepromatous leprosy coexistent with tuberculosis verrucosa cutis in a 29-year-old male, who presented with multiple skin coloured nodules and hyperkeratotic scaly lesions of 3-month duration. Dual infections are associated with high mortality and morbidity. Therefore early diagnosis and management helps to reduce mortality and to mitigate the effects of morbidity.

1. Introduction

Mycobacterium leprae is the causative agent of leprosy that affects the skin and peripheral nerves. On the other hand, tuberculosis is caused by *Mycobacterium tuberculosis* and primarily affects the lungs, but it can involve extrapulmonary sites including the skin. Cutaneous infections are more prevalent in leprosy as compared to tuberculosis and coinfection is uncommon even in countries where mycobacterial infections are endemic [1, 2]. Though many patients with pulmonary tuberculosis and leprosy have been reported in the literature, the association of cutaneous tuberculosis with leprosy has been reported rarely [3–5].

2. Case Report

A 29-year-old male, born to nonconsanguineous parents, presented with multiple skin coloured nodules and hyperkeratotic scaly lesions of 3-month duration. He initially developed asymptomatic skin coloured raised lesions over both the ear lobes. Over the next 2 months he developed multiple similar lesions over the trunk and both the extremities. He also gave history of generalised burning sensation for 15-day duration with low grade fever. There was no history of burning sensation in the eyes, nasal stuffiness, and sensory

or motor weakness. The patient denied any drug intake, fever, myalgia, spontaneous blistering or ulceration, neuritic pain, and testicular pain. None of the family members or neighbours had suffered from leprosy. He denied any past history of infectious diseases but there was no history of immunization including Bacillus Calmette et Guérin (BCG) vaccination. He was a chronic alcoholic.

His general physical examination was normal with no madarosis or lymphadenopathy. Cutaneous examination revealed multiple, soft, succulent, nontender, skin coloured superficial nodules present bilaterally on the forehead, cheeks, ear lobes, forearms, back, and chest with sparing of palms and soles (Figure 1(a)). The surface of these nodules showed follicular plugging. Multiple verrucous plaques were seen over the right ankle (Figure 1(b)). Skin surrounding the plaques was erythematous. Neurological examination revealed thickened bilateral greater auricular, right common peroneal nerve, and tender left posterior tibial nerve. The rest of the musculoskeletal and neurological examination was normal. Routine haematological and biochemical investigations including urine, renal, and liver function test revealed no abnormality. His retroviral serology was negative. Chest X-ray was normal. Slit skin smear from the lesion showed a bacteriological index (BI) of 5+ and the perilesional skin had a BI of 2+.

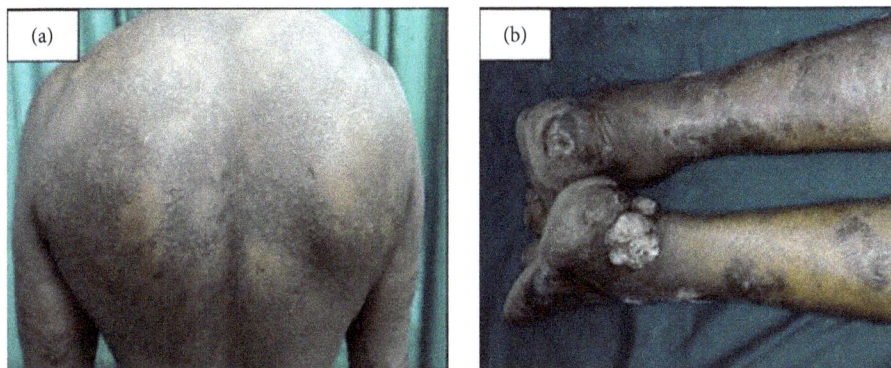

FIGURE 1: (a) Multiple, soft, nontender, skin coloured superficial nodules present bilaterally on the forearms and back. (b) Multiple verrucous plaques were seen over the right ankle.

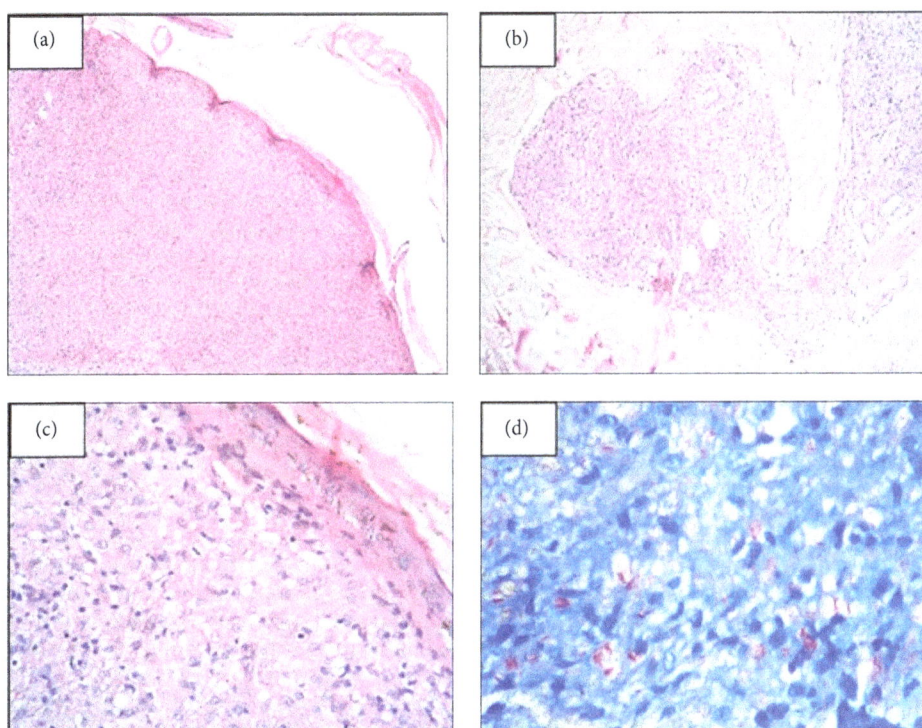

FIGURE 2: (a) and (b) Wedge biopsy done from the forearm and back nodules shows sheets of histiocytes aggregates along with lymphocytes in perivascular and periadnexal location (H&E, 40x and 100x). (c) Collection of epithelioid cells seen in the dermis (H&E, 400x). (d) Strong positivity for acid fast bacilli (Fite Faraco stain, 1000x).

Histopathological examination of the wedge biopsy done from the forearm and back nodules revealed sheets of histiocytes aggregates along with lymphocytes and few polymorphs in perivascular and periadnexal location (Figures 2(a) and 2(b)). There was collection of epithelioid cells (Figure 2(c)). Fite Faraco stain was strongly positive (Figure 2(d)). A diagnosis of borderline lepromatous leprosy with type 2 reaction was made.

A wedge biopsy from the verrucous lesion on the right ankle was taken. Epidermis showed hyperkeratosis and parakeratosis with irregular acanthosis (Figure 3(a)). Dermis showed epithelioid cell granulomas along with lymphocytes and plasma cells (Figures 3(b) and 3(c)). Zeihl-Neelsen stain

for acid fast bacilli was positive (Figure 3(d)). GeneXpert MTB/RIF test based on Nucleic Acid Amplification, which detects MTB-specific region of the rpoB gene and uses real time-PCR (RT-PCR), was done on skin biopsy specimen. The result was positive. However, a culture was not done. Based on clinical and histopathological findings, a diagnosis of tuberculosis verrucosa cutis (TVC) was made.

The patient was treated with rifampicin, isoniazid, pyrazinamide, and ethambutol, in addition to dapsone and clofazimine along with a monthly supervised dose of clofazimine and rifampicin for first 2 months. Then rifampicin and isoniazid with dapsone and clofazimine were continued for further 4 months. After 6 months, treatment of leprosy

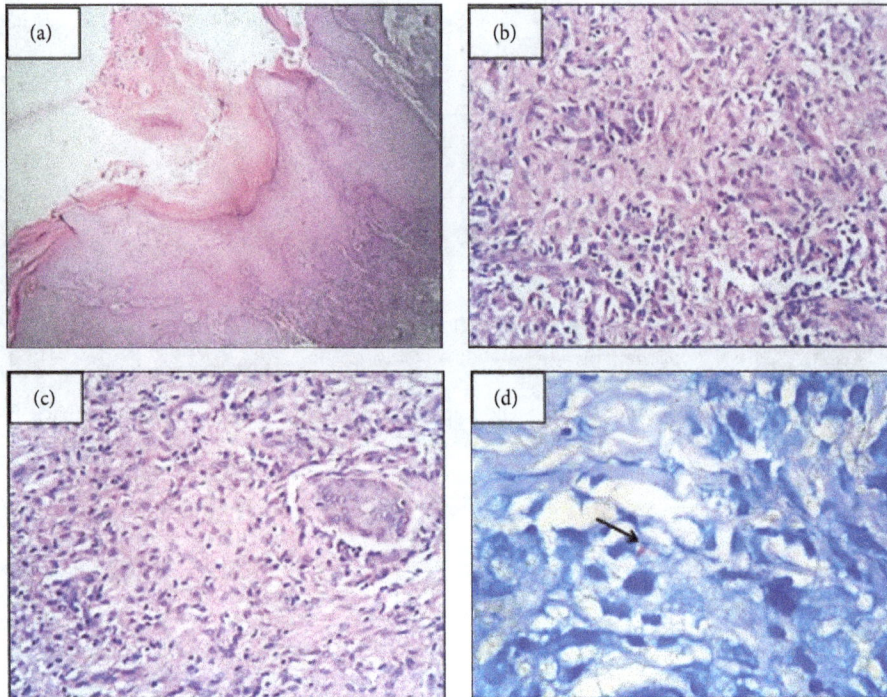

FIGURE 3: (a) Wedge biopsy from the verrucous lesion on the right ankle shows hyperkeratosis and parakeratosis with irregular acanthosis of the epidermis (H&E, 40x). (b) and (c) Dermis shows epithelioid cell granulomas along with lymphocytes and plasma cells (H&E, 400x). (d) Arrow shows positivity for acid fast bacilli (ZN stain, 1000x).

was continued as for multibacillary leprosy. Type 2 reaction was treated with oral anti-inflammatory drugs. The patient tolerated the drugs well with control of type 2 reaction and regression of the TVC lesion.

3. Discussion

Simultaneous occurrence of pulmonary tuberculosis with leprosy is known and its incidence in India varies from 2.5 to 7.7% [6, 7]. The association of cutaneous tuberculosis with leprosy is rare and only 11 cases have been reported in English literature to the best of our knowledge (Table 1).

Although the association between leprosy and tuberculosis has been known for over a century, the exact interaction is still debatable. A number of reasons have been put forth against the simultaneous occurrence of the two infections [8–11]. However studies have suggested that multibacillary (anergic form) leprosy predisposes to tuberculosis [12]. Few reasons have been put forth against the simultaneous occurrence of the two infections. First, both the diseases are caused by Gram-positive, acid fast mycobacteria, which elicit a granulomatous inflammatory reaction as evidenced in histopathological examination [9]. The 65 kilodalton antigens of *Mycobacterium leprae*, *Mycobacterium tuberculosis*, and *Mycobacterium bovis* show more than 95% homology in amino acid sequence [8]. It is evidenced by the partial protection offered by BCG against leprosy and conversion of lepromin intradermal tests after the administration of BCG [8]. Lastly, the tubercular bacilli have higher reproductive rate as compared to lepra bacilli, which prevents both infections to occur simultaneously [9]. However, the issue of the

interaction between the two mycobacterial infections still remains to be clarified. Studies have suggested that leprosy, especially the anergic form, predisposes to tuberculosis [12]. It has been argued that the impaired cell-mediated response to *Mycobacterium leprae* of lepromatous leprosy patients would favor the advance of the more virulent pathogen *Mycobacterium* tuberculosis [12]. It has also been suggested tuberculosis is more severe in coinfections [12]. However, this was not in our case. The patient had paucibacillary TVC as evidenced by few acid fast bacilli. Similar findings have been documented by Trindade and colleagues in which the patients had milder form of tuberculosis [12]. They found that both the patients had normal cellular immune response [12].

It is noted that tuberculosis can occur throughout the spectrum of leprosy [10]. A specific cell-mediated immunity mediated by different subpopulations of CD4/CD8 cells helps the two bacilli to coexist and there exists a partial cross-immunity between the two bacilli [7, 10]. CD4+ T cells along with the cytokines IL-12, IFN-γ, and TNF-α play a pivotal role in the control of tuberculosis and leprae infections [10] Coinfection has been explained by the failure of host's T cells to respond to IL-12 in vivo and as a result host's T cells are unable to produce an appropriate Th 1 cell response [10].

However, the coinfection of leprosy and tuberculosis depends on varied other factors including poor socioeconomic status, malnutrition, immunosuppression due to chemotherapy, and deficient host immune response [11]. The patient's immunity may have been compromised because of chronic alcoholism. Moreover he had no BCG vaccination. BCG vaccination is partly effective against both leprosy and tuberculosis [8, 12]. Another explanation for the evolution of

TABLE 1: Cases of coexistence of leprosy with cutaneous tuberculosis reported in literature.

Authors	Age/gender	Type of leprosy	Type of tuberculosis
Ganapati et al. 1976	30 y/M	Lepromatous leprosy	Lupus vulgaris
Patki et al. 1990	35 y/F	Borderline lepromatous	Lupus vulgaris
Pinto et al. 1991	36 y/M	Borderline tuberculoid	Tuberculosis verrucosa cutis
Dixit et al. 1991	65 y/F	Lepromatous leprosy	Scrofuloderma
Inamadar and Sampagavi 1994	23 y/M	Tuberculoid leprosy	Cutaneous tuberculosis
Ravindra and Sugareddy 2010	10 y/M	Borderline tuberculoid	Tuberculosis verrucosa cutis
Rao et al. 2011	17 y/M	Borderline tuberculoid	Lupus vulgaris
Rajagopala et al. 2013	55 y/M	Tuberculoid leprosy	Cutaneous tuberculosis
Ghunawat et al. 2014	70 y/M	Borderline tuberculoid	Scrofuloderma
Parise-Fortes et al. 2014	59 y/M	Lepromatous leprosy	Cutaneous tuberculosis
Farhana-Quyum et al. 2015	26 y/M	Lepromatous leprosy	Tuberculosis verrucosa cutis

the diseases is that leprosy, especially the anergic form, predisposes to tuberculosis [12]. The patient had multibacillary borderline lepromatous leprosy, a relatively "anergic" form, which might have predisposed him to tuberculosis.

4. Conclusion

Dual infections are associated with high mortality (37.2%) and major morbidity (5.5%) [8]. Therefore the management of these patients requires interdisciplinary management and social support to reduce mortality and to mitigate the effects of morbidity [8].

Competing Interests

The authors declare no competing interests.

References

[1] R. Ganapati, D. H. Deshpande, and R. G. Chulawala, "Some interesting disease combinations. Report on two cases," *Leprosy In India*, vol. 48, no. 4, p. 428, 1976.

[2] A. H. Patki, V. H. Jadhav, and J. M. Mehta, "Leprosy and multicentric lupus vulgaris," *Indian Journal of Leprosy*, vol. 62, no. 3, pp. 368–370, 1990.

[3] J. Pinto, G. S. Pai, and N. Kamath, "Cutaneous tuberculosis with leprosy," *Indian Journal of Dermatology, Venereology and Leprology*, vol. 57, no. 6, pp. 303–304, 1991.

[4] V. B. Dixit, U. S. Pahwa, J. Sen, V. K. Jain, and R. Sen, "Cold abscesses and scrofuloderma in a patient of lepromatous leprosy," *Indian Journal of Leprosy*, vol. 63, no. 1, pp. 101–102, 1991.

[5] A. C. Inamadar and V. V. Sampagavi, "Concomitant occurrence of leprosy, cutaneous tuberculosis and pulmonary tuberculosis-a case report," *Leprosy Review*, vol. 65, no. 3, pp. 282–284, 1994.

[6] K. Ravindra and T. R. Sugareddy, "Coexistence of borderline tuberculoid hansen's disease with tuberculosis verrucosa cutis in a child-a rare case," *Indian Journal of Leprosy*, vol. 82, no. 2, pp. 91–93, 2010.

[7] G. R. Rao, S. Sandhya, M. Sridevi, A. Amareswar, B. L. Narayana, and Shantisri, "Lupus vulgaris and borderline tuberculoid leprosy: an interesting co-occurrence," *Indian Journal of Dermatology, Venereology and Leprology*, vol. 77, no. 1, p. 111, 2011.

[8] S. Rajagopala, U. Devaraj, G. D'Souza, and V. Aithal, "Co-infection with *M. tuberculosis* and *M. leprae-Case* report and systematic review," *Mycobacterial Diseases*, vol. 2, article 118, 2013.

[9] S. Ghunawat, S. Bansal, B. Sahoo, and V. K. Garg, "Borderline tuberculoid leprosy with scrofuloderma: an uncommon association," *Indian Journal of Dermatology, Venereology and Leprology*, vol. 80, no. 4, p. 381, 2014.

[10] M. R. Parise-Fortes, J. C. Lastória, S. A. Marques et al., "Lepromatous leprosy and perianal tuberculosis: a case report and literature review," *Journal of Venomous Animals and Toxins Including Tropical Diseases*, vol. 20, article 38, 2014.

[11] Farhana-Quyum, Mashfiqul-Hasan, and Z. Ahmed, "A case of lepromatous leprosy with co-existing tuberculosis verrucosa cutis (TVC)," *Leprosy Review*, vol. 86, no. 2, pp. 176–179, 2015.

[12] M. Â. B. Trindade, D. Miyamoto, G. Benard, N. Y. Sakai-Valente, D. D. M. Vasconcelos, and B. Naafs, "Leprosy and tuberculosis co-infection: clinical and immunological report of two cases and review of the literature," *American Journal of Tropical Medicine and Hygiene*, vol. 88, no. 2, pp. 236–240, 2013.

15

Corynebacterium striatum Bacteremia Associated with a Catheter-Related Blood Stream Infection

Ueno Daisuke,[1] Tomohiro Oishi,[2] Kunikazu Yamane,[3] and Kihei Terada[2]

[1]*Department of Digestive Surgery, Kawasaki Medical School, Kurashiki, Japan*
[2]*Department of Pediatrics, Kawasaki Medical School, Kurashiki, Japan*
[3]*Department of Public Health, Kawasaki Medical School, Kurashiki, Japan*

Correspondence should be addressed to Ueno Daisuke; daisuke0111@hotmail.co.jp

Academic Editor: Alexandre Rodrigues Marra

A 49-year-old woman visited our emergency department because of exertional dyspnea due to severe left ventricular functional failure. It progressed to disseminated intravascular coagulation and disturbance of consciousness on day 67 of admission. Gram-positive bacilli were detected from two different blood culture samples on day 67 of admission. An API-Coryne test and sequencing (1~615 bp) of the 16S rRNA gene were performed, and the strain was identified as *Corynebacterium striatum*. The bacterium was detected from the removed central venous catheter tip too, and the patient was diagnosed with catheter-related bloodstream infection by *C. striatum*. However, treatment was not effective, and the patient died on day 73 of admission.

1. Introduction

The *Corynebacteria* are a group of aerobic, Gram-positive, catalase-positive, nonsporulating, generally nonmotile rods [1]. The *Corynebacteria* are divided into two groups: *Corynebacterium diphtheriae* and nondiphtherial *Corynebacteria*, collectively referred to as diphtheroids. When isolated from clinical specimens, nondiphtherial *Corynebacteria*, such as *Corynebacterium striatum*, *Corynebacterium amycolatum*, *Corynebacterium minutissimum*, *Corynebacterium xerosis*, and *Corynebacterium freneyi*, were originally thought to be contaminants [2], as these strains are commonly considered as part of the normal flora of human skin and mucous membranes. However, in recent years, they have been reported as emerging opportunistic pathogens in immunocompromised patients with end-stage cancer, hematologic malignancy, and critical condition [2]. There are several reports of *C. striatum* infections including cases of bacteremia, endocarditis, meningitis, pleuropneumonia, osteomyelitis, arthritis, and intrauterine infections [3]. In the present case, we report a catheter-related bloodstream infection caused by *C. striatum*, in a 49-year-old immunocompetent female patient which has multiple organ failures.

2. Case Presentation

A 49-year-old woman was brought to our emergency department because of exertional dyspnea due to severe left ventricular functional failure. Her vital signs were unstable; hence, she was immediately admitted to the intensive care unit (ICU). She had two comorbidities: one was diastole cardiomyopathy, and the other was complete atrioventricular block (c-AVB), already treated with a pacemaker implantation (PM).

Although an implantable cardioverter defibrillator (CRT-D, Cardiac Resynchronization Therapy-Defibrillation), with biventricular pacing function, was replaced with PM for severe left ventricular functional decline, on day 12 of admission, an intra-aortic balloon pump (IABP) was also inserted because of multiple organ failure. The IABP was removed on day 16 of admission. Thereafter, there was no obvious fever, signs of infection, so no antibiotics were administered. However, intermittent hemodialysis was continued due to liver failure and renal failure, and an IABP was necessary again after a worsening of cardiac function on day 66. The illness progressed to disseminated intravascular coagulation (DIC) and disturbance of consciousness on day 67 of admission.

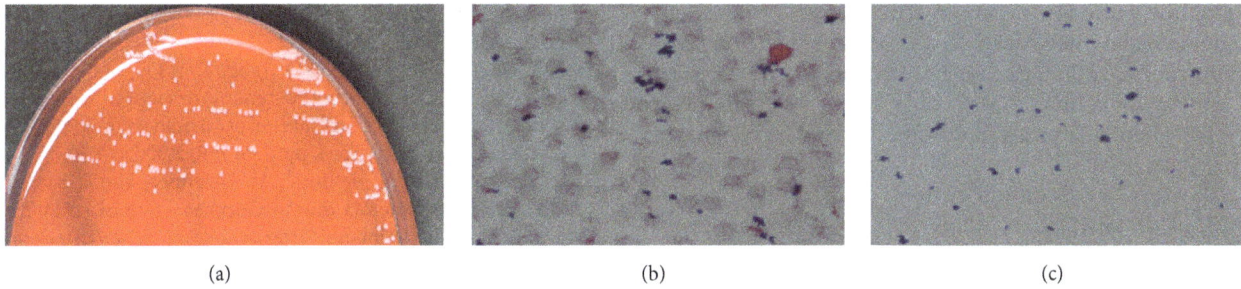

FIGURE 1: (a) White colonies of 1-2 mm diameter of S-type bacteria, observed after incubation of 5% sheep blood agar at 35°C for 24 hours in carbon dioxide gas culture. (b) Gram-positive coccobacillus revealed by Gram staining in blood sample cultures. (c) Detail of a single colony of Gram-positive bacilli in blood sample cultures.

Therefore, two sets of blood samples for blood culture were collected. Gram-positive bacilli were detected in both blood culture samples; each set included aerobic and anaerobic cultures (Figures 1(b) and 1(c)). A central venous catheter inserted in the patient's right internal jugular vein was removed and the catheter tip was sent for a semiquantitative culture analysis on day 68 of admission. No bacteria species could be identified at this time.

Some asynergy in wall motion was detected by echocardiography, but no vegetation was seen. Initially, on day 67 of admission, tazobactam/piperacillin (TAZ/PIPC) (2.25 g every 6 hours) was prescribed. After the results from blood cultures on day 69 of admission, vancomycin (VCM) (1 g every 6 hours) was added to the therapy, while TAZ/PIPC was changed with meropenem (MEPM) (1 g every 6 hours) on day 72. At this time, another two sets of blood samples were collected and blood cultures were negative. However, the patient died on day 73 of admission.

In order to identify the specific strain of infection, the API-Coryne test (BioMèrieux, France) was performed. This method is based on the assessment of biochemical properties. C. striatum/C. amycolatum strain was identified with a probability of 89.7%. The nucleotide sequence (1~615 bp) of the 16s rRNA gene revealed a 99.7% homology to a specific subtype, that is, C. striatum ATCC 6940 (GenBank: NZ_GG667536). The bacterium was detected from the removed central venous catheter tip too. Thus, the patient was diagnosed with a C. striatum catheter-related bloodstream infection. The C. striatum strain was susceptible to VCM, linezolid (LZD), and gentamicin (GM) (Table 1).

3. Discussion

C. striatum colonizes the skin and mucous membranes of both healthy people and hospitalized patients [4]. The majority of cases of C. striatum infection are hospital-acquired as wound infections and a few reports on systemic infections [5], that is, infection confirmed by isolation of C. striatum from a sterile site, are available. However, most of these cases are represented by patients with implanted indwelling devices or who present an immunosuppression [2, 6]. Because her general condition worsened, implanted indwelling devices

TABLE 1: Minimum Inhibitory Concentration of the C. striatum strain.

Drug	MIC (μg/mL)
PCG	>2
CTX	>32
CTRX	>2
CFPM	>2
IPM	>8
MEPM	>8
GM	$\leqq$0.25
EM	>4
CLDM	>2
MINO	8
VCM	0.5
LZD	$\leqq$0.25
CPFX (LVFX)	>4
ST	>38/2

MIC: Minimum Inhibitory Concentration; PCG: benzylpenicillin; CTX: cefotaxime; CTRX: ceftriaxone; CFPM: cefepime; IPM: imipenem; MEPM: meropenem; GM: gentamicin; EM: erythromycin; CLDM: clindamycin; MINO: minocycline; VCM: vancomycin; LZD: linezolid; CPFX: ciprofloxacin; LVFX: levofloxacin; ST: sulfamethoxazole/trimethoprim.

as central venous catheter might cause bacteremia by C. striatum regardless of patient's history.

To our knowledge, this is the second report which found both blood cultures and cultures from a central venous catheter tip positive for the same strain of C. striatum [2]. Since C. striatum may have been isolated from blood sample cultures, it is difficult to distinguish an innocuous contamination from a dangerous infection. Outbreaks caused by multidrug-resistant C. striatum have been reported in patients with prolonged hospitalization, mechanical ventilation, or use of broad-spectrum antibiotics [7, 8].

Approximately 0.2 to 0.4% of native valve endocarditis is caused by Corynebacterium spp., while 9% of early and 4% of late prosthetic valve endocarditis are caused by members of the genus [9, 10]. Although patients with implanted CRT-D may develop infectious endocarditis, obvious vegetation was never observed on echocardiography in these cases [11].

In addition, there is a report of a patient who underwent hemodialysis and developed sepsis caused by a *Corynebacterium* sp. [2]. As the same type of bacteria was detected by the catheter tip culture, the cervical catheter was withdrawn during the hemodialysis, as it was presumed to be the port of entry in this case.

The API-Coryne test is a method to distinguish *C. striatum* from *C. amycolatum*. Although the biochemical properties of *C. amycolatum* and *C. striatum* are similar, only *C. striatum* contains mycolic acid [12]. However, this compound can only be detected by special analyses, for example, gas chromatography; thus *C. striatum* identification was confirmed by 16s rRNA gene analysis.

Since most of reports classified *C. striatum* as susceptible to a wide range of antibiotics [13], it has been suggested that a selective pressure exerted by previous antimicrobial treatment could contribute to its overgrowth. This would eventually lead this strain to become a secondary colonizer in immunocompromised hosts [8].

In general, *C. striatum* is resistant to penicillin but sensitive to other β-lactam antibiotics and to vancomycin. In a previous report, vancomycin was recommended as empirical therapy for serious infections caused by *Corynebacterium* spp. [14]. Although *C. striatum* was susceptible to VCM in this case, the patient might have died because administration of VCM was delayed. Therefore, in this case, appropriate antibiotics could not be judged in vivo. However, the optimal antimicrobial therapy for these infections is still controversial. In vitro susceptibility tests showed that linezolid and tigecycline are active against coryneform bacteria, revealing a potential therapeutic value [15, 16] of these compounds. Currently, there are no guidelines for the treatment of *Corynebacterium* spp. infections. Appropriate susceptibility tests and interpretive criteria are critically needed, in light of the growing emergence of multidrug resistance and its involvement in nosocomial infections.

In conclusion, although *Corynebacterium* could be isolated from a blood culture as a common contaminant, in certain case this observation could conceal a dangerous infection. Patients with a history of exposure to broad-spectrum antibiotics or immunosuppression, as well as critically ill patients with an implanted indwelling device or a central venous catheter, must be considered at high risk of severe infection for this type of bacteria and it is necessary to recognize *C. striatum* as an emerging nosocomial pathogen. In conclusion, we encountered a case of catheter-related bloodstream infection caused by *C. striatum*. Unfortunately, we could not successfully treat the patient because of her poor general condition and comorbidity.

Competing Interests

The authors declare that they have no competing interests.

References

[1] C. B. Severo, L. S. Guazzelli, M. B. Barra, B. Hochhegger, and L. C. Severo, "Multiple pulmonary nodules caused by Corynebacterium striatum in an immunocompetent patient," *Revista do Instituto de Medicina Tropical de Sao Paulo*, vol. 56, no. 1, pp. 89–91, 2014.

[2] F.-L. Chen, P.-R. Hsueh, S.-O. Teng, T.-Y. Ou, and W.-S. Lee, "Corynebacterium striatum bacteremia associated with central venous catheter infection," *Journal of Microbiology, Immunology and Infection*, vol. 45, no. 3, pp. 255–258, 2012.

[3] A. Topić, R. Čivljak, I. Butić, M. Gužvinec, and I. Kuzman, "Relapsing bacteraemia due to Corynebacterium striatum in a patient with peripheral arterial disease," *Polish Journal of Microbiology*, vol. 64, no. 3, pp. 295–298, 2015.

[4] L. Martínez-Martínez, A. I. Suárez, J. Rodríguez-Baño, K. Bernard, and M. A. Muniáin, "Clinical significance of Corynebacterium striatum isolated from human samples," *Clinical Microbiology and Infection*, vol. 3, no. 6, pp. 634–639, 1997.

[5] H. Mizoguchi, M. Sakaki, K. Inoue et al., "Quadricuspid aortic valve complicated with infective endocarditis: report of a case," *Surgery Today*, vol. 44, no. 12, pp. 2388–2391, 2014.

[6] G. Funke and K. A. Bernard, "Corynebacterium gram-positive," in *Manual of Clinical Microbiology*, J. Versalovic, Ed., pp. 413–422, ASM Press, Washington, DC, USA, 2011.

[7] A. H. Brandenburg, A. Van Belkum, C. Van Pelt, H. A. Bruining, J. W. Mouton, and H. A. Verbrugh, "Patient-to-patient spread of a single strain of Corynebacterium striatum causing infections in a surgical intensive care unit," *Journal of Clinical Microbiology*, vol. 34, no. 9, pp. 2089–2094, 1996.

[8] R. B. Leonard, D. J. Nowowiejski, J. J. Warren, D. J. Finn, and M. B. Coyle, "Molecular evidence of person-to-person transmission of a pigmented strain of Corynebacterium striatum in intensive care units," *Journal of Clinical Microbiology*, vol. 32, no. 1, pp. 164–169, 1994.

[9] K. L. Knox and A. H. Holmes, "Nosocomial endocarditis caused by Corynebacterium amycolatum and other nondiphtheriae corynebacteria," *Emerging Infectious Diseases*, vol. 8, no. 1, pp. 97–99, 2002.

[10] P. Riegel, R. Ruimy, R. Christen, and H. Monteil, "Species identities and antimicrobial susceptibilities of Corynebacteria isolated from various clinical sources," *European Journal of Clinical Microbiology and Infectious Diseases*, vol. 15, no. 8, pp. 657–662, 1996.

[11] R. Abi, K. Ez-Zahraouii, M. Ghazouani et al., "A Corynebacterium striatum endocarditis on a carrier of pacemaker," *Annales de Biologie Clinique*, vol. 70, no. 3, pp. 329–331, 2012.

[12] A. Dalal, C. Urban, and S. Segal-Maurer, "Endocarditis due to Corynebacterium amycolatum," *Journal of Medical Microbiology*, vol. 57, no. 10, pp. 1299–1302, 2008.

[13] L. Martinez-Martinez, A. I. Suarez, J. Winstanley, M. C. Ortega, and K. Bernard, "Phenotypic characteristics of 31 strains of Corynebacterium striatum isolated from clinical samples," *Journal of Clinical Microbiology*, vol. 33, no. 9, pp. 2458–2461, 1995.

[14] Y. Otsuka, K. Ohkusu, Y. Kawamura, S. Baba, T. Ezaki, and S. Kimura, "Emergence of multidrug-resistant Corynebacterium striatum as a nosocomial pathogen in long-term hospitalized patients with underlying diseases," *Diagnostic Microbiology and Infectious Disease*, vol. 54, no. 2, pp. 109–114, 2006.

[15] J.-L. Gómez-Garcés, J.-I. Alos, and J. Tamayo, "In vitro activity of linezolid and 12 other antimicrobials against coryneform bacteria," *International Journal of Antimicrobial Agents*, vol. 29, no. 6, pp. 688–692, 2007.

[16] R. Fernandez-Roblas, H. Adames, N. Z. Martín-de-Hijas, D. García Almeida, I. Gadea, and J. Esteban, "In vitro activity of tigecycline and 10 other antimicrobials against clinical isolates of the genus Corynebacterium," *International Journal of Antimicrobial Agents*, vol. 33, no. 5, pp. 453–455, 2009.

16

Pneumocystis Pneumonia Presenting as an Enlarging Solitary Pulmonary Nodule

Krunal Bharat Patel,[1] **James Benjamin Gleason,**[1]
Maria Julia Diacovo,[2] **and Nydia Martinez-Galvez**[1]

[1]*Department of Pulmonary & Critical Care Medicine, Cleveland Clinic Florida, Weston, FL, USA*
[2]*Department of Pathology, Cleveland Clinic Florida, Weston, FL, USA*

Correspondence should be addressed to Krunal Bharat Patel; kbpatelmd@gmail.com

Academic Editor: Sinésio Talhari

Pneumocystis pneumonia is a life threatening infection that usually presents with diffuse bilateral ground-glass infiltrates in immunocompromised patients. We report a case of a single nodular granulomatous *Pneumocystis* pneumonia in a male with diffuse large B-cell lymphoma after R-CHOP therapy. He presented with symptoms of productive cough, dyspnea, and right-sided pleuritic chest pain that failed to resolve despite treatment with multiple antibiotics. Chest X-ray revealed right lower lobe atelectasis and CT of chest showed development of 2 cm nodular opacity with ground-glass opacities. Patient underwent bronchoscopy and biopsy that revealed granulomatous inflammation in a background of organizing pneumonia pattern with negative cultures. Respiratory symptoms resolved but the solitary nodular opacity increased in size prompting a surgical wedge resection which revealed granulomatous *Pneumocystis* pneumonia infection. This case is the third documented report of *Pneumocystis* pneumonia infection within a solitary pulmonary nodule in an individual with hematologic neoplasm. Although *Pneumocystis* pneumonia most commonly occurs in patients with HIV/acquired immunodeficiency syndrome and with diffuse infiltrates, the diagnosis should not be overlooked when only a solitary nodule is present.

1. Introduction

Pneumocystis pneumonia (PcP) is an opportunistic and potentially life threatening fungal infection that occurs in immunocompromised states. It is most commonly encountered in patients with HIV/AIDS and hematopoietic and solid malignancies and those receiving glucocorticoids and chemotherapeutic agents and other immunosuppressive agents [1]. Conventionally, it has been described as a bilateral, diffuse pulmonary disease having a histologic appearance of intra-alveolar eosinophilic foamy exudates containing cysts of *P. jirovecii* [2–4]. Granulomatous PcP accounts for approximately 5% of all PcP cases in AIDS patients, but the incidence in non-HIV patients is unknown due to a paucity of data [5]. A literature search revealed 17 previous cases of granulomatous PcP in patients with hematologic neoplasms [1, 6–9]. Of these 17 published cases, only two patients presented with a solitary pulmonary nodule and only two previous reports of granulomatous PcP have been published with large B-cell lymphoma [6, 7]. Awareness of a solid pulmonary nodule and granulomatous reaction is important as a single nodule could be seen as lymphoma involvement of the lung. In addition, it is important to realize that the diagnostic modality of bronchoalveolar lavage, which is typically done when diffuse infiltrates are present, may be of low yield if the organisms have not infiltrated in the alveolar lumen [7, 9]. Here we describe a case of diffuse large B-cell lymphoma complicated by granulomatous PcP presenting as an enlarging solitary pulmonary nodule.

2. Case Report

A 61-year-old male was diagnosed with stage IIIB diffuse large B-cell lymphoma in August 2013. He underwent treatment with R-CHOP (rituximab, cyclophosphamide, hydroxy-daunorubicin, oncovin, and prednisolone) chemotherapy.

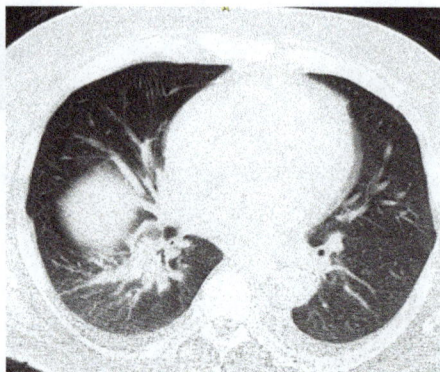

FIGURE 1: Axial image of CT of chest performed on August 17, 2013: pulmonary windows demonstrating atelectatic change or scarring in the right lower lobe.

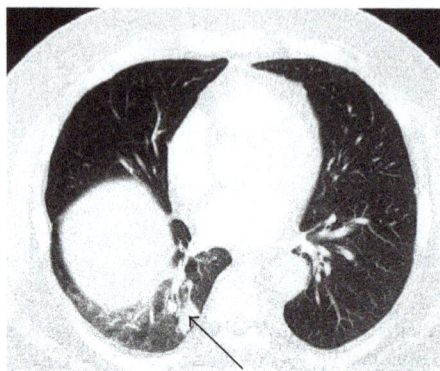

FIGURE 2: Axial image of CT of chest performed on January 31, 2014: pulmonary windows demonstrating a 2.3 cm nodular opacity in the right lower lobe (arrow) with minimal subsegmental atelectatic changes and ground-glass opacity.

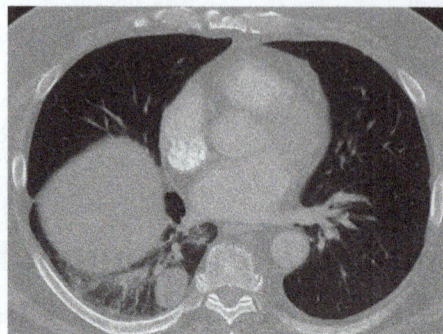

FIGURE 3: Axial image of CT of chest performed on April 15, 2015; pulmonary windows demonstrate an enlarging 3.6 cm nodular opacity in the right lower lobe with minimal subsegmental atelectatic changes and ground-glass opacity.

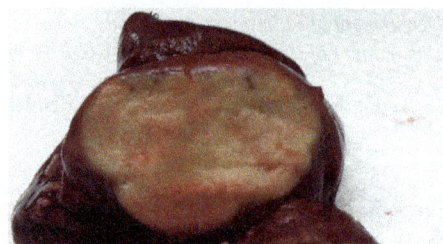

FIGURE 4: Right lower lobe wedge resection gross surgical specimen: the solid nodule measuring 3.6 cm demonstrating smooth lobulated contours and a yellow-tan resilient surface.

Two weeks after completing a total of six cycles of CHOP and eight cycles of rituximab he presented to our office for evaluation of dyspnea on exertion, cough with clear sputum production, night sweats, and right-sided pleuritic chest pain. Review of his chart showed a previous Computed Tomography (CT) imaging of the chest with atelectatic change or scarring within the right lower lobe (Figure 1).

On this visit, chest X-ray showed bibasilar infiltrates/atelectasis and CT of chest showed 2.3 cm nodular opacity in the right lower lobe with minimal subsegmental atelectatic changes and ground-glass opacity (Figure 2). Positron Emission Tomography-Computed Tomography (PET-CT) imaging showed a mildly 18F-fluorodeoxyglucose avid peripheral right lung mass coincident with the previously noted nodular opacity.

Bronchoscopy with bronchoalveolar lavage (BAL) was performed and was negative for infectious (AFB, fungal, and bacterial) and malignant causes. *Pneumocystis jirovecii* was not identified in the fungal smear and gram-stain or subsequent cultures. Because of his atypical presentation *Pneumocystis jirovecii* PCR assay was not performed on the lavage sediment. He was referred for CT guided core needle biopsy and obtained specimens showed granulomatous inflammation in a background of organizing pneumonia pattern. A silver stain was not performed on the core due to limited available sample. The core sample was felt to be nondiagnostic and surgical lung biopsy was recommended but the patient was lost to follow-up. When he returned 1 year later, he was asymptomatic but follow-up CT imaging of the chest revealed an enlarging right lower lobe mass (Figure 3). He underwent video-assisted thoracoscopic surgery (VATS) with right lower lobe wedge biopsy (Figure 4) which disclosed necrotizing granulomatous inflammation with background pulmonary parenchyma with organizing pneumonia and mixed inflammation (Figure 5). Silver stain was performed on the surgical specimens and identified *P. jirovecii* cysts associated with necrosis within the granuloma (Figure 6). He was started on oral trimethoprim/sulfamethoxazole 160 mg/800 mg; however due to intolerance his regimen was changed to atovaquone 750 mg by mouth twice daily for 12 days. He responded well to this treatment and follow-up CT imaging of the chest revealed no further progression of disease.

3. Discussion

PcP is commonly described with the radiologic appearance of diffuse bilateral alveolar and interstitial infiltrates with perihilar distribution along with pathologic findings

FIGURE 5: Microscopy 4x magnification: Hematoxylin and Eosin stain demonstrating confluent necrotizing granulomas with peripheral bands of sclerosis.

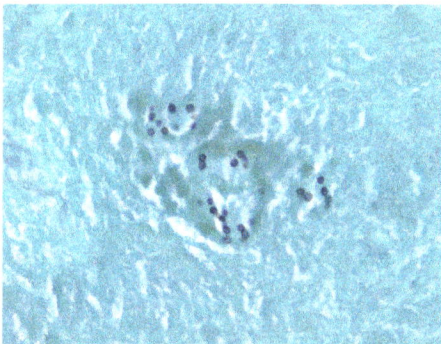

FIGURE 6: Microscopy 800x magnification: Gomori methenamine silver stain demonstrating classic *Pneumocystis jirovecii* cysts (cup-shaped with central dark zone, 5–7 μm) embedded within granuloma necrosis.

of foamy intra-alveolar eosinophilic exudates containing the PcP organisms [2]. Most patients present with the typical symptoms of cough and dyspnea in the setting of immunodeficiency. A granulomatous response has been previously described as an unusual histologic finding and primarily occurs in HIV/AIDS patients.

The pathogenesis of granulomatous reaction in PcP is related to host factors. These include active malignancy, recent corticosteroid use, Immune Reconstitution Inflammatory Syndrome, and prophylaxis with pentamidine rather than PcP genotypes [4]. Patients such as ours, with R-CHOP for lymphoma treatment, are at increased risk of developing PcP and in many cases are overlooked.

Diagnosis of conventional *Pneumocystis* pneumonia has traditionally involved bronchoalveolar lavage. However, a literature review suggests that bronchoscopy is considered to have a very low diagnostic yield, if any, to detect *P. jirovecii* granulomas [9]. Despite this reports of granulomatous PcP being diagnosed by PCR assay of bronchoscopically obtained BAL sediment have been stated [10]. Despite the definitive identification of *P. jirovecii* granulomas in this patient other possible etiologies for enlarging pulmonary nodules after completion of antineoplastic therapy need to be ruled out. These possibilities include large B-cell lymphoma recurrence

(in this case), primary pulmonary malignancy, residua of infection simultaneous to therapy, typical pulmonary bacterial infections, and even endemic mycoses such as histoplasmosis, blastomycosis, and coccidiomycosis [11]. In our case surgical lung biopsy is necessary to rule out these other possibilities and obtain a definitive diagnosis.

To date, our case is the third report of a *Pneumocystis jirovecii* infection within a solitary pulmonary nodule as well as the third report of granulomatous *Pneumocystis jirovecii* in an individual with diffuse large B-cell lymphoma. Additionally, we describe the only case which demonstrated an enlargement of the nodule over a span of 1 year and resolution of symptoms with treatment.

In conclusion, this case demonstrates that granulomatous PcP infections may exhibit rare radiologic manifestations including nodular opacities and affected patients may have subacute or even chronic symptoms. Consequently, granulomatous PcP should be considered in the differential diagnosis of solitary pulmonary nodules in all immunocompromised patients beyond the classically described AIDS affected.

Competing Interests

The authors declare that there are no competing interests regarding the publication of this paper.

References

[1] P. H. Hartel, K. Shilo, M. Klassen-Fischer et al., "Granulomatous reaction to pneumocystis jirovecii: clinicopathologic review of 20 cases," *American Journal of Surgical Pathology*, vol. 34, no. 5, pp. 730–734, 2010.

[2] S. G. Peters and U. B. S. Prakash, "Pneumocystis carinii pneumonia. Review of 53 cases," *The American Journal of Medicine*, vol. 82, no. 1, pp. 73–78, 1987.

[3] A. Y. P. Bondoc and D. A. White, "Granulomatous *Pneumocystis carinii* pneumonia in patients with malignancy," *Thorax*, vol. 57, no. 5, pp. 435–437, 2002.

[4] A. Totet, H. Duwat, G. Daste, A. Berry, R. Escamilla, and G. Nevez, "Pneumocystis jirovecii genotypes and granulomatous pneumocystosis," *Medecine et Maladies Infectieuses*, vol. 36, no. 4, pp. 229–231, 2006.

[5] W. D. Travis, S. Pittaluga, G. Y. Lipschik et al., "Atypical pathologic manifestations of *Pneumocystis carinii* pneumonia in the acquired immune deficiency syndrome. Review of 123 lung biopsies from 76 patients with emphasis on cysts, vascular invasion, vasculitis, and granulomas," *The American Journal of Surgical Pathology*, vol. 14, no. 7, pp. 615–625, 1990.

[6] H. Chang, L.-Y. Shih, C.-W. Wang, W.-Y. Chuang, and C.-C. Chen, "Granulomatous pneumocystis jiroveci pneumonia in a patient with diffuse large b-cell lymphoma: case report and review of the literature," *Acta Haematologica*, vol. 123, no. 1, pp. 30–33, 2009.

[7] H. S. Kim, K. E. Shin, and J.-H. Lee, "Single nodular opacity of granulomatous *Pneumocystis jirovecii* pneumonia in an asymptomatic lymphoma patient," *Korean Journal of Radiology*, vol. 16, no. 2, pp. 440–443, 2015.

[8] N. Kumar, F. Bazari, A. Rhodes, F. Chua, and B. Tinwell, "Chronic *Pneumocystis jiroveci* presenting as asymptomatic

granulomatous pulmonary nodules in lymphoma," *Journal of Infection*, vol. 62, no. 6, pp. 484–486, 2011.

[9] A. Nobile, A. Valenti, J.-D. Aubert, C. Beigelman, I. Letovanec, and M. Bongiovanni, "Granulomatous reaction to *Pneumocystis jirovecii* diagnosed in a bronchoalveolar lavage: a case report," *Acta Cytologica*, vol. 59, pp. 284–288, 2015.

[10] A. E. Wakefield, R. F. Miller, L. A. Guiver, and J. M. Hopkin, "Granulomatous *Pneumocystis carinii* pneumonia: DNA amplification studies on bronchoscopic alveolar lavage samples," *Journal of Clinical Pathology*, vol. 47, no. 7, pp. 664–666, 1994.

[11] J. R. Wingard, J. W. Hiemenz, and M. A. Jantz, "How I manage pulmonary nodular lesions and nodular infiltrates in patients with hematologic malignancies or undergoing hematopoietic cell transplantation," *Blood*, vol. 120, no. 9, pp. 1791–1800, 2012.

17

Unusual Presentation of Cutaneous Leishmaniasis: Ocular Leishmaniasis

Masoud Doroodgar,[1] **Moein Doroodgar,**[1] **and Abbas Doroodgar**[2]

[1]*School of Medicine, Shahid Beheshti University of Medical Sciences, Tehran, Iran*
[2]*Department of Medical Parasitology, Kashan University of Medical Sciences, Kashan, Iran*

Correspondence should be addressed to Abbas Doroodgar; adoroudgar@gmail.com

Academic Editor: Paola Di Carlo

The leishmaniases are parasitic diseases that are transmitted to humans by infected female sandflies. Cutaneous leishmaniasis (CL) is one of 3 main forms of the disease. CL is the most common form of the disease and is endemic in many urban and rural parts of Iran and usually caused by two species of *Leishmania*: *L. major* and *L. tropica*. We report a case of unusual leishmaniasis with 25 lesions on exposed parts of the body and right eyelid involvement (ocular leishmaniasis). The patient was a 75-year-old male farmer referred to health care center in Aran va Bidgol city. The disease was diagnosed by direct smear, culture, and PCR from the lesions. PCR was positive for *Leishmania major*.

1. Introduction

Leishmaniasis is a disease caused by protozoan parasites of the genus *Leishmania* and transmitted by the bite of infected female phlebotomine sandflies. The disease can be seen in three forms: cutaneous, mucocutaneous, and visceral leishmaniasis [1–3]. Leishmaniasis is endemic in 98 countries with more than 350 million people at risk. Leishmaniasis is associated with environmental changes such as deforestation, building of dams, irrigation schemes, and urbanization [4]. The cutaneous leishmaniasis (CL) with 1.5 million new cases per year is the most common form of the disease and causes skin lesions, mainly ulcers, on exposed parts of the body [3, 4].

In the old and new world, up to 90% of cases of CL occur in Afghanistan, Algeria, Iran, Saudi Arabia, and Syrian Arab Republic and in Bolivia, Brazil, Colombia, Nicaragua, and Peru [3]. Both form of rural and urban CL; zoonotic CL (ZCL) and anthroponotic CL (ACL) were seen in Iran. CL with about annually 20,000 new cases is considered one of the most important parasitic diseases in Iran. In addition, sometimes there are a few unusual and atypical clinical forms [5–10].

Here a case of unusual leishmaniasis (ocular leishmaniasis) from endemic area of Aran va Bidgol (Isfahan province,

central Iran) with 25 lesions on exposed parts of the body and eight lesions on the face and right eyelid involvement (OL) is reported. The disease was diagnosed by direct smear, culture of lesion, and RAPD-PCR technique for identifying the leishman agent causative. The PCR product was compared to reference stocks: *L. major* (MHOM/IR/75/ER) and *L. tropica* (MHOM/IR/IR/99) and the results were obtained. The data related to the patient was analyzed by descriptive statistics and bands of PCR product were compared to the standard marker (XIV) strains.

2. Case Report

A 75-year-old man with complaint of lesions extended on the hands, legs, face, and upper lid of right eye was referred to a health center of Kashan.

He was a farmer in Aran va Bidgol city from Isfahan province in the center of Iran. The patient about his infection said, sandflies have bitten him when referring to the farm for irrigation on the nights in the season of sandflies activity.

Based on questioning, the patient described the appearance of 25 multiple nodular, ulcerative, and crusted lesions on his body. In physical examination the size of lesions was varied from a few millimeters to several centimeters. He had

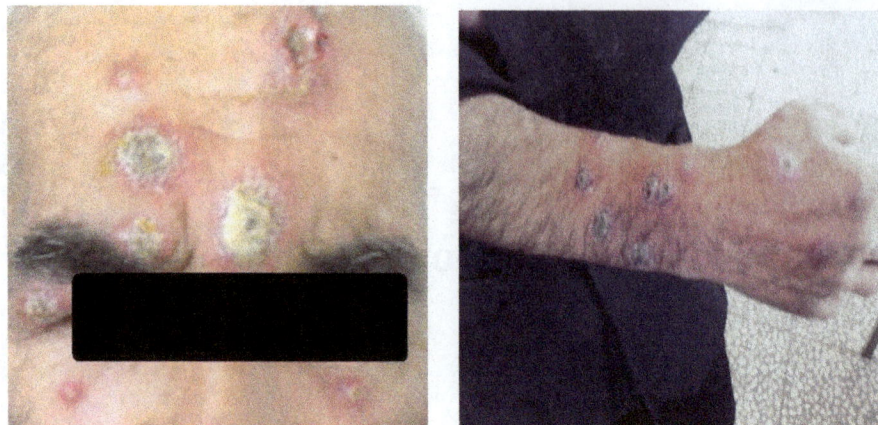

FIGURE 1: Patient with eight lesions on the face, right eyelid, and some lesions on the hands.

no particular medical history and systemic symptoms. There were eight lesions on the face that one of them was on the upper eyelid right eye (Figure 1).

In fact, the patient suffered from ocular leishmaniasis in addition to having multiple CL lesions. He had no fever and lesions were painless and his general condition was good.

Direct smears were prepared from the edge of skin lesions on different parts of body by using vaccinostyle and were fixed with pure methanol. Samples were stained by Giemsa 10% and examined under a light microscope and amastigote forms of *Leishmania* species were observed and CL was confirmed (Figure 2).

To identify the leishman agent causative of the disease materials of skin lesions cultured on RPMI-1640 medium plus 10% FBS, DNA was extracted and PCR was performed. PCR was positive for *Leishmania major* (Figure 3).

The patient was treated intramuscularly by meglumine antimoniate (Glucantime).

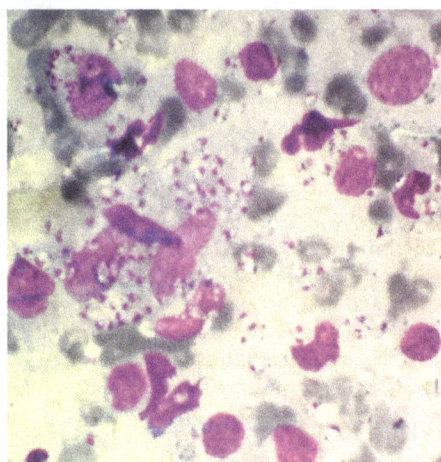

FIGURE 2: Direct smear was positive for leishman bodies (Giemsa stain).

3. Discussion

This report describes an unusual case of cutaneous leishmaniasis. The patient is residing and working in a rural area in the city of Aran va Bidgol (Isfahan province, located in the center of Iran). Many farms are located near or on the wild burrows in this county. According to the development of farms and human residency in wild rodents living area in the desert region of Aran va Bidgol, CL is the most common and the disease has been endemic. In recent years Aran va Bidgol county has been reported as an important zoonotic CL focus in Isfahan province [11]. Natural leishmanial infection caused by *L. major* in great gerbil (*Rhombomys opimus*) as reservoir and *Phlebotomus papatasi* sandfly as vector was confirmed in Aran va Bidgol [11].

In the case reported in the present study, the patient had no positive history of traveling to leishmaniasis endemic areas and there were 25 lesions on his body. Of these, 8 lesions were on the face that one of them was on the upper eyelid right

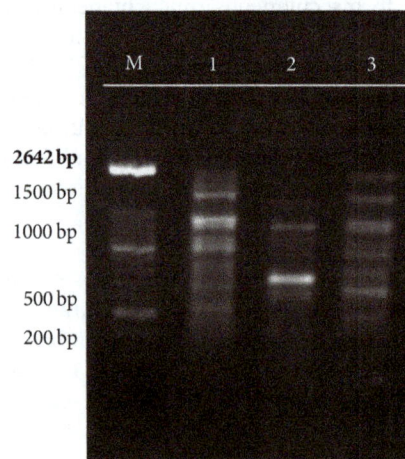

FIGURE 3: RAPD-PCR technique results by OPA4 primer in isolated strain and standards: M- marker (XIV 100 bp), (1) unknown strain, (2) *L. tropica* (MHOM/IR/IR/99), and (3) *L. major* (MHOM/IR/75/ER).

eye and he was suffering from ocular leishmaniasis. Untreated ocular leishmaniasis may cause ophthalmologic side effects and can cause irreparable damage. In Iran, Modarres Zadeh et al. reported four cases of ocular leishmaniasis from 1950 to 2005. In Iran two of them ended in blindness [12]. *Leishmania major* with about 75% frequency is causative agent of zoonotic CL and is endemic in many rural areas of the Iran. CL caused by *L. major* is reported in 17 out of 31 provinces in Iran. Isfahan is one of the involved provinces [13, 14]. In the present study, RAPD-PCR technique showed that causative agent was *L. major*. Ocular leishmaniasis is caused by different *Leishmania* species [12]. At the present time, most cases of atypical and OL lesions of cutaneous leishmaniasis which are reported from Iran are caused by *L. major*. Hajjaran et al. reported four unusual CL cases in which lesions are more located on hands, feet, and backs [8]. Moravvej et al. described four cases of unusual cutaneous leishmaniasis in which ulcers were located all over body, face, around eyes, chin, around upper lip, chest, and back [10]. Nasiri et al. described a case of CL on lower lip [15]. Ayatollahi et al. described a case of unusual cutaneous leishmaniasis involving a solitary lesion on the right eyelid (ocular leishmaniasis) [7]. Sadeghian et al. described a case of ocular leishmaniasis on lower and upper right eyelid margins [16]. Abrishami et al. reported a case of ocular leishmaniasis on right lower lid [17]. Jafari et al. described a case of OL on upper eyelid [18]. Nikandish et al. reported OL on the right eye [19]. In other parts of the world, several cases of unusual OL cases have been reported [20–26]. OL is a rare disease and involved 2.5% of cases with CL [6, 12]. There is still no vaccine to prevent the disease and the drugs of treatment for all forms of leishmaniasis are pentavalent antimony compounds [27, 28].

Although cutaneous leishmaniasis is a self-limited disease [29], untreated OL can potentially be very serious for eyes. Since the early diagnosis and treatment of diseases can prevent the ophthalmologic side effects, ocular leishmaniasis should be considered and studied further in endemic areas of CL.

Competing Interests

The authors have no conflict of interests related to this work.

Acknowledgments

The authors thank and appreciate the patient for his cooperation and all who have collaborated with this case report.

References

[1] World Health Organization, *Control of the Leishmaniases*, World Health Organization, Geneva, Switzerland, 2010, http://whqlibdoc.who.int/trs/WHO_TRS_949_eng.pdf.

[2] M. Service, *Medical Entomology for Students*, Cambridge University Press, Cambridge, UK, 4th edition, 2009.

[3] M. P. Barrett and S. L. Croft, "Management of trypanosomiasis and leishmaniasis," *British Medical Bulletin*, vol. 104, no. 1, pp. 175–196, 2012.

[4] World Health Organization, "Leishmaniasis Fact sheet," 2016, http://www.who.int/mediacentre/factsheets/fs375/en/.

[5] Ministry of Health and Medical Education, *Care Guide Cutaneous Leishmaniasis in Iran*, Center for Communicable Diseases Control, Tehran, Iran, 2012 (Persian), http://health.behdasht.gov.ir/?fkeyid=&siteid=435&pageid=53871&catid=289&dview=1189.

[6] S. Veraldi, S. Bottini, N. Currò, and R. Gianotti, "Leishmaniasis of the eyelid mimicking an infundibular cyst and review of the literature on ocular leishmaniasis," *International Journal of Infectious Diseases*, vol. 14, supplement 3, pp. e230–e232, 2010.

[7] J. Ayatollahi, A. Ayatollahi, and S. H. Shahcheraghi, "Cutaneous leishmaniasis of the eyelid: a case report," *Case Reports in Infectious Diseases*, vol. 2013, Article ID 214297, 2 pages, 2013.

[8] H. Hajjaran, M. Mohebali, A. A. Akhavan, A. Taheri, B. Barikbin, and N. S. Soheila, "Unusual presentation of disseminated cutaneous leishmaniasis due to Leishmania major: case reports of four Iranian patients," *Asian Pacific Journal of Tropical Medicine*, vol. 6, no. 4, pp. 333–336, 2013.

[9] H. Mortazavi, M. Mohebali, Y. Taslimi et al., "Hoarseness as the presenting symptom of visceral leishmaniasis with mucocutaneous lesions: a case report," *Iranian Journal of Parasitology*, vol. 10, no. 2, pp. 296–300, 2015.

[10] H. Moravvej, M. Barzegar, S. Nasiri, E. Abolhasani, and M. Mohebali, "Cutaneous leishmaniasis with unusual clinical and histological presentation: report of four cases," *Acta Medica Iranica*, vol. 51, no. 4, pp. 274–278, 2013.

[11] A. Doroodgar, F. Sadr, M. R. Razavi, M. Doroodgar, M. Asmar, and M. Doroodgar, "A new focus of zoonotic cutaneous leishmaniasis in Isfahan Province, Central Iran," *Asian Pacific Journal of Tropical Disease*, vol. 5, supplement 1, pp. S54–S58, 2015.

[12] M. Modarres Zadeh, K. Manshai, M. Shaddel, and H. Oormazdi, "Ocular leishmaniasis review article," *Iranian Journal of Ophthalmology*, vol. 19, no. 3, pp. 1–5, 2006.

[13] M. R. Shirzadi, S. B. Esfahania, M. Mohebalia et al., "Epidemiological status of leishmaniasis in the Islamic Republic of Iran, 1983–2012," *Eastern Mediterranean Health Journal*, vol. 21, no. 10, pp. 736–742, 2015.

[14] M. R. Shirzadi, "Neglected tropical diseases innovative and intensified disease management leishmaniasis control," in *Proceedings of the WHO Headquarters Report of the Consultative Meeting on Cutaneous Leishmaniasis*, 2007.

[15] S. Nasiri, N. Mozafari, and F. Abdollahimajd, "Unusual presentation of cutaneous leishmaniasis: lower lip ulcer," *Archives of Clinical Infectious Diseases*, vol. 7, no. 2, pp. 66–68, 2012.

[16] G. Sadeghian, M. A. Nilfroushzadeh, S. H. Moradi, and S. H. Hanjani, "Ocular leishmaniasis: a case report," *Dermatology Online Journal*, vol. 11, no. 2, article 19, 2005.

[17] M. Abrishami, M. Soheilian, A. Farahi, and Y. Dowlati, "Successful treatment of ocular leishmaniasis," *European Journal of Dermatology*, vol. 12, no. 1, pp. 88–89, 2002.

[18] A. K. Jafari, M. Akhyani, M. Valikhani, Z. S. Ghodsi, B. Barikbin, and S. Toosi, "Bilateral cutaneous leishmaniasis of upper eyelids: a case report," *Dermatology Online Journal*, vol. 12, article no. 20, 2006.

[19] M. Nikandish, V. Mashayekhi Goyonlo, A. R. Taheri, and B. Kiafar, "Ocular leishmaniasis treated by intralesional amphotericin B," *Middle East African Journal of Ophthalmology*, vol. 23, no. 1, pp. 153–155, 2016.

[20] M. P. Oliveira-Neto, V. J. Martins, M. S. Mattos, C. Pirmez, L. R. Brahin, and E. Benchimol, "South american cutaneous leishmaniasis of the eyelids: report of five cases in Rio de Janeiro State, Brazil," *Ophthalmology*, vol. 107, no. 1, pp. 169–172, 2000.

[21] M. S. Gurel, M. Ulukanligil, and H. Ozbilge, "Cutaneous leishmaniasis in Sanliurfa: epidemiologic and clinical features of the last four years (1997–2000)," *International Journal of Dermatology*, vol. 41, no. 1, pp. 32–37, 2002.

[22] M. Charif Chefchaouni, R. Lamrani, A. Benjelloune, M. El Lyacoubi, and A. Berraho, "Cutaneous leishmaniasis of the lid," *Journal Francais d'Ophtalmologie*, vol. 25, no. 5, pp. 522–526, 2002.

[23] E. Mencía-Gutiérrez, E. Gutiérrez-Díaz, J. L. Rodríguez-Peralto, and J. Monsalve-Córdova, "Old World eyelid cutaneous leishmaniasis: a case report," *Dermatology Online Journal*, vol. 11, no. 3, p. 29, 2005.

[24] A. Ul Bari and S. B. Rahman, "Many faces of cutaneous leishmaniasis," *Indian Journal of Dermatology, Venereology and Leprology*, vol. 74, no. 1, pp. 23–27, 2008.

[25] F. A. Ayele, Y. A. Wolde, T. Hagos, and E. Diro, "Ocular leishmaniasis presenting as chronic ulcerative blepharoconjunctivitis: a case report," *Journal of Clinical & Experimental Ophthalmology*, vol. 6, article 395, 2015.

[26] A. Satici, B. Gurler, G. Aslan, and I. Ozturk, "Ocular involvement in cutaneous leishmaniasis four cases with blepharoconjunctivitis," *European Journal of Epidemiology*, vol. 19, no. 3, pp. 263–266, 2004.

[27] R. Kumar and C. Engwerda, "Vaccines to prevent leishmaniasis," *Clinical & Translational Immunology*, vol. 3, no. 3, article no. e13, 2014.

[28] A. K. Haldar, P. Sen, and S. Roy, "Use of antimony in the treatment of leishmaniasis: current status and future directions," *Molecular Biology International*, vol. 2011, Article ID 571242, 23 pages, 2011.

[29] P. R. Machado, J. Ampuero, L. H. Guimarães et al., "Miltefosine in the treatment of cutaneous leishmaniasis caused by *Leishmania braziliensis* in Brazil: a randomized and controlled trial," *PLOS Neglected Tropical Diseases*, vol. 4, no. 12, p. e912, 2010.

18

A Case of Fluoroquinolone-Resistant Leprosy Discovered after 9 Years of Misdiagnosis

Onivola Raharolahy,[1] **Lala S. Ramarozatovo,**[1] **Irina M. Ranaivo,**[1] **Fandresena A. Sendrasoa,**[1] **Malalaniaina Andrianarison,**[1] **Mala Rakoto Andrianarivelo,**[2] **Emmanuelle Cambau,**[3] **and Fahafahantsoa Rapelanoro Rabenja**[1]

[1]*USFR Dermatologie, Centre Hospitalier Universitaire Joseph Raseta Befelatanana, 101 Antananarivo, Madagascar*
[2]*Centre d'Infectiologie Charles Mérieux, Université d'Antananarivo, 101 Antananarivo, Madagascar*
[3]*APHP, Hôpital Lariboisière, Bactériologie, Centre National de Référence des Mycobactéries et de la Résistance des Mycobactéries aux Antituberculeux, 75475 Paris Cedex 10, France*

Correspondence should be addressed to Mala Rakoto Andrianarivelo; mala@cicm-madagascar.com

Academic Editor: Sinésio Talhari

We report a case of misdiagnosed leprosy in a 21-year-old Malagasy male, who, improperly treated, developed secondary mycobacterial resistance to fluoroquinolone. The patient contracted the infection 9 years prior to the current consultation, displaying on the right thigh a single papulonodular lesion, which progressively spread to the lower leg, back, and face. Initial administration of ciprofloxacin and prednisolone led to temporary and fluctuating improvement. Subsequent long-term self-medication with ciprofloxacin and corticosteroid did not heal the foul and nonhealing ulcers on the legs and under the right sole. Histopathological findings were compatible with lepromatous leprosy. Skin biopsy was positive for acid-fast bacilli and PCR assay confirmed the presence of a fluoroquinolone-resistant strain of *Mycobacterium leprae* (*gyrA* A91V). After 6 months of standard regimen with rifampicin, clofazimine, and dapsone, clinical outcome significantly improved. Clinical characteristics and possible epidemiological implications are discussed.

1. Introduction

Leprosy is a chronic infectious disease caused by *Mycobacterium leprae* that commonly affects skin and peripheral nerves. The diagnosis of leprosy is not always easy due to the great diversity of clinical manifestations, which depend mainly on the patient's cellular immunity to *Mycobacteria* [1], but also on his immune status and genetic factors [2]. Whereas the prevalence of leprosy has been significantly reduced in most endemic areas, its incidence has remained steady for the past decade. In Madagascar, where leprosy is considered a major public health concern [3], more than 1,000 new cases were reported annually from 2005 to 2014. Yet there has been progress in the worldwide fight against leprosy ever since WHO promoted multidrug therapy for multibacillary and paucibacillary leprosy. Major challenges still remain including the emergence of drug-resistant strains

of *M. leprae*. In this report, we describe a case of misdiagnosed typical lepromatous leprosy caused by a secondary fluoroquinolone-resistant strain in a patient with probable drug-induced immunosuppression.

2. Case Report

A 21-year-old Malagasy male student, with no significant medical history, reported to our Dermatology Ward in May 2015, with extensive papulonodular lesions and nonhealing ulcers on his lower limbs. The patient had contracted the infection 9 years earlier, initially displaying on his right thigh a single papulonodular lesion, which progressively spread to his arms and legs and to his back and face within 5 years. Living in a remote area, the patient sought medical attention in a small private health centre. He was prescribed

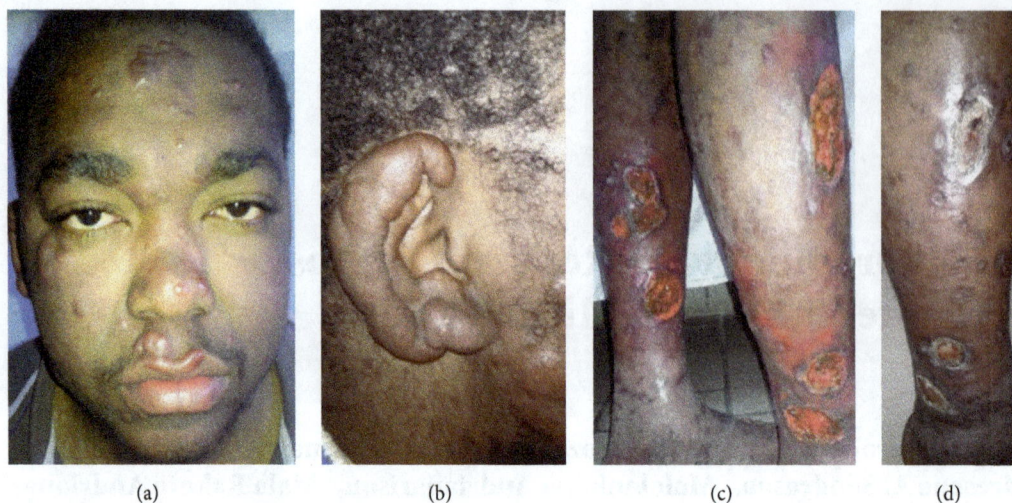

FIGURE 1: (a) Infiltrated papulonodular lesions on the face. (b) Infiltrated earlobe. (c) Multiple round and oval ulcers on legs. (d) Ulcers with sharply defined borders, margin erythema, and septic, purulent base.

ciprofloxacin 1 g per day associated with prednisolone 10 mg per day for one week. This treatment resulted in moderate yet fluctuating improvement before the patient presented foul and nonhealing ulcers on his legs and under his right sole, as well as recurrent hemorrhagic rhinitis. This was followed from 2001 on by long-term self-administration of ciprofloxacin 1 g per day and prednisolone 10 mg per day, as well as topical eosin and betamethasone ointment.

Upon our examination, the patient appeared to be in fairly good condition without fever. His hemodynamic parameters were normal. He presented with multiple infiltrated erythematous papulonodular lesions on his face, nose, and upper lip (Figure 1(a)) and earlobe (Figure 1(b)). These painless lesions had symmetrically spread to his trunk, back, and limbs. His legs and right sole presented foul, round, and oval ulcers having a greatest diameter of 3.5 cm (Figure 1(c)) and with sharply defined borders, a discreet marginal erythema, and a dirty, purulent base masked by a colored antiseptic product (Figure 1(d)). Purplish stretch marks were visible on his flanks and underarms, as well as the presence of a buffalo neck. He had multiple enlarged lymph nodes, but palpable nerve trunk pain was absent, motricity was not deficient, and the blinking reflex appeared unaffected. However, we detected hypoesthesia on the outside edge of his left sole. Cardiopulmonary auscultation was normal.

Biological tests showed marked inflammation as evidenced by accelerated erythrocyte sedimentation rate at 71 mm in the first hour, elevated C-reactive protein at 24 mg/L, and polyclonal hypergammaglobulinemia at 18 g/L on blood protein electrophoresis, despite a normal blood cell count. Blood sugar, creatinine, and liver enzymes were within normal ranges. HIV, hepatitis B, and hepatitis C serology proved negative. Chest radiography was normal. Arteriovenous Doppler ultrasound was performed to rule out vascular etiology for nonhealing ulcers. Histopathological findings were compatible with lepromatous leprosy, showing polymorphic infiltration of foamy lymphohistiocytic cells

into the skin, often located around adnexal structures, but without Virchow's cells, nor any sign of vasculitis. Ziehl-Neelsen staining performed on a skin biopsy revealed a positive high score (5+) of acid-fast bacilli. Infection with *Mycobacterium leprae* was confirmed by PCR assay (Geno-Type® LepraeDR, Hain Lifescience). Quinolone resistance due to A91V mutation on the *gyrA* gene encoding the A subunit of DNA gyrase was identified by a technique previously described [4] (Figure 2). However, this strain was shown to be sensitive to rifampicin (no *rpoB* mutation) and dapsone (no *folP*1 mutation).

After 6 months of standard multidrug therapy regimen for multibacillary leprosy, a combination of rifampicin, clofazimine, and dapsone, most cutaneous lesions disappeared, and ulcers on the lower limbs healed. The bacillary index fell to 2+, although some infiltrated nodular lesions still remained. As of this date, no new cases have been reported among the persons who have been in close contact with the patient.

3. Discussion

Polar lepromatous leprosy is described as a highly contagious, multibacillary, cutaneous, and mucosal form of leprosy with frequent visceral involvement. This condition occurs when *M. leprae* multiplies and spreads into the blood due to the lack of the host's cellular immune response against the bacillus [1]. In addition, our patient presented apparent peripheral signs of corticoid impregnation, which may have explained the diffuse clinical features of lepromatous leprosy and the presence of longstanding nonhealing ulcers. The systemic administration of corticosteroid over a 4-year period without etiological treatment has worsened the lack of cellular immune response.

Typical lepromatous lesions are papulonodular "leproma," which are symmetric in shape, and located on the face, particularly over the eyebrows, and on the earlobes and chin.

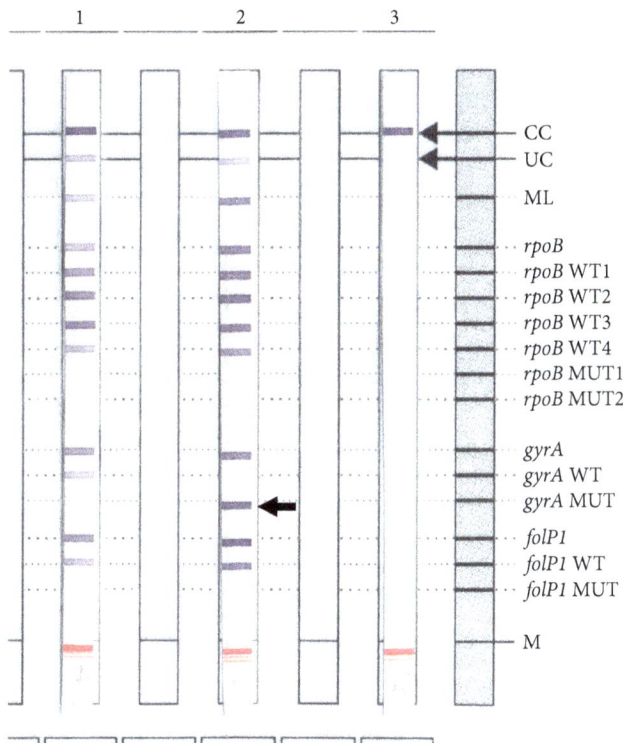

FIGURE 2: GenoType LepraeDR DNA strip test to assess drug resistance of *Mycobacterium leprae*. Lane 1, positive control using *M. leprae* wild-type strain with *rpoB*, *gyrA*, and *folP1* alleles. Lane 2, *M. leprae* strain of the case with *gyrA* mutation (A91V) and resistant to fluoroquinolone (arrow). Lane 3, negative control.

Peripheral edema of the foot and hypoesthesia in the limbs may also be found. Our patient, examined at an advanced stage of the disease, presented all the signs mentioned. Even though Malagasy physicians practice medicine in a country where leprosy is endemic, very few typically recognize the cutaneous signs of the infection, thus leading to misdiagnosis and erroneous treatment. Unfortunately, leprosy often only refers to macular hypochromic and hypoesthetic lesions in daily practice.

Ulcers are an unusual clinical symptom of leprosy in the advanced stages of the disease. They are mainly due to a loss of sensation in connection with peripheral neuropathy and rarely due to a complication of erythema nodosum leprosy [5]. Lucio's phenomenon, a reaction that causes ulcers in leprosy, may be ruled out in our present study following histopathological findings. Lucio's phenomenon is a type of dermal leukocytoclastic vasculitis characterized by necrotic skin ulcers, preferentially affecting the lower extremities and usually associated with ongoing diffuse lepromatous leprosy [6].

Drug resistance in *M. leprae* has become a major public health concern worldwide [7]. It can be detected using molecular methods, as in our present case. Although rarely encountered [8, 9], quinolone-resistant *M. leprae* cases cannot be neglected, since quinolones are used as part of second-line treatment against drug-resistant strains, usually applied following secondary resistance observed in relapse

cases [10]. The resistance mutation (A91V) is the one most commonly observed and here is likely a result of selection from continuous self-medicated doses of quinolones leading to secondary drug resistance. Limiting the overconsumption and supply of antibiotics by enforcing the requirement for medical prescription is the best approach for the prevention of atypical primary resistance.

In conclusion, there is a need to sustain leprosy expertise, even after its elimination at the global level. Clinicians must have access to up-to-date information on recognizing the symptoms of leprosy to avoid unnecessary delay in diagnosis and treatment. This will help reduce the risk of the disease from spreading. This approach can be explained in training programs to sensitize health workers throughout our country. Molecular diagnostic tests are now available and can be performed locally to accurately detect drug resistance to leprosy.

Consent

In this report, written informed consent related to publication of patient figure was obtained.

Competing Interests

All authors reported no competing interests.

Acknowledgments

This work was supported by the Fondation Mérieux, Lyon, France.

References

[1] J. C. Lastória and M. A. M. M. de Abreu, "Leprosy: review of the epidemiological, clinical, and etiopathogenic aspects-part 1," *Anais Brasileiros de Dermatologia*, vol. 89, no. 2, pp. 205–218, 2014.

[2] J. Gaschignard, E. Scurr, and A. Alcaïs, "Leprosy, a pillar of human genetics of infectious diseases," *Pathologie Biologie*, vol. 61, no. 3, pp. 120–128, 2013.

[3] World Health Organization, "Global leprosy update, 2014: need for early case detection," *Weekly Epidemiological Record*, vol. 90, no. 36, pp. 389–400, 2015.

[4] E. Cambau, A. Chauffour-Nevejans, L. Tejmar-Kolar, M. Matsuoka, and V. Jarlier, "Detection of antibiotic resistance in leprosy using GenoType LepraeDR, a novel ready-to-use molecular test," *PLoS Neglected Tropical Diseases*, vol. 6, no. 7, Article ID e1739, 2012.

[5] S. Chauhan, S. D'Cruz, H. Mohan, R. Singh, J. Ram, and A. Sachdev, "Type II lepra reaction: an unusual presentation," *Dermatology Online Journal*, vol. 12, no. 1, article 18, 2006.

[6] F. Jurado, O. Rodriguez, J. Novales, G. Navarrete, and M. Rodriguez, "Lucio's leprosy: a clinical and therapeutic challenge," *Clinics in Dermatology*, vol. 33, no. 1, pp. 66–78, 2015.

[7] E. Cambau, P. Bonnafous, E. Perani, W. Sougakoff, B. Ji, and V. Jarlier, "Molecular detection of rifampin and ofloxacin resistance for patients who experience relapse of multibacillary leprosy," *Clinical Infectious Diseases*, vol. 34, no. 1, pp. 39–45, 2002.

[8] S. Maeda, M. Matsuoka, N. Nakata et al., "Multidrug resistant *Mycobacterium leprae* from patients with leprosy," *Antimicrobial Agents and Chemotherapy*, vol. 45, no. 12, pp. 3635–3639, 2001.

[9] E. Cambau, E. Perani, I. Guillemin, P. Jamet, and B. Ji, "Multidrug-resistance to dapsone, rifampicin, and ofloxacin in *Mycobacterium leprae*," *The Lancet*, vol. 349, no. 9045, pp. 103–104, 1997.

[10] D. P. Legendre, C. A. Muzny, and E. Swiatlo, "Hansen's disease (Leprosy): current and future pharmacotherapy and treatment of disease-related immunologic reactions," *Pharmacotherapy*, vol. 32, no. 1, pp. 27–37, 2012.

19

Atypical Mycobacterial Infection after Abdominoplasty Overseas

Prabin Sharma,[1] **Laia Jimena Vazquez Guillamet,**[1] **and Goran Miljkovic**[2]

[1]*Department of Internal Medicine, Yale New Haven Health System, Bridgeport Hospital, Bridgeport, CT 06610, USA*
[2]*Department of Infectious Diseases, Yale New Haven Health System, Bridgeport Hospital, Bridgeport, CT 06610, USA*

Correspondence should be addressed to Prabin Sharma; prabin.sharma@bpthosp.org

Academic Editor: Jean-François Faucher

Increasing number of medical tourists travel internationally for cosmetic procedures. *Lipotourism* is a form of medical tourism becoming popular among patients of developed countries due to the cost efficiency of cosmetic procedures when performed in developing nations. There is a paucity of data on quality, safety, and risks involved with these surgeries. Many cases of infections have been documented in patients following cosmetic surgeries in developing countries. We present a case of a 34-year-old female who underwent abdominoplasty in Dominican Republic that was complicated with development of multiple abdominal wall abscesses due to infection from rapidly growing mycobacteria (RGM). In the absence of clear treatment guidelines, she was treated with a combination of intermittent surgical drainage and prolonged antibiotic course. This case is of interest as more than one species of RGM was isolated from the same patient. Our case highlights the fact that identification of these organisms can be difficult requiring referral of samples to specialized laboratories and treatment duration can last several months, which is determined by clinical and microbiological response.

1. Introduction

Travel to developing nations for cheaper surgical procedures is getting popular in the form of medical tourism. Modernization of technology, medicine, and medical facilities in low-income countries, access to information via Internet, and efficient air travel are facilitating this phenomenon [1]. Majority of these surgical procedures are for cosmetic reasons and body fat removal; thus, this practice is often termed *lipotourism* [2]. Surgeries performed in these settings are often complicated with skin and surgical site infections. Legal protection of medical tourists is usually absent due to inadequate malpractice laws in the destination countries [1]. Rapidly growing mycobacteria (RGM) has been associated with skin and surgical site infections in patients returning from cosmetic surgical procedures overseas [3–5]. We present another case of such infection caused by *M. chelonae-abscessus* complex and *M. fortuitum* complex.

2. Case Presentation

A 34-year-old female with past medical history significant for abdominoplasty in Dominican Republic three weeks prior to presentation came to our hospital with complaints of redness and swelling in the epigastric region. She developed abdominal discomfort a few days after she left the hospital and this progressed slowly over the weeks. Pertinent negative history included absence of nausea, vomiting, diarrhea, fever, chills, chest pain, shortness of breath, or changes in bowel habits. She also denied recent illness, sick contacts, or exposures.

On arrival to the Emergency Department, her vitals were stable with blood pressure of 99/65 mm Hg, pulse rate of 100 beats per minute, and respiratory rate of 20 per minute. Her body temperature was 36.8°C and she saturated 98% in room air. Physical examination revealed an erythematous tender indurated area in the epigastrium approximately 2 cm in diameter. Complete blood count revealed a hemoglobin of 9.1 g/dl and white blood cell count of 13.7×10^9 per

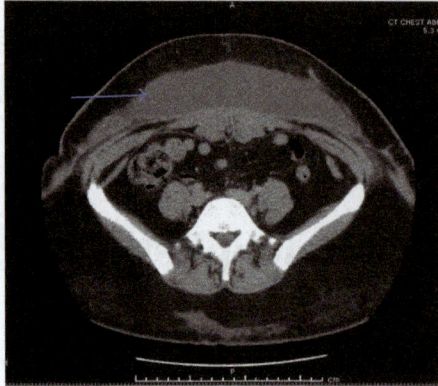

FIGURE 1: CT abdomen and pelvis with intravenous contrast showing large subcutaneous collection in the anterior abdominal wall (blue arrow) suggestive of abscess.

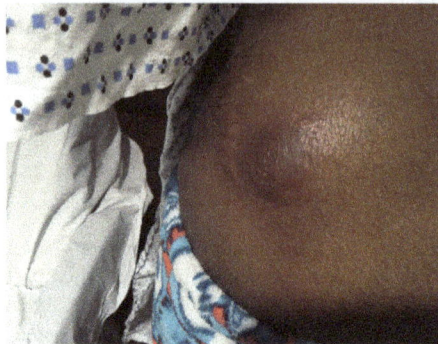

FIGURE 2: Soft, fluctuant, erythematous, and tender swelling in the lateral aspect of left hip.

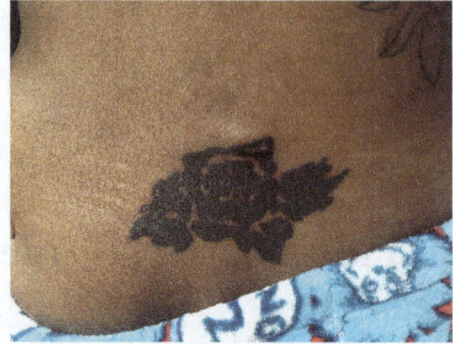

FIGURE 3: Soft, fluctuant, erythematous, and tender swelling in the lower central back (upper border of the tattoo).

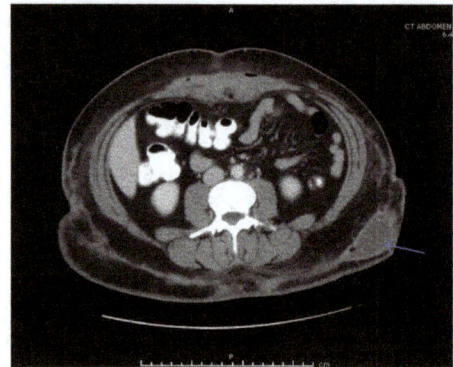

FIGURE 4: CT abdomen and pelvis with intravenous contrast showing subcutaneous rim-enhancing lesion in the left flank (blue arrow) suggestive of an abscess.

liter (L) with 73% neutrophils. Both Erythrocyte Sedimentation Rate (ESR) and C-Reactive Protein (CRP) were elevated at 33 mm/hr and 2.3 mg/dL, respectively. Comprehensive metabolic panel was within normal limits. Computed Tomography (CT) of the abdomen and pelvis with contrast noted a large subcutaneous collection in the anterior abdominal wall suggestive of abdominal wall seroma (Figure 1). It also showed multiple areas of increased attenuation over the subcutaneous tissues of the abdomen, lower back, and bilateral flanks. Patient underwent CT guided drainage with placement of a drain in the anterior abdominal wall. During the procedure a sample of cloudy, straw colored fluid was sent for aerobic, anaerobic, and acid-fast bacilli (AFB) cultures. Ziehl-Neelsen stain was positive and rapid growth was detected in the AFB culture media. Samples were sent to Yale New Haven Hospital Laboratory for further identification. After 16 s rRNA sequencing analysis, the isolate was identified as *Mycobacterium fortuitum* complex. Patient was started on oral levofloxacin and doxycycline and discharged home with outpatient follow-up.

Two weeks later, she returned with two new soft tender swellings in her left lateral hip (Figure 2) and low mid back (Figure 3). A repeat CT abdomen and pelvis revealed significant resolution of the anterior abdominal wall fluid collection and subcutaneous rim-enhancing collection in the left flank suggestive of developing abscesses along with multiple other developing abscesses (Figure 4). She underwent incision and drainage and surgical debridement of the abdominal wall abscesses. Each abscess was incised at the pointed area with maximal threat of tissue breakdown. Incision was followed by immediate egress of pus under pressure. It was yellow, thick, and creamy, and a culture swab was taken of this for aerobic and anaerobic infection. Each wound was opened further and the wound cavity was cleaned by pulse irrigation. The wounds were then dressed using Iodoform gauze and ABD pads and secured with a Tegaderm with Mastisol used to keep the Tegaderm in place. She was started on empiric intravenous (IV) antibiotics (meropenem and amikacin) and moxifloxacin. Susceptibilities for *M. fortuitum* complex were ordered at the National Jewish Health Laboratory in Denver. New fluid samples collected during the second drainage were sent to the State of Connecticut's laboratory for identification.

After two weeks of intravenous antibiotics, IV amikacin was discontinued to avoid its adverse effects including interstitial nephritis, renal tubular necrosis, and ototoxicity. Doxycycline was added to the treatment with moxifloxacin and intravenous meropenem. The National Jewish Health laboratory identified *Mycobacterium senegalense* (one of the species that belongs to *Mycobacterium fortuitum* complex) by rpoB gene sequencing. The Mycobacterium was sensitive to amikacin, kanamycin, cefoxitin, imipenem, ciprofloxacin, doxycycline, moxifloxacin, tigecycline, clarithromycin, and azithromycin. It was noted to be resistant to sulfamethoxazole-trimethoprim, augmentin, and linezolid. After a total of twenty-one days of IV antibiotics, patient was discharged home on clarithromycin, doxycycline, and moxifloxacin. Final cultures from the second debridement identified *M. chelonae-abscessus group* using chemotaxonomic testing (high performance liquid chromatography (HPLC)); susceptibilities were not obtained. Patient has been on a regular follow-up with the infectious disease physician for seven months with slow progressive resolution of abdominal lesions.

3. Discussion

International travel in search of affordable health care or medical tourism is becoming very popular. Our patient travelled from United States to Dominican Republic with the aim of getting a cosmetic procedure for body fat removal. *Lipotourism* is a terminology used to describe practice of such travel for cosmetic surgeries for removal of body fat [5]. This practice has its financial benefits at the cost of other untoward risks. Data on quality, safety, and risks involved with these surgeries is lacking. Infections with RGM have been reported in cosmetic surgeries performed in the developing nations including Latin America and Caribbean. Increasing number of cases are also reported in Europe due to lipotourism to Eastern and Southern Europe [1, 2]. Most of the prior reports have found *M. abscessus* to be responsible for these infections.

Nontuberculous Mycobacteria (NTM) or atypical mycobacteria encompass a group of acid-fast organisms of mycobacteria species apart from *Mycobacterium tuberculosis* and *Mycobacterium leprae*. With advance in isolation and identification methods, there have been increasing incidence and reports of infections caused by this bacterial species ranging from skin and soft tissue infections to pulmonary and disseminated disease. Depending on the growth rate, NTM can be classified into rapidly growing mycobacteria (RGM) and slowly growing mycobacteria (SGM). RGM obtain their name from rapid growth in culture media within seven days. This group is subdivided into six different complexes based on genetic relatedness and pigmentation: *Mycobacterium fortuitum, Mycobacterium chelonae/abscessus, Mycobacterium mucogenicum, Mycobacterium smegmatis, early pigmenting RGM, and nonpigmented RGM* [6, 7].

Mycobacterium fortuitum, Mycobacterium chelonae, and *Mycobacterium abscessus* are three species of RGM responsible for the majority of clinical cases of skin and soft tissue infections in the United States [6]. Patients affected by *M. chelonae* usually have a predisposing immune suppression, while patients affected by *M. fortuitum* are immunocompetent patients that have suffered a trauma or an open laceration. *M. abscessus* can affect both normal hosts and immunocompromised patients [7]. Clinical findings of RGM are usually nonspecific and variable. Because of this variability in presentation, a high index of suspicion is required to diagnose skin infections caused by RGM. *M. chelonae* and M. abscessus usually present with multiple skin lesions. Severe and disseminated cutaneous disease is most common with *M. chelonae*. Classic presentation of skin infection caused by *M. fortuitum* is a single subcutaneous nodule at the site of trauma or surgery [6].

NTM are environmental bacteria that are found in natural and treated waters, soils, aerosols, and animals. Biofilms protect these mycobacteria from eradication by ordinary disinfection processes [6]. NTM are responsible for a wide array of infections, ranging from skin and soft tissue infections to osteomyelitis, pulmonary infections, and disseminated disease. Humans get infected by exposure to environmental reservoirs [8]. Skin and soft tissue infections result from colonization of mycobacteria by direct inoculation acquired via trauma, surgery, drug injections, and animal bites [3, 4, 6]. We believe that our patient was infected during her cosmetic procedure, since it has been shown that water supplies in hospitals can act as a reservoir leading to contamination of surgical instruments, irrigation solutions, and injectable medicines [6].

Diagnosis is established by biopsy of the skin lesions and abscess followed by cultures and histopathology. Gram stains and regular cultures usually do not yield any results and specific stains and cultures for mycobacteria are required [6, 9, 10]. RGM are specially sensitive to decontamination and discoloration procedures; therefore, it is difficult to rule out RGM infection with a negative smear [8]. Our patient had two different species of RGM isolated from different body locations, collected weeks apart. These varying results may reflect a true infection by different pathogenic RGM or simply an error in identification. We believe that she had a true infection and she was colonized by both bacteria species during her surgery in Dominican Republic. Our theory is further supported by the fact that the second set of cultures was obtained from lesions that were already developing on the first abdominal imaging. Also, the absence of any prior surgical soft tissue infections by RGM at our institution makes us less suspicious about an acquired infection while at our facility. Thus, this case reports coinfection by different rapidly growing mycobacteria after abdominoplasty. However, we want to acknowledge the possibility of an identification error since different techniques were used and HPLC has more limitations compared to molecular sequencing (discussion about identification techniques and its limitations is beyond the purpose of this article) [8].

Treatment usually requires a multidisciplinary approach and includes a combination of antibiotics with surgical drainage of abscess. There is no consensus in treatment and there are no prior well-controlled trials to guide treatment. RGM are susceptible to oral antibiotics: macrolides (clarithromycin, azithromycin), fluoroquinolones (ciprofloxacin, levofloxacin, and moxifloxacin), tetracyclines (doxycycline, minocycline), linezolid, and trimethoprim-sulfamethoxazole [10–12]. *M. fortuitum* is more susceptible to drugs than *M. chelonae* or *M. abscessus*. Due to emergence of resistance and failure of treatment, monotherapy with a single agent is not recommended. Options for parenteral therapy include amikacin, imipenem, and levofloxacin [13, 14]. Treatment duration and route of administration are variable depending on site, severity of infection, and microbiological and clinical response. It is important to monitor drug toxicity while administering these antibiotics with regular follow-up of liver function, renal panel, and assessment of auditory and vestibular function [10]. Our patient has completed seven months of oral antibiotics with good response.

In summary, we present a case of a 34-year-old woman who acquired a soft tissue infection caused by RGM after an abdominoplasty overseas. In medical tourists presenting with infections following cosmetic surgery performed overseas, RGM should always be included in microbiological workup. Factors pointing towards the diagnosis of RGM include lack of response to conventional antibiotic regimen, recurrent wound infections, wound dehiscence, and poor wound healing as seen in our patient. Identification of these organisms can be difficult and referral of samples to specialized laboratories may be needed. Even though there are no clear guidelines, our patient responded well to a combination of antibiotic treatment and surgical debridement. Treatment can last several months and must be determined by clinical and microbiological response. What is unique about our case is the isolation of two different RGM species, which could have presented a treatment challenge in terms of antibiotic sensitivities. With this case, it is also important to raise awareness among physicians as well as general public about the risks involved with medical procedures performed in developing countries to avoid these complications.

Consent

Informed consent was obtained.

Competing Interests

The authors declare that they have no competing interests.

Authors' Contributions

Prabin Sharma saw the patient, reviewed the literature, and drafted the manuscript. Laia Jimena Vazquez Guillamet drafted and reviewed the manuscript. Goran Miljkovic saw the patient and reviewed the manuscript.

References

[1] L. E. Franzblau and K. C. Chung, "Impact of Medical Tourism on Cosmetic Surgery in the United States," *Plastic and Reconstructive Surgery Global Open*, vol. 1, no. 7, article e63, 2013.

[2] H. I. Bax, J. van Ingen, R. S. Dwarkasing, and A. Verbon, "[Lipotourism, not without risks: a complication of cosmetic surgery abroad]," *Nederlands Tijdschrift Voor Geneeskunde*, vol. 158, Article ID A7926, 2014.

[3] US Centers for Disease Control and Prevention, "Rapidly growing mycobacterial infection following liposuction and liposculpture—Caracas, Venezuela, 1996–1998," *Morbidity and Mortality Weekly Report (MMWR)*, vol. 47, pp. 1065–1067, 1998.

[4] E. Y. Furuya, A. Paez, A. Srinivasan et al., "Outbreak of *Mycobacterium abscessus* wound infections among 'lipotourists'

from the United States who underwent abdominoplasty in the Dominican Republic," *Clinical Infectious Diseases*, vol. 46, no. 8, pp. 1181–1188, 2008.

[5] J. Murillo, J. Torres, L. Bofill et al., "Skin and wound infection by rapidly growing: an unexpected complication of liposuction and liposculpture," *Archives of Dermatology*, vol. 136, no. 11, pp. 1347–1352, 2000.

[6] T. M. Gonzalez-Santiago and L. A. Drage, "Nontuberculous mycobacteria: skin and soft tissue infections," *Dermatologic Clinics*, vol. 33, no. 3, pp. 563–577, 2015.

[7] B. A. Brown-Elliott and R. J. Wallace, "Infections caused by *Mycobacterium bovis* and nontuberculous mycobacteria other than *Mycobacterium avium* complex," in *Mandell, Douglas, and Bennett's Principles and Practice of Infectious Diseases*, J. E. Bennett, R. Dolin, and M. J. Blaser, Eds., pp. 2844–2852, Saunders, Philadelphia, Pa, USA, 8th edition, 2015.

[8] C. Daley and D. Griffith, "Nontuberculous mycobacterial infections," in *Murray and Nadel's Textbook of Respiratory Medicine*, V. C. Broaddus, R. J. Mason, J. D. Ernst et al., Eds., pp. 629–645, Saunders, 6th edition, 2016.

[9] R. C. Lamb and G. Dawn, "Cutaneous non-tuberculous mycobacterial infections," *International Journal of Dermatology*, vol. 53, no. 10, pp. 1197–1204, 2014.

[10] D. E. Griffith, T. Aksamit, B. A. Brown-Elliott et al., "An official ATS/IDSA statement: diagnosis, treatment, and prevention of nontuberculous mycobacterial diseases," *American Journal of Respiratory and Critical Care Medicine*, vol. 175, no. 4, pp. 367–416, 2007.

[11] B. A. Brown-Elliott, K. A. Nash, and R. J. Wallace Jr., "Antimicrobial susceptibility testing, drug resistance mechanisms, and therapy of infections with nontuberculous mycobacteria," *Clinical Microbiology Reviews*, vol. 25, no. 3, pp. 545–582, 2012.

[12] J. M. Swenson, R. J. Wallace Jr., V. A. Silcox, and C. Thornsberry, "Antimicrobial susceptibility of five subgroups of Mycobacterium fortuitum and Mycobacterium chelonae," *Antimicrobial Agents and Chemotherapy*, vol. 28, no. 6, pp. 807–811, 1985.

[13] B. A. Brown, R. J. Wallace Jr., G. O. Onyi, V. De Rosas, and R. J. Wallace III, "Activities of four macrolides, including clarithromycin, against Mycobacterium fortuitum, Mycobacterium chelonae, and M. chelonae-like organisms," *Antimicrobial Agents and Chemotherapy*, vol. 36, no. 1, pp. 180–184, 1992.

[14] S. H. Kasperbauer and M. A. De Groote, "The treatment of rapidly growing mycobacterial infections," *Clinics in Chest Medicine*, vol. 36, no. 1, pp. 67–78, 2015.

20

Neurologic Adverse Events Associated with Voriconazole Therapy: Report of Two Pediatric Cases

Sevliya Öcal Demir,[1] Serkan Atici,[1] Gülşen Akkoç,[1] Nurhayat Yakut,[1] Nilay Baş İkizoğlu,[2] Ela Erdem Eralp,[2] Ahmet Soysal,[1] and Mustafa Bakir[1]

[1]Marmara University School of Medicine, Department of Pediatrics, Division of Pediatric Infectious Diseases, 34912 Istanbul, Turkey
[2]Marmara University School of Medicine, Department of Pediatrics, Division of Pediatric Pulmonology, 34912 Istanbul, Turkey

Correspondence should be addressed to Ahmet Soysal; asoysal@marmara.edu.tr

Academic Editor: Lawrence Yamuah

Although voriconazole, a triazole antifungal, is a safe drug, treatment with this agent is associated with certain adverse events such as hepatic, neurologic, and visual disturbances. The current report presents two cases, one a 9-year-old boy and the other a 17-year-old girl, who experienced neurologic side effects associated with voriconazole therapy. Our aim is to remind readers of the side effects of voriconazole therapy in order to prevent unnecessary investigations especially for psychological and ophthalmologic problems. The first case was a 9-year-old boy with cystic fibrosis and invasive aspergillosis that developed photophobia, altered color sensation, and fearful visual hallucination. The second case was a 17-year-old girl with cystic fibrosis and allergic bronchopulmonary aspergillosis, and she experienced photophobia, fatigue, impaired concentration, and insomnia, when the dose of voriconazole therapy was increased from 12 mg/kg/day to 16 mg/kg/day. The complaints of the two patients disappeared after discontinuation of voriconazole therapy. Our experience in these patients reminded us of the importance of being aware of the neurologic adverse events associated with voriconazole therapy in establishing early diagnosis and initiating prompt treatment. In addition, although serum voriconazole concentration was not measured in the present cases, therapeutic drug monitoring for voriconazole seems to be critically important in preventing neurologic side effects in pediatric patients.

1. Introduction

Voriconazole is a broad-spectrum triazole antifungal agent, which is the drug of first choice in the treatment of invasive aspergillosis in adult patients [1]. In European Union, the drug received approval for use in children aged 2 to 11 years in 2005. The increased use of the agent in pediatric population revealed that the compound, particularly its oral formulation, was found to have considerably variable pharmacokinetics in children [2]. Currently, an intravenous dose of 8 mg/kg taken twice daily (9 mg/kg twice daily at day 1) and an oral dose of 9 mg/kg for the oral suspension formulation taken twice daily have been adopted by the European Medicines Agency (EMA) for children aged 2 to <12 years and aged 12 to 14 years weighing <50 kg, and these doses are under further investigation in clinical phase II trials conducted by the manufacturer [3, 4].

Although voriconazole is a safe and often well-tolerated drug, it was found to be associated with some adverse effects such as neurotoxicity, visual disturbances, and dermatologic reactions [5, 6]. Reversible visual disturbances including altered color sensation, photophobia, and blurred vision were reported as the most common side effects accounting for 20 to 30% of adverse reactions in patients [7, 8]. Hallucinations and encephalopathy deserve further investigations for psychological disorders, as these are relatively uncommon adverse reactions associated with voriconazole therapy.

The current report presents two patients with visual and neurological symptoms that occurred during voriconazole therapy. Although the reactions are well-known side effects of voriconazole therapy, we found only a few reports in the literature [9–11], and, thus, the present paper highlighted these known but neglected adverse effects of voriconazole.

2. Case 1

A 9-year-old boy was admitted to the hospital due to acute exacerbation of cystic fibrosis. In the first sputum culture, there was growth of *Pseudomonas aeruginosa*, methicillin-sensitive *Staphylococcus aureus*, and methicillin-resistant *Staphylococcus aureus*, and antibacterial therapy was initiated based on the antibiotic susceptibility testing. However, no sufficient clinical improvement was achieved despite use of appropriate doses and duration of antibacterial therapy. The sputum culture performed at day 10 of the hospitalization period showed growth of *Aspergillus fumigatus* for which intravenous voriconazole therapy was initiated at a loading dose of 9 mg/kg twice daily at day 1 followed by the maintenance dose of 8 mg/kg twice daily. In the first day of the treatment, the patient developed photophobia and he continuously winked his eyes approximately for 10 minutes during each voriconazole infusion. At day 2, the patient winked his eyes approximately for 15 minutes during voriconazole infusion, and the patient additionally suffered from seeing ant colonies, and he reported that his mother had dressed with clothes with pink and red flowers, although the mother was actually dressed in black. The patient kept his eyes closed to avoid these hallucinations. These symptoms were considered as drug reactions, as the patient did not have a previous history of psychological problems or did not previously exhibit similar symptoms. Therefore, the treatment was switched to caspofungin and all symptoms disappeared. There were no further complaints one month after discontinuation of voriconazole therapy.

3. Case 2

A 17-year-old female patient with cystic fibrosis and allergic bronchopulmonary aspergillosis (ABPA) was admitted to our outpatient clinics due to increased sputum production and cough for the last fifteen days. Pulmonary auscultation revealed wheezing, while repeated measurement of total serum IgE was found to be elevated from 536 IU/mL to 1508 IU/mL and sputum cultures showed no growth. Based on these findings, we considered exacerbation of ABPA, and the dose of voriconazole therapy was increased from 200 mg twice daily to a maximum daily dose of 600 mg in order to reduce antigenic burden by combating fungal infection of the airway. However, the patient suffered from fatigue and impaired concentration a week after, and she developed photophobia and anxiety, which persisted approximately for four hours following oral dose of voriconazole. These symptoms were considered to be suggestive of a drug reaction. Voriconazole therapy was discontinued and all symptoms disappeared.

4. Discussion

Voriconazole is the drug of first choice in the treatment of invasive aspergillosis. Voriconazole trough concentrations >1 μg/mL were reported to be associated with good clinical response to therapy and improved survival. However, due to nonlinear pharmacokinetics of voriconazole in children,

achieving this concentration in this group may be challenging. Data suggest that children <12 years have approximately a 50% reduction in bioavailability for voriconazole compared to adults, which suggests that higher doses are required for children to provide the same effects [12, 13]. Currently, the dose of voriconazole used in children ranges from 3.4 to 23 mg/kg/d [14].

A strong correlation has been suggested between higher voriconazole trough concentrations and neurologic side effects, although this still remains controversial [11, 15]. Zonios et al. [9] suggested that there might be an increased risk of hallucination in patients with levels greater than the mean voriconazole level. Likewise, Imhof et al. [11] also reported a significant association between elevated serum voriconazole levels (sVL) and occurrence of neurological symptoms within 3 and 22 days (median 7 days) after the initiation of voriconazole therapy or dosage adjustment [11]. Our first case experienced visual disturbances and hallucination during voriconazole infusion at a loading dose of 9 mg/kg. The incidence of hallucinations associated with voriconazole therapy was reported to range from 4.3% to 16.6% in various studies [9, 16], whereas reversible visual disturbances occurred in 20 to 30% of patients. On the other hand, we must be aware of the fact that differentiation of visual hallucination from visual disturbances can be challenging. Beside hallucination and visual impairment, Imhof et al. reported nonspecific signs of encephalopathy during voriconazole treatment such as fatigue, impaired concentration, loss of memory, insomnia, anxiety, irritability, and dysarthria [11]. Except dysarthria, all of these signs were reported by the second case after voriconazole dose has been increased to a maximum daily dose of 600 mg/d. Due to the fact that voriconazole levels (VL) are not measured at our institution, VL of our cases were not available. Hepatotoxicity, renal toxicity, arrhythmia, or rash was not observed during the follow-up period. In a large cohort of immunocompromised children, Pieper et al. [17] reported their eight-year experience on the adverse effects of voriconazole therapy; elevated hepatic transaminases, serum bilirubin, and alkaline phosphatase levels, skin eruptions, and neurological adverse effects were observed in 53.5, 23.6, 10.9, 5.6, and 4.8% of the courses of voriconazole therapy, respectively. Photophobia was noted in eight cases, visual hallucination in one, insomnia in one, vertigo in one, and lack of concentration in one [17].

No specific treatment was required for neurological symptoms associated with voriconazole therapy, and discontinuation of drug was sufficient to control symptoms in the present cases as was reported in a prospective study by Zonios et al. [9]. In addition, switching therapy from intravenous formulation to oral formulation could be sometimes sufficient or mild symptoms can be observed at the beginning of the voriconazole therapy, which later disappear despite continuation of the therapy [9]. Therefore, making an attempt to initiate an oral formulation of voriconazole before discontinuing intravenous formulation can be considered in some critically ill patients. In our first case that received intravenous voriconazole therapy, due to the deterioration in medical condition of the patient and concerns of their parents, we switched to another antifungal agent, caspofungin, instead of proceeding with oral voriconazole therapy.

In conclusion, neurologic adverse effects associated with voriconazole therapy should be kept in mind in order to early recognize and initiate prompt treatment for these conditions and to avoid unnecessary investigations. Although serum voriconazole levels were not evaluated in the present study, monitoring of serum voriconazole levels might increase efficiency and safety of therapy particularly in pediatric patients.

Competing Interests

The authors declare no competing interests.

References

[1] T. J. Walsh, E. J. Anaissie, D. W. Denning et al., "Treatment of aspergillosis: clinical practice guidelines of the infectious diseases society of America," *Clinical Infectious Diseases*, vol. 46, no. 3, pp. 327–360, 2008.

[2] I. H. Bartelink, T. Wolfs, M. Jonker et al., "Highly variable plasma concentrations of voriconazole in pediatric hematopoietic stem cell transplantation patients," *Antimicrobial Agents and Chemotherapy*, vol. 57, no. 1, pp. 235–240, 2013.

[3] Vifend: EPAR—Product Information. European Medicines Agency (EMA), 2014, http://www.ema.europa.eu/docs/en_GB/document_library/EPAR_-_Product_Information/human/002669/WC500144015.pdf.

[4] Label Information for VİFEND, NDA no. 021266, Highlight of prescribing information, US Food and Drug Administration (FDA), http://www.accessdata.fda.gov/drugsatfda_docs/label/2011/021266s035,021267s040,021630s026lbl.pdf.

[5] B. J. Kullberg, J. D. Sobel, M. Ruhnke et al., "Voriconazole versus a regimen of amphotericin B followed by fluconazole for candidaemia in non-neutropenic patients: a randomised non-inferiority trial," *The Lancet*, vol. 366, no. 9495, pp. 1435–1442, 2005.

[6] R. Ally, D. Schurmann, W. Kreisel et al., "A randomized, double-blind, double-dummy, multicenter trial of voriconazole and fluconazole in the treatment of esophageal candidiasis in immunocompromised patients," *Clinical Infectious Diseases*, vol. 33, pp. 1447–1454, 2001.

[7] L. B. Johnson and C. A. Kauffman, "Voriconazole: a new triazole antifungal agent," *Clinical Infectious Diseases*, vol. 36, no. 5, pp. 630–637, 2003.

[8] L. Purkins, N. Wood, P. Ghahramani, K. Greenhalgh, M. J. Allen, and D. Kleinermans, "Pharmacokinetics and safety of voriconazole following intravenous- to oral-dose escalation regimens," *Antimicrobial Agents and Chemotherapy*, vol. 46, no. 8, pp. 2546–2553, 2002.

[9] D. I. Zonios, J. Gea-Banacloche, R. Childs, and J. E. Bennett, "Hallucinations during voriconazole therapy," *Clinical Infectious Diseases*, vol. 47, no. 1, pp. e7–e10, 2008.

[10] M. Fernández-Ruiz, F. López-Medrano, E. Gutiérrez, and J. M. Aguado, "Complex visual hallucinations induced by voriconazole," *Medicina Clinica*, vol. 133, no. 4, pp. 156–157, 2009.

[11] A. Imhof, D. J. Schaer, U. Schwarz, and U. Schanz, "Neurological adverse events to voriconazole: evidence for therapeutic drug monitoring," *Swiss Medical Weekly*, vol. 136, no. 45-46, pp. 739–742, 2006.

[12] M. J. Dolton, J. E. Ray, S. C.-A. Chen, K. Ng, L. G. Pont, and A. J. McLachlan, "Multicenter study of voriconazole pharmacokinetics and therapeutic drug monitoring," *Antimicrobial Agents and Chemotherapy*, vol. 56, no. 9, pp. 4793–4799, 2012.

[13] Y. Hamada, Y. Seto, K. Yago, and M. Kuroyama, "Investigation and threshold of optimum blood concentration of voriconazole: a descriptive statistical meta-analysis," *Journal of Infection and Chemotherapy*, vol. 18, no. 4, pp. 501–507, 2012.

[14] E. H. Doby, D. K. Benjamin Jr., A. J. Blaschke et al., "Therapeutic monitoring of voriconazole in children less than three years of age: a case report and summary of voriconazole concentrations for ten children," *Pediatric Infectious Disease Journal*, vol. 31, no. 6, pp. 632–635, 2012.

[15] A. E. Boyd, S. Modi, S. J. Howard, C. B. Moore, B. G. Keevil, and D. W. Denning, "Adverse reactions to voriconazole," *Clinical Infectious Diseases*, vol. 39, no. 8, pp. 1241–1244, 2004.

[16] T. J. Walsh, P. Pappas, D. J. Winston et al., "Voriconazole compared with liposomal amphotericin B for empirical antifungal therapy in patients with neutropenia and persistent fever," *The New England Journal of Medicine*, vol. 346, no. 4, pp. 225–234, 2002.

[17] S. Pieper, H. Kolve, T. Meine, G. Goletz, and A. H. Groll, "Safety and outcome of treatment with voriconazole in a large cohort of immunocompromised children and adolescents," *GMS Infectious Diseases*, vol. 3, article Doc01, 2015.

21

Haemophilus parainfluenzae Mural Endocarditis: Case Report and Review of the Literature

Luca T. Giurgea[1] and Tim Lahey[2]

[1]*Department of Medicine, Dartmouth-Hitchcock Medical Center, Lebanon, NH 03756, USA*
[2]*Section of Infectious Disease and International Health, Department of Medicine, Dartmouth-Hitchcock Medical Center, Lebanon, NH 03756, USA*

Correspondence should be addressed to Luca T. Giurgea; luca.t.giurgea@dartmouth.edu

Academic Editor: Larry M. Bush

Haemophilus parainfluenzae, which uncommonly causes endocarditis, has never been documented to cause mural involvement. A 62-year-old immunocompetent female without predisposing risk factors for endocarditis except for poor dentition presented with fever, emesis, and dysmetria. Echocardiography found a mass attached to the left ventricular wall with finger-like projections. Computed tomography showed evidence of embolic phenomena to the brain, kidneys, spleen, and colon. Cardiac MRI revealed involvement of the chordae tendineae of the anterior papillary muscles. Blood cultures grew *Haemophilus parainfluenzae*. The patient was treated successfully with ceftriaxone with resolution of symptoms, including neurologic deficits. After eleven days of antibiotics a worsening holosystolic murmur was discovered. Worsening mitral regurgitation on echocardiography was only found three weeks later. Nine weeks after presentation, intraoperative evaluation revealed chord rupture but no residual vegetation and mitral repair was performed. Four weeks after surgery, the patient was back to her baseline. This case illustrates the ability of *Haemophilus parainfluenzae* to form large mural vegetations with high propensity of embolization in otherwise normal cardiac tissue among patients with dental risk factors. It also underscores the importance of physical examination in establishing a diagnosis of endocarditis and monitoring for progression of disease.

1. Introduction

Endocarditis is a rare but serious infection with hospital mortality averaging 18% but dependent upon causative pathogen, lesion type, and patient comorbidities [1]. Mural endocarditis, seen in 4% of cases of endocarditis, is defined as inflammation of the nonvalvular endocardial surface in any of the four chambers of the heart [2]. It is thought to arise from seeding of either congenitally or iatrogenically abnormal endocardium. *Staphylococcus aureus* and streptococci are the most common causes of mural endocarditis, whereas mural endocarditis from the HACEK organisms (*Haemophilus* species, *Aggregatibacter* species, *Cardiobacterium hominis*, *Eikenella corrodens*, and *Kingella* species) has not been reported [2, 3], even though 1.4% of total endocarditis cases are attributed to HACEK organisms [4].

2. Case Description

A 62-year-old female with a history of migraines and hypertension presented with nausea, malaise, and vertigo. Twelve days prior to admission, she developed discomfort and pressure in the epigastric region. Five days later, she developed night sweats, chills, and emesis and presented to an outside hospital. She was given intravenous fluids with potassium and sent home. Her symptoms persisted and, two days prior to admission, she developed vertigo and light headedness. She presented back to the outside hospital. Vital signs were within normal limits. Laboratory data revealed a leukocytosis of $13.3 \times 10^3/\mu L$ and mildly elevated troponin. Computed tomography (CT) of the head showed a 2 cm right occipital region of diminished attenuation of uncertain acuity. Blood cultures were drawn and she was transferred to our hospital. On presentation, she also complained of bifrontal headache different from her usual migraine, flashes of light, and subtle left peripheral vision loss. She had no history of congenital cardiac disease, rheumatic fever, or IV drug use. Neurological examination was remarkable for somnolence, generalized weakness, mildly decreased left peripheral vision, and dysmetria. Cardiovascular exam revealed no murmur or gallop. Abdominal exam was unremarkable. Poor dentition was noted. Blood and urine cultures were drawn and ceftriaxone and vancomycin were started. On hospital day (HD) 2, dysmetria worsened and she spiked a fever of 39°C. Splinter hemorrhages were noted. Transthoracic echocardiography (TTE) showed a mobile mass in the left ventricle. Magnetic resonance imaging (MRI) of the head showed cerebellar, parietal, and occipital lesions. CT of the abdomen and pelvis revealed colonic inflammation, hepatomegaly, and multiple renal and splenic infarcts. HIV testing was negative. After 23 hours, blood cultures from this hospital grew small gram negative coccobacilli. Vancomycin was discontinued. By HD 3, cultures from the outside hospital grew gram negative coccobacilli as well. Transesophageal echocardiography (TEE) showed a complex echogenic mass of 1.5 cm by 1.7 cm in the left ventricle, which extended into the left ventricular outflow tract with finger-like projections. A small filamentous vegetation was noted on the anterior leaflet of the mitral valve. By HD 4, dysmetria and malaise improved. The isolate growing in blood cultures was identified by biochemical testing as *Haemophilus parainfluenzae* susceptible to ceftriaxone. Subsequent cultures on antibiotics remained negative. Cardiac MRI showed two mobile nodular structures located near the chordae tendineae of the anterior papillary muscle along its posterior aspect and near the anterior mitral valve leaflet. Repeat MRI of the brain with diffusion weighted imaging showed new infarcts within the cerebellum and cerebral hemispheres. On HD 11 she developed a faint systolic murmur, which worsened rapidly. By HD 12, it became a holosystolic murmur loudest at the apex, radiating to the axilla. Surgery was considered but repeat TEE demonstrated a substantial decrease in vegetation size and only mild mitral regurgitation which was unchanged from the prior study. The patient was discharged to complete four weeks of ceftriaxone. At follow-up two months later, she was doing well without any neurological deficits and no signs or symptoms of heart failure. Repeat TEE showed resolution of vegetations but residual severe mitral regurgitation. She underwent mitral valve repair without further complications. At follow-up 4 weeks after surgery, she was back to her baseline health, without any dyspnea on exertion or neurologic sequelae.

3. Discussion

Haemophilus parainfluenzae is a rare cause of subacute endocarditis, particularly in North America [1, 5]. *H. parainfluenzae* is responsible for 0.5% of total endocarditis cases and 36% of HACEK endocarditis cases [4]. Poor dentition is seen in as many as 20% of patients afflicted with HACEK endocarditis, with nearly twice that many patients also having recently undergone a dental procedure [6, 7]. The vegetations in *Haemophilus* spp. endocarditis are classically large and have

a high risk of embolization, at 35.7% among all *Haemophilus* spp. but up to 60% in cases of endocarditis specifically attributed to *Haemophilus parainfluenzae* [6, 7]. The risk of embolization is associated with large vegetation size and hyphal morphology of vegetations in *Haemophilus* endocarditis [8]. In a study of all cause endocarditis, vegetations greater than 10 mm exhibited 2.8 greater odds of embolization [9]. More than half of patients with *Haemophilus parainfluenzae* endocarditis have no predisposing valvular disease, although congenital and iatrogenic abnormalities of the myocardium are common as among all cases of endocarditis [8]. The mitral valve is most commonly affected in *Haemophilus* endocarditis followed by the aortic valve [7]. *Haemophilus* can be difficult to grow in vitro and susceptibilities may be unavailable. Due to significant presence of ampicillin resistance, ceftriaxone is often used unless susceptibilities dictate otherwise. Therapy usually involves 4 weeks of intravenous antibiotics in native valve endocarditis and 6 weeks in prosthetic valve endocarditis [10].

A rare presentation of endocarditis, mural endocarditis can involve the endocardium in both atria and ventricles [11] and most commonly involves previously abnormal endocardium affected by mural thrombi, myocardial abscesses, pacemaker lead sites, congenital defects, hypertrophic subaortic stenosis, jet lesions, ventricular aneurysms, or pseudoaneurysm [3]. Immunocompromise from chemotherapy, steroids, and other immunosuppressant medications underlies many cases of mural endocarditis, particularly those caused by fungal organisms [3]. Organisms commonly implicated in mural endocarditis include staphylococci, streptococci, *Enterococcus* spp., *Salmonella* spp., *Klebsiella* spp., *Bacteroides fragilis*, *Candida* spp., and *Aspergillus* spp. [3]. Despite cases series [4, 6–8] on HACEK endocarditis including one published by Chambers et al. in 2013 on 77 patients and one published by Das et al. in 1997 on 45 patients, we are aware of no reports of mural endocarditis attributed to HACEK organisms.

The patient in this case had a very small mitral vegetation and initial echocardiography only showed trace mitral regurgitation, so it was unsurprising that there were no auscultatory findings early on [12]. Although not specifically addressed in larger studies, other case reports of mural endocarditis have also reported absence of murmur [13, 14]. Our patient developed severe mitral regurgitation after discharge and was found to have chordae tendineae rupture along with an audible murmur. Cardiac MRI did show involvement of the chordae tendineae by the mural vegetation. It is interesting to note that despite echocardiography's documented superior sensitivity in diagnosing mitral regurgitation in comparison with physical examination [12], the development and worsening of a murmur on cardiac auscultation in this patient heralded deterioration of mitral valve function not immediately identifiable on echocardiography.

4. Conclusion

Haemophilus parainfluenzae is an uncommon cause of endocarditis that affects patients with poor dentition and causes large vegetations with a high propensity for embolization. It can affect both normal and abnormal valves and can rarely cause mural vegetations which may be silent on cardiac examination. Careful auscultation for changes in murmurs can reveal deterioration of affected valve function, which may appear unchanged on echocardiography. Antibiotic therapy alone can be effective but early surgical intervention should be considered for patients with large vegetations or persistent embolization despite appropriate therapy.

Competing Interests

The authors declare that there is no conflict of interests regarding the publication of this paper.

References

[1] D. R. Murdoch, R. G. Corey, B. Hoen et al., "Clinical presentation, etiology, and outcome of infective endocarditis in the 21st century: the international collaboration on endocarditis-prospective cohort study," *Archives of Internal Medicine*, vol. 169, no. 5, pp. 463–473, 2009.

[2] S. Morpeth, D. Murdoch, C. H. Cabell et al., "Non-HACEK gram-negative bacillus endocarditis," *Annals of Internal Medicine*, vol. 147, no. 12, pp. 829–835, 2007.

[3] R. A. Kearney, H. J. Eisen, and J. E. Wolf, "Nonvalvular infections of the cardiovascular system," *Annals of Internal Medicine*, vol. 121, no. 3, pp. 219–230, 1994.

[4] S. T. Chambers, D. Murdoch, A. Morris et al., "HACEK infective endocarditis: characteristics and outcomes from a large, multinational cohort," *PLoS ONE*, vol. 8, no. 5, Article ID e63181, 2013.

[5] D. H. Bor, S. Woolhandler, R. Nardin, J. Brusch, and D. U. Himmelstein, "Infective Endocarditis in the U.S., 1998–2009: a Nationwide study," *PLoS ONE*, vol. 8, no. 3, Article ID e60033, 2013.

[6] M. Das, A. D. Badley, F. R. Cockerill, J. M. Steckelberg, and W. R. Wilson, "Infective endocarditis caused by HACEK microorganisms," *Annual Review of Medicine*, vol. 48, pp. 25–33, 1997.

[7] C. Darras-Joly, O. Lortholary, J.-L. Mainardi, J. Etienne, L. Guillevin, and J. Acar, "Haemophilus endocarditis: report of 42 cases in adults and review," *Clinical Infectious Diseases*, vol. 24, no. 6, pp. 1087–1094, 1997.

[8] J. G. Jemsek, S. B. Greenberg, L. O. Gentry, D. E. Welton, and K. L. Mattox, "Haemophilus parainfluenzae endocarditis. Two cases and review of the literature in the past decade," *The American Journal of Medicine*, vol. 66, no. 1, pp. 51–57, 1979.

[9] M. Rizzi, V. Ravasio, A. Carobbio et al., "Predicting the occurrence of embolic events: an analysis of 1456 episodes of infective endocarditis from the Italian Study on Endocarditis (SEI)," *BMC Infectious Diseases*, vol. 14, article 230, 2014.

[10] L. M. Baddour, W. R. Wilson, A. S. Bayer et al., "Infective endocarditis in adults: diagnosis, antimicrobial therapy, and management of complications: a scientific statement for healthcare professionals from the American Heart Association," *Circulation*, vol. 132, no. 15, pp. 1435–1486, 2015.

[11] N. A. Buchbinder and W. C. Roberts, "Active infective endocarditis confined to mural endocardium. A study of six necropsy patients," *Archives of Pathology*, vol. 93, no. 5, pp. 435–440, 1972.

[12] C. A. Roldan, B. K. Shively, and M. H. Crawford, "Value of the cardiovascular physical examination for detecting valvular heart disease in asymptomatic subjects," *The American Journal of Cardiology*, vol. 77, no. 15, pp. 1327–1331, 1996.

[13] A. Adel, E. Jones, J. Johns, O. Farouque, and P. Calafiore, "Bacterial mural endocarditis. A case series," *Heart Lung and Circulation*, vol. 23, no. 8, pp. e172–e179, 2014.

[14] P. Mullen, C. Jude, M. Borkon, J. Porterfield, and T. J. Walsh, "Aspergillus mural endocarditis. Clinical and echocardiographic diagnosis," *Chest*, vol. 90, no. 3, pp. 451–452, 1986.

22

Severe Thrombocytopenic Purpura in a Child with Brucellosis: Case Presentation and Review of the Literature

Alexandros Makis, Aikaterini Perogiannaki, and Nikolaos Chaliasos

Child Health Department, Faculty of Medicine, University of Ioannina, Ioannina, Greece

Correspondence should be addressed to Alexandros Makis; amakis@cc.uoi.gr

Academic Editor: Lawrence Yamuah

Brucellosis is still endemic and a significant public health problem in many Mediterranean countries, including Greece. It is a multisystemic disease with a broad spectrum of clinical manifestations including hematological disorders, such as anemia, pancytopenia, leucopenia, and thrombocytopenia. Thrombocytopenia is usually moderate and attributed to bone marrow suppression or hypersplenism. Rarely, autoimmune stimulation can cause severe thrombocytopenia with clinically significant hemorrhagic manifestations. We present the case of a girl with severe thrombocytopenic purpura as one of the presenting symptoms of *Brucella melitensis* infection. Treatment with intravenous immunoglobulin and the appropriate antimicrobial agents promptly resolved the thrombocyte counts. A review of similar published cases is also presented.

1. Introduction

Brucellosis is a zoonotic infection, which is endemic in Northwestern Greece [1] and is caused by Gram-negative bacteria that belong to the genus *Brucella*. *Brucella melitensis* is the most virulent form of the disease for humans. As far as the pediatric population is concerned, the infection is transmitted by direct contact with the contaminated animals or their fluids and by consumption of unpasteurized milk or other dairy products.

Several hematological manifestations such as anemia, leucopenia, thrombocytopenia, pancytopenia, leukocytosis, and thrombocytosis have been reported at diagnosis as well as during the course of the disease [2]. The pathophysiology of these abnormalities remains unclear but several mechanisms have been suggested including direct bone marrow infiltration, hypersplenism, hemophagocytosis, and activation of the immune system with production of autoantibodies.

Thrombocytopenia caused by *Brucella* is usually mild with no hemorrhagic complications and subsides after appropriate antibiotic treatment for the disease [1, 3]. Less often, immune mediated severe platelet depletion can occur at diagnosis or during the course of the disease, with significant bleeding manifestations. Isolated thrombocytopenia has been reported as the first symptom of the disease, initially misdiagnosed as primary immune thrombocytopenic purpura (ITP) [4]. The purpose of this paper is to describe the case of an immune mediated severe thrombocytopenia in a small child during the course of brucellosis and to present the relevant literature review.

2. Case Report

A 5.5-year-old girl presented with six-day fever up to 38.5°C with spikes mostly in the afternoon, accompanied by pain at the right wrist joint and right elbow joint. The girl's parents are stockbreeders and homemade dairy products had been offered to the child. Three days prior to her admission in our department, she was examined in another hospital, where no remarkable findings from the joints or other systems were noted. As shown in Table 1, laboratory tests were white blood cells 7.2×10^9/L, platelets 180×10^9/L, hemoglobin 131 g/L, erythrocyte sedimentation rate (ESR) 19 mm/h, C-reactive protein (CRP) 10 mg/L, monotest negative, alanine aminotransferase (AST) 62 U/L, positive Wright agglutination reaction (title 1/1280), and negative Rose Bengal. Based on the symptoms and the positive Wright reaction, treatment for brucellosis was initiated. Trimethoprim/sulfamethoxazole

TABLE 1: Hematological parameters and treatment at admission and during the course of the disease.

Treatment	3 days before admission TMP/SMX, rifampicin	Admission IVIG, amikacin, rifampicin	Day 5	Day 10	Week 6
			TMP/SMX, rifampicin		
WBC ($\times 10^9$/L)	7.2	7.5	8.7	7.2	9.9
Ht	0.37	0.33	0.38	0.37	0.38
Hb (g/L)	131	120	126	121	129
Plt ($\times 10^9$/L)	180	1	218	503	315

TMP/SMX: trimethoprim/sulfamethoxazole; WBC: white blood cell count; Ht: hematocrit; Hb: hemoglobin; Plt: platelets.

(TMP/SMX) (10 mg/kg/day) and rifampicin (15 mg/kg/day) were administered orally.

On the third day of treatment, generalized purpuric lesions were noted accompanied with severe thrombocytopenia (platelets 3×10^9/L) and the child was referred to our hospital. On admission the child was febrile (38.8°C) and generalized petechial/purpuric rash, bruising, wet purpura on the palate, and gingival bleeding were noted, while the spleen and the liver were palpable 2 cm below the subcostal margin at the midclavicular line. Examination of the joints and the other systems did not reveal any pathological signs.

Laboratory tests showed white blood cells 7.5×10^9/L (neutrophils 45%, lymphocytes 52%, and monocytes 3%), platelets 1×10^9/L, hemoglobin 120 g/L, ESR 15 mm/h, CRP 7 mg/L, AST 64 U/L, urea 4.1 mmol/L, creatinine 92 μmol/L, and total bilirubin 12 μmol/L. Wright agglutination reaction was positive (title 1/1280), as well as the specific IgM, IgA antibodies against Brucella melitensis. The specific IgG antibodies were negative. Blood cultures were sterile. Direct and indirect Coombs were negative. The quantification of immunoglobulins IgG, IgM, and IgA and complements C3 and C4 was within normal range. Antinuclear antibodies, anti-double stranded DNA antibodies, and rheumatoid factor were negative, while the antiplatelet antibody test was positive. Clotting time and fibrinogen were normal (Table 1).

Due to the very low platelet count and the mucous membrane hemorrhage, treatment with intravenous immunoglobulin (IVIG) (1 gr/kg/day for two days) was initiated, combined with antibiotic therapy with amikacin intravenously (15 mg/kg/day for seven days) and oral rifampicin. TMP/SMX treatment was stopped due to the suspicion of drug-induced thrombocytopenia.

The patient responded with a gradual increase in the number of platelets up to 218×10^9/L five days after treatment. At this stage, oral TMP/SMX administration was reinitiated, without any negative effect on the platelet count. On the contrary, a rise in platelet number up to 503×10^9/L was observed. Fever resolved at the second day of treatment and no new bleeding manifestations appeared. The patient was discharged with rifampicin and TMP/SMX as maintenance therapy for a total six-week treatment. She completed the treatment without further complications and during the regular follow-up platelet counts were normal (Table 1).

3. Discussion

Thrombocytopenia is one of the hematological manifestations of brucellosis in children with a variable percentage of 5–40% in several studies [1–3, 5, 6]. The pathogenic pathways of Brucella-related thrombocytopenia have not been fully elucidated, with hypersplenism, hemophagocytosis, bone marrow suppression, and antiplatelet antibodies production being the most possible mechanisms. It is usually moderate without clinically significant bleeding problems. Less often, severe isolated thrombocytopenia occurs, possibly immune mediated, mimicking ITP (Table 2).

In Greece, several cases of severe thrombocytopenia have been described over the years. In 1998, Benecos et al. from our department reported a case of a boy who presented with severe thrombocytopenic purpura with petechiae, epistaxis, oral bleeding, and positive antiplatelet antibodies. He was initially treated as ITP with IVIG with good clinical and hematological response. A few days later prolonged fever occurred with persistent hepatomegaly and positive blood culture for Brucella melitensis and the child was successfully treated with streptomycin and TMP/SMX [7]. Tsirka et al. reported an 11-year-old boy with anemia, leukopenia, and severe thrombocytopenic purpura, who was treated as ITP with IVIG with an initial good response. Surprisingly, a few days later a blood culture was positive for Brucella melitensis and treatment with gentamicin, doxycycline, and rifampicin was successfully implemented [8]. Tsolia et al. presented 39 children diagnosed with brucellosis over a period of 15 years in central Greece, two of whom had severe thrombocytopenic purpura and received oral antibiotic therapy with a good outcome [3].

In Turkey brucellosis remains a major public health problem, with approximately 15000 cases per year. Pediatric patients represent 20–25% of all cases [9]. Authors from several areas of the country have reported cases of isolated severe thrombocytopenia as the presenting feature of brucellosis that responded well to appropriate antibiotic treatment combined with corticosteroids or IVIG. Fever was noticed in most cases, with positive blood culture for Brucella [10–13].

Apart from these case reports, large series of pediatric patients with brucellosis have been studied in Turkey with interesting findings regarding Brucella-related severe thrombocytopenia. Akbayram et al. reported five cases presenting with isolated thrombocytopenia out of 187 children (2.6%) diagnosed with brucellosis in one hospital in Turkey between

TABLE 2: Cases of children with brucellosis and severe thrombocytopenia.

Country	Authors	Year	Number of cases	Treatment	Outcome
	Benecos et al.	1998	1	IVIG, TMP/SMX, streptomycin	Good
Greece	Tsirka et al.	2002	1	IVIG, gentamycin, doxycycline, rifampicin	Good
	Tsolia et al.	2002	2	TMP/SMX, rifampicin	Good
	Sevinc et al.	2000	1	Corticosteroids, TMP/SMX, rifampicin, ciprofloxacin	Good
	Yalaz et al.	2004	1	Doxycycline, rifampicin	Good
	Ulug et al.	2011	1	TMP/SMX, rifampicin	Good
Turkey	Akbayram et al.	2011	5	Doxycycline and rifampicin (>8 years) or TMP/SMX and rifampicin (<8 years)	Good
	Citak et al.	2010	5	IVIG, TMP/SMX, rifampicin	Good
	Aypak et al.	2016	11	Doxycycline and rifampicin (>8 years) or TMP/SMX and rifampicin (<8 years)	Good
	Karaman et al.	2016	15	Doxycycline and rifampicin (>8 years) or TMP/SMX and rifampicin (<8 years)	Good
	Benjamin and Annobil	1992	4	Rifampicin, TMP/SMX, doxycycline, streptomycin	Good
Saudi Arabia	Al-Eissa and Al-Nasser	1993	5	Rifampicin, TMP/SMX, doxycycline, streptomycin	Good
	Benjamin	1995	2	Rifampicin, TMP/SMX, doxycycline	Good
Lebanon	Farah et al.	2010	1	IVIG, TMP/SMX, gentamicin	Good
Israel	Marom et al.	2000	1	Rifampicin, TMP/SMX	Good
Iran	Kamali Aghdam et al.	2016	1	IVIG, rifampicin, TMP/SMX	Good

TMP/SMX: trimethoprim/sulfamethoxazole.

2004 and 2010. All patients had a complete recovery and their platelet counts returned to normal after the administration of a combination of doxycycline and rifampicin or TMP/SMX and rifampicin [14]. During the same period in another hospital, Citak et al. retrospectively assessed the records of 146 children with brucellosis. Among them, 5 (3.4%) presented with immune thrombocytopenia, which was severe and manifested with a variety of symptoms and positive blood cultures for the bacteria. Apart from the appropriate antibiotic treatment, IVIG was administered with excellent response [6]. Aypak et al. evaluated the hematological findings in 69 children who were diagnosed with brucellosis over a one-year period [2010-2011] and 15.9% of them presented with thrombocytopenia restored after antibiotic treatment without the need of corticosteroids or IVIG [2]. In a most recent study with large numbers of patients from Eastern Turkey, Karaman et al. presented the hematological findings of 622 children with brucellosis over a 6-year period. Isolated severe thrombocytopenia was found in 16 patients (2.5%), which resolved with antibiotics or IVIG [5].

In countries of the Middle East where brucellosis is a significant health problem, isolated severe thrombocytopenia has been reported as a presenting symptom in several cases. In a series of 115 children with brucellosis in Saudi Arabia, four of them had severe thrombocytopenia and proper oral antibiotic therapy led to quick recovery [15]. In another study, clinically significant thrombocytopenia was found in 5 children from a population of 110 children with brucellosis and it was successfully treated with antibiotics [16]. Benjamin described two cases of children with fever, thrombocytopenic purpura, and mucosal bleeding which resolved promptly with the initiation of antimicrobial therapy. Thrombocytopenia was attributed to peripheral destruction since large platelets in the peripheral blood and proliferation of megakaryocytes in the bone marrow were identified: an image resembling ITP [17]. In 2010, Farah et al. in Lebanon reported a case of severe thrombocytopenic purpura as the sole manifestation of brucellosis in an 8-year-old boy. Giant platelets were found in his peripheral blood smear and bone marrow aspiration showed elevated megakaryocytes with no evidence of hemophagocytosis. He was successfully treated with gentamicin, TMP/SMX, and IVIG [18]. In a similar case from Iran, with isolated Brucella-related thrombocytopenia, administration of rifampicin, TMP/SMX, and IVIG solved the problem [19], while in another case from Israel sole antibiotic treatment was given because the hemorrhagic features were mild [20].

As it is apparent from reports in the literature, it is necessary for the general pediatrician to consider brucellosis in the differential diagnosis of thrombocytopenia, particularly in endemic areas. Children with the initial diagnosis of ITP who do not respond to treatment or present with fever, arthralgia, or hepatosplenomegaly should be also investigated for brucellosis, especially when there is a history of nonpasteurized dairy products consumption, a family history of brucellosis, or a preceding trip in endemic countries.

As far as our case is concerned, we faced some difficulties which raised certain concerns. The patient was admitted with extremely low platelet count and bleeding lesions of the mucous membranes. Consequently, the risk of internal or intracranial bleeding and the need for immediate intervention were urgent. Therefore, IVIG and intravenous treatment with aminoglycoside were administered, which led to a rapid and significant increase in platelet count.

Another discussion topic is the possibility of the involvement of the drugs already administered to the patient in the induction of thrombocytopenia. Rifampicin is a drug that could cause thrombocytopenia, but it is usually mild and clinically insignificant, whereas TMP/SMX can occasionally cause severe drop in platelet count with significant bleeding. Therefore, we decided to stop TMP/SMX treatment. Given that the patient had to continue double antimicrobial treatment beyond the acute phase for a total of six weeks, it was decided to continue the use of rifampicin. To exclude possible drug-induced thrombocytopenia from TMP/SMX, the drug was reintroduced after the stabilization of the patient's condition and this had no effect on the platelet count.

In conclusion, in regions where brucellosis is endemic, it should be included in the differential diagnosis in cases of ITP. There should be an individualized approach to each patient but in any case the administration of IVIG or corticosteroids is of great significance, while the final and main resolution occurs with appropriate antimicrobial therapy.

Competing Interests

The authors declare that there is no conflict of interests regarding the publication of this paper.

References

[1] E. Galanakis, K. L. Bourantas, S. Leveidiotou, and P. D. Lapatsanis, "Childhood brucellosis in north-western Greece: a retrospective analysis," European Journal of Pediatrics, vol. 155, no. 1, pp. 1–6, 1996.

[2] A. Aypak, C. Aypak, and Y. Bayram, "Hematological findings in children with brucellosis," Pediatrics International, vol. 57, no. 6, pp. 1108–1111, 2016.

[3] M. Tsolia, S. Drakonaki, A. Messaritaki et al., "Clinical features, complications and treatment outcome of childhood brucellosis in central Greece," Journal of Infection, vol. 44, no. 4, pp. 257–262, 2002.

[4] M. Yilmaz, O. Tiryaki, M. Namiduru et al., "Brucellosis-induced immune thrombocytopenia mimicking ITP: a report of seven cases," International Journal of Laboratory Hematology, vol. 29, no. 6, pp. 442–445, 2007.

[5] K. Karaman, S. Akbayram, G. İ. Bayhan et al., "Hematologic findings in children with brucellosis: experiences of 622 patients in eastern Turkey," Journal of Pediatric Hematology/Oncology, vol. 38, no. 6, pp. 463–466, 2016.

[6] E. C. Citak, F. E. Citak, B. Tanyeri, and D. Arman, "Hematologic manifestations of brucellosis in children: 5 years experience of an anatolian center," Journal of Pediatric Hematology/Oncology, vol. 32, no. 2, pp. 137–140, 2010.

[7] P. Benecos, T. Spingou, E. Galanakis, and P. D. Lapatsanis, "Thrombocytopenic purpura secondary to brucellosis," European Journal of Pediatrics, vol. 157, no. 8, article no. 698, 1998.

[8] A. Tsirka, I. Markesinis, V. Getsi, and S. Chaloulou, "Severe thrombocytopenic purpura due to brucellosis," *Scandinavian Journal of Infectious Diseases*, vol. 34, no. 7, pp. 535–536, 2002.

[9] Z. Yumuk and D. O'Callaghan, "Brucellosis in Turkey—an overview," *International Journal of Infectious Diseases*, vol. 16, no. 4, pp. e228–e235, 2012.

[10] A. Sevinc, N. O. Kutlu, I. Kuku, U. Ozgen, I. Aydogdu, and H. Soylu, "Severe epistaxis in brucellosis-induced isolated thrombocytopenia: a report of two cases," *Clinical and Laboratory Haematology*, vol. 22, no. 6, pp. 373–375, 2000.

[11] M. Yalaz, M. T. Arslan, and Z. Kurugöl, "Thrombocytopenic purpura as only manifestation of brucellosis in a child," *Turkish Journal of Pediatrics*, vol. 46, no. 3, pp. 265–267, 2004.

[12] M. Ulug, F. Yapici, and N. Can-Ulug, "Unusual clinical presentations of brucellosis in childhood," *Brazilian Journal of Infectious Diseases*, vol. 15, no. 4, pp. 406–407, 2011.

[13] R. Sac, N. Yarali, B. Tavil, M. F. Azik, A. Kara, and B. Tunc, "Severe persistent thrombocytopenia as a sole manifestation of brucellosis," *Indian Journal of Pediatrics*, vol. 80, no. 1, pp. 85–86, 2013.

[14] S. Akbayram, M. Dogan, C. Akgun, E. Peker, M. Parlak, and A. F. Oner, "An analysis of children with brucellosis associated with isolated thrombocytopenia," *Clinical and Applied Thrombosis/Hemostasis*, vol. 17, no. 6, pp. E36–E38, 2011.

[15] B. Benjamin and S. H. Annobil, "Childhood brucellosis in Southwestern Saudi Arabia: a 5-year experience," *Journal of Tropical Pediatrics*, vol. 38, no. 4, pp. 167–172, 1992.

[16] Y. Al-Eissa and M. Al-Nasser, "Haematological manifestations of childhood brucellosis," *Infection*, vol. 21, no. 1, pp. 23–26, 1993.

[17] B. Benjamin, "Acute thrombocytopenic purpura in childhood brucellosis," *Annals of Tropical Paediatrics*, vol. 15, no. 3, pp. 189–192, 1995.

[18] R. A. Farah, P. Hage, A. Al Rifai, and C. Afif, "Immune thrombocytopenic purpura associated with brucellosis. Case report and review of the literature," *Journal Medical Libanais*, vol. 58, no. 4, pp. 241–243, 2010.

[19] M. Kamali Aghdam, K. Davari, and K. Eftekhari, "Recurrent epistaxis and bleeding as the initial manifestation of brucellosis," *Acta Medica Iranica*, vol. 54, no. 3, pp. 218–219, 2016.

[20] R. Marom, D. Miron, H. Gabriel, and Y. Horowitz, "Thrombocytopenic purpura as sole manifestation of brucellosis in children," *Harefuah*, vol. 139, no. 7-8, pp. 278–326, 2000.

23

Candida glabrata Pneumonia in a Patient with Chronic Obstructive Pulmonary Disease

Onur Yazici,[1] Mustafa Cortuk,[2] Hasan Casim,[3] Erdogan Cetinkaya,[2] Ali Mert,[4] and Ali Ramazan Benli[5]

[1]Department of Chest Disease, Adnan Menderes University, Aydın, Turkey
[2]Department of Chest Disease, Karabuk University, Karabuk, Turkey
[3]Department of Chest Disease, Karabuk University Training and Research Hospital, Karabuk, Turkey
[4]Department of Infectious Diseases, İstanbul Medipol University, İstanbul, Turkey
[5]Department of Family Medicine, Karabuk University, Karabuk, Turkey

Correspondence should be addressed to Mustafa Cortuk; mcortuk@yahoo.com

Academic Editor: Sandeep Dogra

Pneumonia remains an important cause of morbidity and mortality among infectious diseases. *Streptococcus pneumoniae* and viruses are the most common cause of pneumonia. Candidiasis in such patients has been associated with haemodialysis, fungal colonization, exposure to broad-spectrum antibiotics, intensive care unit (ICU) hospitalization, and immunocompromised patients. The most common cause of infection is *C. albicans*. The case presented here is of a 66-year-old male patient diagnosed with *C. glabrata*. The patient suffered from chronic obstructive pulmonary disease.

1. Introduction

Pneumonia is a common respiratory tract disease and is one of the leading causes of mortality. Streptococcal and viral pneumonia are determined to be among the most common causes of community-acquired pneumonia in adults. In individuals with normal immunity, *Candida* species rarely cause pneumonia. The most common pathogen among the *Candida* species is *C. albicans*, particularly in subjects with reduced immunity or patients necessitating intensive care management [1].

C. glabrata is known as a nonpathogen *Candida* species. *C. glabrata* rarely acts as an infectious agent when compared to other *Candida* species and it is present within normal respiratory flora [2]. Few cases have been reported in which *C. glabrata* was determined to be an infectious agent causing pneumonia [3–6].

In this case report, *C. glabrata* pneumonia was diagnosed in a patient who has chronic obstructive pulmonary disease (COPD) and has been taking thyroid replacement therapy.

2. Case Presentation

A 66-year-old male patient was admitted with cough, purulent and blood-mixed sputum, and increased shortness of breath. His medical history included COPD for the last 5 years and total thyroidectomy performed 3 years ago with the diagnosis of multinodular goiter. When questioned about prescriptions, he was under inhaled formoterol, ipratropium bromide, and levothyroxine sodium, administered orally at $100\,\mu g$/day. He had not been hospitalized in the last year. Physical examination revealed blood pressure of 110/70 mmHg and pulse of 89/minute; his temperature was $36.8°C$ and fingertip-measured oxygen saturation (SpO_2) was 89% on room air. He presented with decreased breath sounds and prolongation of expiratory time. In addition, rales were present on auscultation of the mid and lower zones of the lungs. Laboratory investigation revealed C-reactive protein of 85 mg/dL, leukocytosis, with a white blood cell (WBC) count of 12.000/mm^3, and increased erythrocyte sedimentation rate (35 mm/hour). The chest X-ray showed increased bronchovascular shadows of the lungs. Treatment

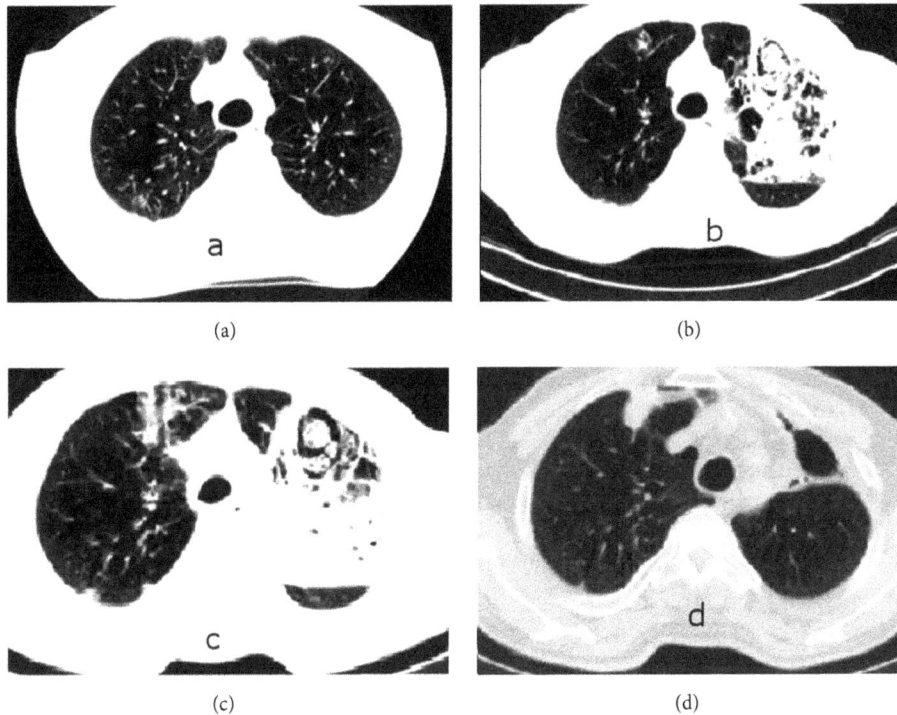

Figure 1: Chest tomography views on 4th day (a), 18th day (b and c), and 6th month (d) of hospitalization.

of an inhaler bronchodilator, intravenous theophylline, and 40 mg/day methylprednisolone was started. An antibiotic combination of intravenous ampicillin sulbactam (4 g/day) and oral levofloxacin (500 mg/day) was administered. On the 4th day of treatment, the administered antibiotics were discontinued due to a deterioration in clinical features together with progression of infection parameters and cefoperazone sodium/sulbactam sodium combination (4 g/day) and moxifloxacin (400 mg/day) were started as new antibiotics. Computerized tomography (CT) of the chest was performed where emphysema and a small infiltration of right upper lobe posterior part were identified (Figure 1(a)). As the patient's clinical condition was getting worse and the infection parameters were not improving despite the treatment, a chest X-ray was obtained, which showed an increase of nonhomogeneous density on the left upper lobe. Additionally, flexible bronchoscopy was performed with normal findings except increased bronchial submucosal vascularity on the tenth day of being admitted to the hospital. *Streptococcus mitis* and *Candida* species were produced in the bronchoalveolar lavage obtained by left upper lobe. Therefore, the antibiotics were discontinued and linezolid 800 mg/day and fluconazole 200 mg/day were started intravenously. Meanwhile, an increase in blood sugar level was detected, which was considered to be related to intravenous corticosteroid. Therefore, the corticosteroid dosage was reduced and discontinued on the 12th day, after which the blood sugar level returned to normal. Since SpO$_2$ continued to remain below 88% despite administration of 5 L/min oxygen and tachycardia and tachypnea were present, the patient was admitted to

the intensive care unit and bilevel positive airway pressure (BPAP) treatment was applied. Despite this treatment, no improvement was observed in the patient. A further chest CT was obtained which showed a pneumonic appearance with patchy necrotic areas in the left upper lobe (Figures 1(b) and 1(c)). Flexible bronchoscopy was performed again on the 25th day of being admitted to the hospital and it revealed a view consistent with diffuse white *Candida* plaques in sites starting from the vocal cords and covering the entire trachea and both bronchial systems (Figure 2(a)). Bronchial biopsies and lavage of the left upper lobe were obtained. The bronchial biopsy revealed no fungus or similar pathology in the tissue. Because *Candida* spp. is reproduced in bronchoalveolar lavage taken at both 10th and 25th days, and *Candida* plaque is compatible with macroscopic appearance on bronchoscopy done at 25th day, it has been thought to be resistant *Candida* spp. and voriconazole treatment has been started. The bronchoalveolar lavage sample that *Candida* spp. reproduced on *Candida* plaques that are taken from BAL sample was sent to "Refik Saydam National Public Health Agency" for classification and antibiogram. Fluconazole resistant *C. glabrata* reproduced on the fungi culture that is done in this institution. The MIC90S value was reported as ≥32 μg/mL for fluconazole and 1 μg/mL and for voriconazole. We could not obtain *Candida* specific antibodies and mannan antigen tests that are used for the diagnosis of *Candida* infections, because it is not performed in our hospital. The fluconazole was discontinued and intravenous voriconazole 400 mg/day was started. Following this treatment, the clinical status of the patient gradually ameliorated, hemoptysis stopped, and infection parameters improved. The patient, who no longer required BPAP, was admitted to the clinical ward. Intravenous voriconazole was continued for 23 days. Control bronchoscopy performed on the 15th day of voriconazole treatment revealed almost complete recovery of the previously observed *Candida* plaques. Following significant improvement of his general status and dyspnea, the patient was discharged from the hospital with a prescription for oral voriconazole. Blood and urine cultures obtained during the hospitalization did not manifest any *Candida* growth. During ambulatory treatment with voriconazole, *E. coli* grew once in the urine culture and this was treated with ertapenem administered for 10 days. The voriconazole treatment was continued for 6 months. The appearance of air-fluid level at the left upper lobe and traction of the trachea to the left were identified during treatment. Left upper lobectomy was recommended because of this radiological appearance, but the patient refused surgery and so was continued to be followed up clinically and radiologically. The clinical situation of the patient did not worsen. Radiological and bronchoscopic recovery (Figure 2(b)) was seen on the last obtained CT (Figure 1(d)). Therefore, the idea of surgery was abandoned and the ambulatory follow-up of the patient currently continues uneventfully.

3. Discussion

Candida species exist as opportunistic pathogens in the microflora of the human body [7]. *Candida* infections are encountered especially in patients hospitalized in intensive care units (ICU) and these infections prolong ICU stay and increase the mortality rate [8]. When *Candida* is produced, particularly in cases obtained from the respiratory tract, the most important problem is due to either colonization or invasive pulmonary candidiasis. Since *Candida* is an element of microflora, to differentiate from colonization, it is necessary to be identified in the tissue, in general.

Pulmonary fungal infections are being increasingly identified as infectious agents in immunocompromised subjects. In the article by Chen et al., in which pulmonary fungal infections were compiled, *C. glabrata* was reported in 4 out of 140 patients [9].

Candida pneumonia is caused either by candidemia via the hematogenous route or by aspiration from the oropharynx. Kobayashi et al. reported the case of a 71-year-old patient who was being fed through nasogastric catheter [3]. In this case, the probable contamination route was considered to be aspiration. Another 78-year-old patient, reported by Speletas et al., had chronic myeloid leukemia and was using imatinib mesylate [6]. In this patient, candidemia was not reported. Hamilton et al. reported a case of *Candida glabrata* pneumonia with candidemia in an immunocompetent patient [5]. Bankier et al. reported a case of *C. Glabrata* infection in a nonimmunocompromised patient [4]. To the best of our knowledge, no other case has been reported except those mentioned above.

Franquet et al. reported that there is no specific radiologic image on *Candida* pneumonia. It has been reported that, in the study, computerized tomography (CT) findings included multiple nodules and air-space consolidation and nodules surrounded by discrete areas of ground-glass opacity (CT halo sign) can be seen [10]. In our case consolidation and cavitation were also shown on the CT of left upper lobe and a nodule of right upper lobe. Although there are many respiratory signs and symptoms from the respiratory system on the admission day, the patients suffered from COPD for the last 5 years.

In the current case, the patient suffered from COPD and thyroid replacement therapy. There was no history of central catheter utilization or admission to hospital or intensive care unit. There was no history of vomiting and aspiration. Although the lower respiratory tract infection is a common complication of COPD that is being presented in the case, general immune deficiency has not been determined. Although colonization by *Candida* of multiple nonsterile sites has been declared, prolonged use of antibacterial antibiotics has been linked to increased risk of invasive candidiasis [11]. In our case, *Candida* plaques were seen under the vocal cords which were excepted as sterile normally. Also, on the laboratory parameter, CRP sedimentation and WBC were found to be high on the day when the patient is hospitalized and these parameters got worse despite the antibiotics. The status of the patient deteriorated from the beginning and no response was observed from the administered nonspecific treatments. Since the second bronchoscopy, which was performed while the patient was under empirical fluconazole treatment, revealed *Candida* plaques in the entire bronchial system starting from the vocal cords, the fluconazole treatment was discontinued before the culture results were obtained and voriconazole was started. Thereafter, the culture result was received as *C. glabrata* and its resistance against fluconazole was verified by antibiogram. Previous publications have frequently identified the resistance of *C. glabrata* to azole group antifungals [12].

To differentiate a pulmonary infection caused by *Candida* from colonization, the microbiological agent should be identified in tissue, in general. In the current case, we showed wide *Candida* plaque on the bronchoscopy, but, unfortunately, we could not identify it microscopically in the tissue. Nevertheless *C. glabrata* were identified by bronchoalveolar lavage twice. Although *Aspergillus* type fungi were intensively sought in both the biopsy specimens and the cultures, due to a similar radiological appearance, they were not identified.

4. Conclusion

C. glabrata is quite a rare cause of pneumonia. Although it is quite rare, it may also be the cause in ambulatory patients. It should be kept in mind especially in cases where the clinical condition does not improve despite treatment with azole group antifungal agents and *Candida* species are detected in respiratory tract isolates. It should also be kept in mind that successful treatment is possible with voriconazole.

Consent

Written informed consent was obtained from the patient.

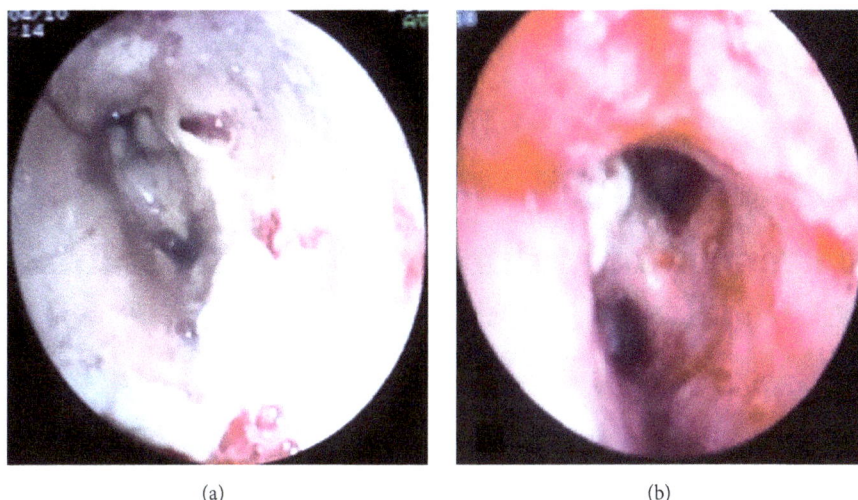

(a)   (b)

FIGURE 2: The appearance of the left main bronchus in the bronchoscopic examination performed before (a) and after (b) the 15th day of voriconazole treatment.

Competing Interests

No competing interests were declared by the authors.

References

[1] S. Li and Y.-Z. An, "Retrospective analysis of invasive fungal infection in surgical intensive care unit," *Zhonghua Yi Xue Za Zhi*, vol. 90, no. 6, pp. 382–385, 2010.

[2] L. D. Haley, "Yeasts of medical importance," *American Journal of Clinical Pathology*, vol. 36, pp. 227–234, 1961.

[3] T. Kobayashi, Y. Miyazaki, K. Yanagihara et al., "A probable case of aspiration pneumonia caused by *Candida glabrata* in a non-neutropenic patient with candidemia," *Internal Medicine*, vol. 44, no. 11, pp. 1191–1194, 2005.

[4] A. Bankier, D. Fleischmann, M. Wiesmayr, K. Laczika, and P. Hübsch, "*Candida glabrata* pneumonia in a non-immunosuppressed patient: diagnostic imaging with digital luminescence radiography and CT," *Aktuelle Radiologie*, vol. 4, no. 4, pp. 192–194, 1994.

[5] L. A. Hamilton, N. R. Lockhart, and M. R. Crain, "Candida glabrata and Candida tropicalis in an immunocompetent patient: a case report," *Journal of Pharmacy Practice*, vol. 28, no. 3, pp. 284–287, 2015.

[6] M. Speletas, T.-A. Vyzantiadis, F. Kalala et al., "Pneumonia caused by *Candida krusei* and *Candida glabrata* in a patient with chronic myeloid leukemia receiving imatinib mesylate treatment," *Medical Mycology*, vol. 46, no. 3, pp. 259–263, 2008.

[7] E. Azoulay, J.-F. Timsit, M. Tafflet et al., "Candida colonization of the respiratory tract and subsequent pseudomonas ventilator-associated pneumonia," *Chest*, vol. 129, no. 1, pp. 110–117, 2006.

[8] N. Adigüzel, Z. Karakurt, G. Güngör et al., "Mortality rates and risk factors associated with nosocomial *Candida* infection in a respiratory intensive care unit," *Tuberküloz ve Toraks*, vol. 58, no. 1, pp. 35–43, 2010.

[9] K.-Y. Chen, S.-C. Ko, P.-R. Hsueh, K.-T. Luh, and P.-C. Yang, "Pulmonary fungal infection: emphasis on microbiological spectra, patient outcome, and prognostic factors," *Chest*, vol. 120, no. 1, pp. 177–184, 2001.

[10] T. Franquet, N. L. Müller, K. S. Lee, A. Oikonomou, and J. D. Flint, "Pulmonary candidiasis after hematopoietic stem cell transplantation: thin-section CT findings," *Radiology*, vol. 236, no. 1, pp. 332–337, 2005.

[11] P. G. Pappas, J. H. Rex, J. D. Sobel et al., "Guidelines for treatment of candidiasis," *Clinical Infectious Diseases*, vol. 38, no. 2, pp. 161–189, 2004.

[12] I. I. Balkan, A. Savas, A. Geduk, M. Yemisen, B. Mete, and R. Ozaras, "*Candida glabrata* perinephric abscess," *The Eurasian Journal of Medicine*, vol. 43, no. 1, pp. 63–65, 2011.

24

Surgical Management of Multiple Valve Endocarditis Associated with Dialysis Catheter

R. Zea-Vera,[1] M. Sanchez,[1] E. Castañeda,[1,2] and L. Soto-Arquiñigo[1,3]

[1]*Universidad Peruana Cayetano Heredia, San Martin de Porres, Lima, Peru*
[2]*Cardiovascular Surgery Department, Hospital Cayetano Heredia, San Martin de Porres, Lima, Peru*
[3]*Infectious Disease Department, Hospital Cayetano Heredia, San Martin de Porres, Lima, Peru*

Correspondence should be addressed to L. Soto-Arquiñigo; leslie.soto@upch.pe

Academic Editor: Gernot Walder

Endocarditis associated with dialysis catheter is a disease that must be suspected in every patient with hemodialysis who develops fever. Multiple valve disease is a severe complication of endocarditis that needs to be managed in a different way. There is very limited data for treatment and every case must be considered individually. We present a patient with this complication and describe the medical treatment and surgical management. We report the case of a 15-year-old patient with acute renal failure that develops trivalvular endocarditis after the hemodialysis catheter was placed, with multiple positive blood culture for *Staphylococcus aureus*. Transesophageal echocardiography was done and aortic and tricuspid valvular vegetations and mitral insufficiency were reported. Patient was successfully treated by surgery on the three valves, including aortic valve replacement. There is limited data about the appropriate treatment for multiple valvular endocarditis; it is important to consider this complication in the setting of hemodialysis patients that develop endocarditis and, despite the appropriate treatment, have a torpid evolution. In countries where endovenous drug abuse is uncommon, right sided endocarditis is commonly associated with vascular catheters. Aggressive surgical management should be the treatment of choice in these kinds of patients.

1. Introduction

Endocarditis is the inflammation of the endocardium, the inner lining of cardiac chambers, and valves; even though there are other causes of endocarditis, infectious etiology is the most common.

First, there is disruption of endocardium through multiple mechanisms, the most common being turbulent flow due to congenital heart diseases in developed countries and rheumatic heart disease in underdeveloped ones; other causes are intracardiac devices and some bacteria with high virulence such as *Staphylococcus aureus* [1].

Then platelets and fibrin deposit within this lesion and a sterile thrombus form. When bacteremia ensues, for example, after dental treatment, there can be bacterial growth within the thrombus due to adhesins [2]. Finally when the vegetation "matures" further fibrin deposit stabilizes the thrombus.

Reported mortality varies from 15 to 30% and has been stable in the past years; nonetheless there has been a variation in risk factors; recently prevalence of endocarditis associated with invasive procedures, higher population age, and diabetes prevalence has increased [3].

In the present case report we present a patient with acute renal injury that develops multiple valve endocarditis (tricuspid, mitral, and aortic) associated with a dialysis catheter, and we also present a literature review highlighting medical treatment and surgical management of infectious endocarditis.

2. Case Presentation

A 15-year-old male patient comes to the emergency department with a 4-week history of lower extremity edema and arthralgia of knees and ankles that increases in intensity and restricts deambulation.

Approximately 4 hours before presenting to the emergency room, the patient reports an episode of macroscopic hematuria. At the emergency department, he referred to

TABLE 1: Laboratory results.

Exam	Result	Laboratory normal values
Glucose	91 mg/dL	75–110 mg/dL
Urea	308.5 mg/dL	19–43 mg/dL
Creatinine	19.4 mg/dL	0.8–1.5 mg/dL
Hemoglobin	5.6 g/dL	11–15 g/dL
Leukocytes	$8.740 \times 10^3/mm^3$	$5–10 \times 10^3/mm^3$
Platelets	$23\,200 \times 10^3/mm^3$	$150–400 \times 10^3/mm^3$
Sodium	140 mEq/L	135–148 mEq/L
Potassium	5.11 mEq/L	3.5–5.3 mEq/L
Arterial blood gases	pH: 7.00 pCO_2: 20.5 mmHg pO_2: 132 mmHg HCO_3: 4.9	
Urine analysis	>100 RBC per field 3 WBC per field	<3 RBC per field <5 WBC per field

TABLE 2: Culture results.

Hospitalization day (HD)	Culture	Result
11	Blood 1	*Staphylococcus epidermidis*
13	Blood 2	MRSA
17	Blood 3	MRSA
21	Blood 4	MRSA
15	Urine	Negative
34	Peritoneal fluid	Negative

sleepiness, adequate appetite, and 2-3 kg of weight loss in the last month. The patient denied fever or chills, diarrhea, movement disorders, or other symptoms.

2.1. Clinical Findings. Upon physical examination he is found to be alert and fully oriented. Blood pressure was 109/60 mmHg, heart rate was 103 beats per minute and 19 respirations per minute, temperature was 37.4°C, and O_2 saturation was 95% at room air. Skin paleness and edema of lower extremities were noticed on inspection. The rest of the physical examination was within normal limits.

Laboratory results on admission can be seen on Table 1. Electrocardiogram was within normal limits. Because of abnormal urea, creatinine, and hemoglobin results, hemodialysis was indicated.

2.2. Diagnostic Assessment. Within one week after hemodialysis, the patient presented febrile episodes with multiple positive blood culture for methicillin-resistant *Staphylococcus aureus* (MRSA) (Table 2). Upon physical examination, a holosystolic murmur was heard at the tricuspid focus and Janeway lesions in toes where observed (Figure 1). Transesophageal echocardiography reported aortic and tricuspid valvular vegetations as well as mitral insufficiency.

2.3. Therapeutic Intervention. Antibiotic therapy with vancomycin for infectious endocarditis was initiated due to the

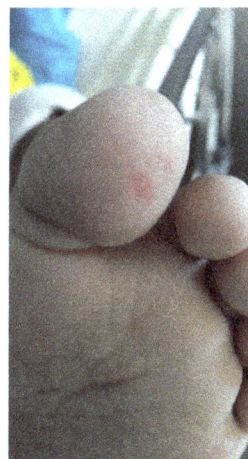

FIGURE 1: Janeway lesion on patient's left toe.

increased risk of coagulase-negative *Staphylococcus*. Later this treatment was maintained when positive cultures for MRSA (Table 3) were available. Because of new onset heart failure and failure to respond to antibiotic therapy, surgical intervention was decided. Before the surgical procedure, the infected catheter was removed and a peritoneal catheter was placed in order to continue renal replacement therapy.

A median sternotomy approach was used; extracorporeal circulation was initiated. After aortic clamping and cardiac arrest with cardioplegia, an incision was made in the right atrium. Vegetations on the right atrium, superior vena cava entrance, inferior vena cava, and tricuspid valve leaflets were removed.

The surgical team proceeded to open the interauricular septum and vegetations on the mitral valve were also removed. After this, the aortic artery was opened and aortic vegetations as well as the valves were removed. The aortic annulus was enlarged with pericardial patch and an aortic valve mechanical prosthesis number 19 (Bicarbon Slimline, Sorin Group, Saluggia, Italy) was implanted.

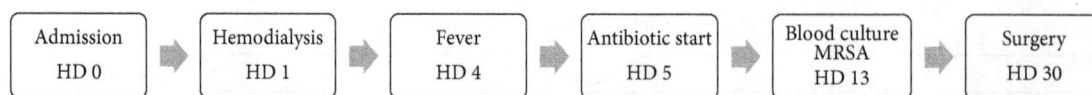

FIGURE 2: Hospital course.

TABLE 3: Antibiogram: MRSA.

Antibiotics	Interpretation
Amikacin	Resistant
Ciprofloxacin	Resistant
Clindamycin	Resistant
Chloramphenicol	Sensible
Erythromycin	Resistant
Gentamicin	Resistant
Levofloxacin	Resistant
Oxacillin	Resistant
Penicillin	Resistant
Rifampicin	Sensible
Tetracycline	Sensible

TABLE 4: Peritoneal fluid cytology.

Cytology	Results	Normal values
Color	Yellow	Yellow
Aspect	Turbid	Transparent
Leukocytes	6900/mm^3	<500/mm^3
Polymorphonuclear cells	70%	<25%
Red blood cells	5	0.10–2.00/mm^3

Finally the aorta and right atrium were closed in standard fashion and aortic clamping and cardiopulmonary bypass were discontinued. Pacemaker wires were placed in the right atrium and right ventricle and the sternum was closed.

2.4. Follow-Up and Outcomes. The postoperatory valve culture reported MRSA and the pathology report described, "dense infiltrates with large areas of necrosis and multiple germ colonies in relationship with infectious endocarditis."

The patient presented a perioperative myocardial infarction. At the time, echocardiogram reported the following: inferior and anteroseptal hypokinesia with ejection fraction of 40%. Captopril adjusted to creatinine clearance and carvedilol 6.25 mg PO twice a day were started to prevent cardiac remodeling.

Later during hospitalization, he also developed spontaneous bacterial peritonitis, suggested by a high level of leukocytes demonstrated in the peritoneal fluid cytology (Table 4), possibly due to peritoneal dialysis catheter infection.

The catheter was removed and treatment with meropenem 1 g daily was started and continued for 3 weeks. Peritoneal fluid culture was negative (Table 2). The treatment with vancomycin 1 g every 72 hours was stopped after 42 days. Eventually the patient showed good clinical response with remission of disease and was discharged home (Figure 2).

At 6-month follow-up the patient is on oral anticoagulation with an INR within therapeutic ranges. Renal function has improved and he no longer needs dialysis support. From a cardiologic stand-point no new symptoms were reported, EKG remains in normal sinus rhythm with nonspecific ST and T wave changes; lastly follow-up echocardiography has not been performed.

3. Discussion

Infectious endocarditis incidence varies from 3 to 10 per 100 000 at risk patients [3], around 60–70% are males [4], and patient age as well as male to female ratio has increased. A recent study in the United States found an increased incidence from 11 to 16 cases per 100 000 at risk people [5]. Mackie et al. also reported increased incidence throughout an 11-year period in Canada [4].

This rise is most likely related to higher predisposition to endocarditis in the general population such as higher population age, higher survival of patients with congenital heart diseases, more patients on hemodialysis, and more intracardiac devices used [6]. Currently healthcare associated endocarditis cases account for 25–30% and are mainly acute [7]. In developing countries the most important predisposing factor is still rheumatic heart disease, making up to one-third of the cases [8].

The percentage of infective endocarditis caused by *Staphylococcus aureus* is increasing; meanwhile Streptococcus viridans and culture negative endocarditis have decreased [9]. Coagulase-negative *Staphylococcus* are part of the normal skin flora but are also the most common cause of early onset prosthetic valve endocarditis; the high association is due to the ability to produce biofilms, high frequency of abscess formation, and increased antibiotic resistance.

In this context the present case illustrates a very difficult clinical situation, where a young patient hospitalized for a renal insufficiency syndrome requiring hemodialysis develops acute multiple valve endocarditis due to MRSA. While hemodialysis is a well-known risk factor for healthcare-related infective endocarditis, the conjunction of the two situations and the potential high mortality risk of endocarditis made endocarditis a prime concern for therapeutic intervention. On its side, the exact etiology of the renal syndrome remained unclear but ultimately improved over time.

3.1. Clinical Presentation. Sir William Osler said the following on his, now classic, Gulstonian Lectures: "Few diseases present greater difficulties in the way of diagnosis than malignant endocarditis, difficulties which in many cases are practically insurmountable" [10].

Even though diagnostic tools have certainly improved, the variable clinical presentation requires high suspicion in anyone with sepsis of unknown origin or fever in the presence of risk factors, such as hemodialysis in this case; these patients have an increased calculated incidence up to 308 per 100 000 patient years, and the most common presenting sign is fever [11, 12].

Most common physical findings are fever and a new onset cardiac murmur; also classic findings such as Osler nodes and Janeway lesions are rare (<5%); thereby further laboratory and echocardiographic assessment is necessary.

Laboratory findings are also nonspecific and usually show elevated inflammatory markers and can show normochromic and normocytic anemia. Hematuria can be present in up to 25% of patients [7].

Right sided endocarditis is commonly associated with endovenous drug abuse, but in developing countries such as Peru, endovenous drug abuse is uncommon due to economic and cultural reasons [13]. In this population right sided endocarditis is more commonly associated with dialysis catheters.

3.2. Diagnosis. Diagnostic criteria have been developed to help clinician and researchers in decision making; the Duke criteria were first proposed in 1994 and later modified in 2000 [14]. Even though Duke's criteria are helpful for clinicians, they are meant to help classification in clinical research and thereby should never replace clinical judgment [3].

Echocardiography plays a major role in endocarditis diagnosis; currently it is recommended to perform transthoracic echocardiography as an initial imaging study in any patient with suspicion of endocarditis.

Transesophageal echocardiography should be performed when an optimal echocardiographic window is not possible (e.g., previous thoracic or cardiovascular surgery, morbid obesity, and chronic lung disease) or when there is high clinical suspicion even if transthoracic echocardiography is negative [15].

3.3. Management. Current American and English guidelines do not recommend antibiotic prophylaxis for all patients undergoing dental procedures, yet the American Heart Association does suggest that it is reasonable to give prophylaxis to those patients with highest risk for endocarditis [16, 17]. Studies on the impact of these new guidelines on endocarditis prevalence and pathogenesis present conflicting results [4, 5].

Management should be by a multidisciplinary team involving cardiology, echocardiography, infectious diseases, and cardiothoracic surgery, and other specialties should be available if required, such as nephrology, spinal surgery, neurology, and neurosurgery [18].

Empirical antibiotic treatment has been proposed by the British Society for Antimicrobial Chemotherapy depending on clinical data, yet involvement of local infectious disease experts is recommended due to different causing agents and resistance patterns [19]. Further treatment should be according to blood culture results [12].

Currently around 50% of patients undergo surgery [7]; indications for surgery are heart failure, uncontrolled infection, and prevention of embolism. It is important to note that surgery is not done in all patients with indications, mostly due to clinical status.

The most common indication for surgery is heart failure, and it's present in approximately 45–60% of cases, timing for surgery in the presence of acute aortic or mitral valve regurgitation varies depending on haemodynamic effects.

Another indication is uncontrolled infection, which refers to persistent infection despite adequate antibiotic treatment; also because infection by highly virulent or resistant organisms is difficult to control medically, it can be managed surgically. Finally, embolism prevention, complicating 20–50% of cases, usually presents within the first 2 weeks of antibiotic treatment and with stroke symptoms; surgery depends on vegetation characteristics [20]. Surgery for recurrent embolism is suggested.

In the present case early surgery (26 days after fever onset) was indicated for both cardiac dysfunction and uncontrolled infection, most probably due to extensive vegetations inhabited by bacterial biofilm-like aggregates (see pathology description).

Early surgery, defined as replacement or repair of a valve in the initial hospitalization, has shown to be associated with better in-hospital survival [21]; this association has also been found on patients in chronic hemodialysis [11]. Nevertheless, early mortality following operation of active endocarditis remains not trivial [22]. It was up to 40% and 50%, respectively, 3 and 6 months after surgery for multiple valve infections versus 10% and 20% for single valve infection.

In this case report we presented a patient with acute renal failure that develops trivalvular endocarditis after placement of hemodialysis catheter and was successfully treated by early surgery on the three valves. In countries where intravenous drug use is uncommon the increased use of hemodialysis catheters should present a new group of high risk patients. Finally, the present case illustrates the good side of the medal as both his cardiac and renal conditions are improving after 6 months of follow-up.

Consent

Written informed consent was obtained from the patient's parents for the publication of this case report.

Competing Interests

The authors state that they have no competing interests.

References

[1] S. W. Kerrigan, N. Clarke, A. Loughman, G. Meade, T. J. Foster, and D. Cox, "Molecular basis for *Staphylococcus aureus*-mediated platelet aggregate formation under arterial shear in vitro," *Arteriosclerosis, Thrombosis, and Vascular Biology*, vol. 28, no. 2, pp. 335–340, 2008.

[2] C. Golias, A. Batistatou, G. Bablekos et al., "Physiology and pathophysiology of selectins, integrins, and IgSf cell adhesion molecules focusing on inflammation. A paradigm model on infectious endocarditis," *Cell Communication and Adhesion*, vol. 18, no. 3, pp. 19–32, 2011.

[3] T. J. Cahill and B. D. Prendergast, "Infective endocarditis," *The Lancet*, vol. 387, no. 10021, pp. 882–893, 2016.

[4] A. S. Mackie, W. Liu, A. Savu, A. J. Marelli, and P. Kaul, "Infective endocarditis hospitalizations before and after the 2007 American heart association prophylaxis guidelines," *Canadian Journal of Cardiology*, vol. 32, no. 8, pp. 942–948, 2016.

[5] S. Pant, N. J. Patel, A. Deshmukh et al., "Trends in infective endocarditis incidence, microbiology, and valve replacement in the United States from 2000 to 2011," *Journal of the American College of Cardiology*, vol. 65, no. 19, pp. 2070–2076, 2015.

[6] F. Carrasco, M. Anguita, M. Ruiz et al., "Clinical features and changes in epidemiology of infective endocarditis on pacemaker devices over a 27-year period (1987–2013)," *Europace*, vol. 18, no. 6, pp. 836–841, 2016.

[7] D. R. Murdoch, G. R. Corey, B. Hoen et al., "Clinical presentation, etiology, and outcome of infective endocarditis in the 21st century: the International Collaboration on Endocarditis-Prospective Cohort Study," *Archives of Internal Medicine*, vol. 169, no. 5, pp. 463–473, 2009.

[8] F. Romaní, J. Cuadra, F. Atencia, F. Vargas, and C. Canelo, Endocarditis infecciosa: análisis retrospectivo en el Hospital Nacional Arzobispo Loayza, 2002–2007 [Internet], Revista Peruana de Epidemiología, 2009, http://www.redalyc.org/articulo.oa?id=203120363004.

[9] L. Slipczuk, J. N. Codolosa, C. D. Davila et al., "Infective endocarditis epidemiology over five decades: a systematic review," *PLoS ONE*, vol. 8, no. 12, Article ID e82665, 2013.

[10] W. Osler, "The gulstonian lectures, on malignant endocarditis," *British Medical Journal*, vol. 1, no. 1264, pp. 577–579, 1885.

[11] D. Kamalakannan, R. M. Pai, L. B. Johnson, J. M. Gardin, and L. D. Saravolatz, "Epidemiology and clinical outcomes of infective endocarditis in hemodialysis patients," *Annals of Thoracic Surgery*, vol. 83, no. 6, pp. 2081–2086, 2007.

[12] J.-L. Tao, J. Ma, G.-L. Ge et al., "Diagnosis and treatment of infective endocarditis in chronic hemodialysis patients," *Chinese Medical Sciences Journal*, vol. 25, no. 3, pp. 135–139, 2010.

[13] Informe Ejecutivo Encuesta Nacional sobre Consumo de Drogas en la Población General del Perú 2010—DEVIDA [Internet], http://www.devida.gob.pe/2012/12/informe-ejecutivo-encuesta-nacional-sobre-consumo-de-drogas-en-poblacion-general-peru-2010/.

[14] J. S. Li, D. J. Sexton, N. Mick et al., "Proposed modifications to the Duke criteria for the diagnosis of infective endocarditis," *Clinical Infectious Diseases*, vol. 30, no. 4, pp. 633–638, 2000.

[15] L. M. Baddour, W. R. Wilson, A. S. Bayer et al., "On behalf of the American Heart Association Committee on Rheumatic Fever, Endocarditis, and Kawasaki Disease of the Council on Cardiovascular Disease in the Young, Council on Clinical Cardiology, Council on Cardiovascular Surgery and Anesthesia, and Stroke Council. Infective endocarditis in adults: diagnosis, antimicrobial therapy, and management of complications: a scientific statement for healthcare professionals from the American Heart Association," *Circulation*, vol. 132, no. 15, pp. 1435–1486, 2015.

[16] Centre for Clinical Practice at NICE (UK), *Prophylaxis Against Infective Endocarditis: Antimicrobial Prophylaxis Against Infective Endocarditis in Adults and Children Undergoing Interventional Procedures*, National Institute for Health and Clinical Excellence, London, UK, 2008, http://www.ncbi.nlm.nih.gov/books/NBK51789/.

[17] W. Wilson, K. A. Taubert, M. Gewitz et al., "Prevention of infective endocarditis," *Circulation*, vol. 116, no. 15, pp. 1736–1754, 2007.

[18] J. Chambers, J. Sandoe, S. Ray et al., "The infective endocarditis team: recommendations from an international working group," *Heart*, vol. 100, no. 7, pp. 524–527, 2014.

[19] F. K. Gould, D. W. Denning, T. S. J. Elliott et al., "Guidelines for the diagnosis and antibiotic treatment of endocarditis in adults: a report of the working party of the british society for antimicrobial chemotherapy," *Journal of Antimicrobial Chemotherapy*, vol. 67, no. 2, Article ID dkr450, pp. 269–289, 2012.

[20] G. Habib, P. Lancellotti, M. J. Antunes et al., "2015 ESC Guidelines for the management of infective endocarditis," *European Heart Journal*, vol. 36, no. 44, pp. 3075–3128, 2015.

[21] T. Lalani, C. H. Cabell, D. K. Benjamin et al., "Analysis of the impact of early surgery on in-hospital mortality of native valve endocarditis: use of propensity score and instrumental variable methods to adjust for treatment-selection bias," *Circulation*, vol. 121, no. 8, pp. 1005–1013, 2010.

[22] K. Meszaros, S. Nujic, G. H. Sodeck et al., "Long-term results after operations for active infective endocarditis in native and prosthetic valves," *Annals of Thoracic Surgery*, vol. 94, no. 4, pp. 1204–1210, 2012.

25

Challenges in Treating Secondary Syphilis Osteitis in an Immunocompromised Patient with a Penicillin Allergy: Case Report and Review of the Literature

Robert Ali,[1] Julio Perez-Downes,[1] Firas Baidoun,[1] Bashar Al Turk,[1] Carmen Isache,[1] Girish Mohan,[2] and Charles Perniciaro[2]

[1]Department of Internal Medicine, University of Florida-Jacksonville, 655 W 8th Street, Jacksonville, FL 32209, USA
[2]Department of Pathology, University of Florida-Jacksonville, 655 W 8th Street, Jacksonville, FL 32209, USA

Correspondence should be addressed to Robert Ali; robert.ali@jax.ufl.edu

Academic Editor: Antonella Marangoni

Syphilis is a sexually transmitted infection that remains fairly commonplace. The introduction of penicillin aided in curbing the incidence of disease; however, with the advent of the human immunodeficiency virus (HIV), syphilis is now on a resurgence with sometimes curious presentations. We present a case of a 36-year-old Caucasian gentleman with untreated HIV who complained of a skin eruption and joint pains for 6 weeks, prompting the diagnosis of secondary syphilis osteitis. Skin lesions were reminiscent of "malignant" syphilis. CD4 count was 57 cells/μL. RPR was elevated with 1 : 64 titer and positive confirmatory TP-PA. Radiography of the limbs revealed polyostotic cortical irregularities corroborated on bone scintigraphy. The patient had an unknown penicillin allergy and was unwilling to conduct a trial of penicillin-based therapy. He was subsequently treated with doxycycline 100 mg twice daily for 6 weeks and commenced antiretroviral therapy, noting dramatic improvement in both the skin lesions and joint pains. Unfortunately, he defaulted on follow-up, precluding serial RPR and bone imaging. Penicillin allergies have proven to be quite a conundrum in such patients, without much recourse for alternative therapy. Doxycycline with/without azithromycin is other options worth considering.

1. Introduction

Syphilis is a sexually transmitted disease which is still prevalent in the world. It is caused by the spirochete *Treponema pallidum*, and it is transmitted mainly by contact with a syphilitic sore. These sores are most commonly present in the genitals and can be located both internally and externally [1]. Syphilis can be classified into several stages according to the clinical manifestations of the disease. These include early syphilis, which typically occurs within the first year of infection and can be divided into primary, secondary, and early latent syphilis, as well as latent syphilis, which is characterized as asymptomatic infection with a positive serology [2]. Other presentations of syphilis also include central nervous system involvement, causing neurosyphilis, as well as extensive vascular involvement with syphilitic aortitis [2].

Due to the advent of antibiotics and the increased awareness and health campaigns throughout the United States and the world, the incidence of syphilis has decreased significantly over the past decades [3]. In addition, better screening methods, early identification, and more access to healthcare have allowed early treatment, further reducing the clinical presentation, and diagnosis of the late manifestations of syphilis [3]. Despite such advancements, secondary syphilis is still prevalent in high risk populations, mainly individuals with the human immunodeficiency virus (HIV), people who engage in high risk sexual activity, and those who do not regularly use protection [3]. In this case, we present the uncommon finding of secondary syphilis in an immune-compromised individual, with diffuse bone involvement and concurrent allergies to penicillin, necessitating treatment with doxycycline.

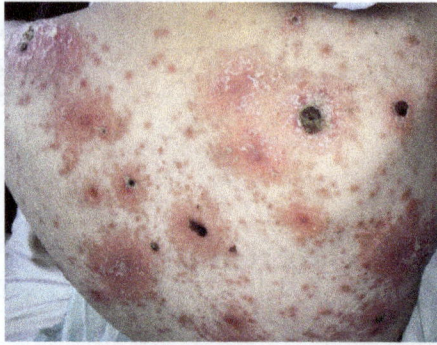

FIGURE 1: Photograph of the patient's back demonstrating an erythematous skin eruption with patches of desquamation, plaques, and papules.

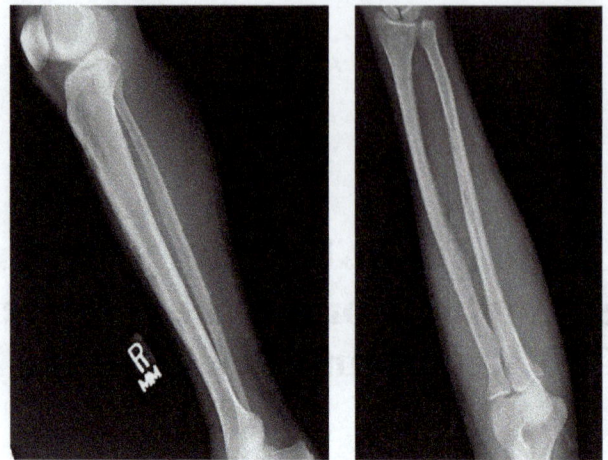

(a)   (b)

FIGURE 2: Plain radiographs of right tibia/fibula (a) and left forearm (b) showing multifocal region of cortical irregularities scattered throughout the diaphysis.

2. Case

A 36-year-old Caucasian, homosexual male with known human immunodeficiency virus (HIV) infection for the past 15 years presented with a disseminated skin eruption over 6 weeks. The patient had been without antiretroviral medications for the past 8 years, defaulted on follow-up, and was uncertain of his last CD4 count or viral load.

The eruption was composed of annular, scalene papules and plaques, some of which were ulcerated (Figure 1). Lesions were distributed on the trunk, extremities, and face. A few lesions demonstrated a thick, ostraceous crust consistent with the skin eruption described in "malignant" syphilis [5].

Constitutional symptoms included night sweats, decreased appetite, and fatigue. The patient also complained of joint pains at both hands and feet. He denied recent travel, walks in the woods, and recent environmental changes. He could not recall any sick contacts.

Of note, he was allergic to penicillin. The allergy was ascribed since childhood and he could not recall the specific reaction but did emphasize that he was strongly advised against taking any penicillin-containing antibiotics. He denied recent sexual interaction but stated that he contracted HIV via anal intercourse.

The patient looked unwell on general examination. He had pink, but dry mucous membranes and was mildly tachycardic with otherwise unremarkable vital signs. White, adherent plaques were noted in the mouth. The diffuse skin eruption was noted as above. Joint swelling and tenderness were also noted at the wrist and ankles. Cardiovascular, respiratory, abdominal, and neurological examinations were noncontributory.

Initial hematologic workup was significant for mild pancytopenia, leukocyte count $3.4 \times 10^3/\text{mm}^3$, hemoglobin 10.2 g/dL, and platelet count $123 \times 10^3/\text{mm}^3$. The CD4 count was 57 cells/μL and HIV RNA was 365,000 copies/mL. Antinuclear antibody and rheumatoid factor assays were both negative.

Evaluation for additional sexually transmitted infections revealed a negative acute hepatitis panel but a positive rapid plasma reagin (RPR) with a titer of 1 : 64. Confirmatory testing with *Treponema pallidum* antibody (TP-PA) testing

was positive. A call to the department of health confirmed no previously reported syphilis infection. Subsequent lumbar puncture was not consistent with infection, specifically a negative VDRL. Blood cultures and wound swabs were negative, and the sedimentation rate was 132 mm/hr.

Punch biopsies were performed on the skin lesions at the left forearm and the left thigh. The histopathologic features were those of psoriasiform lichenoid dermatitis, typical for secondary syphilis. Plasma cells were not readily identified in the infiltrate. Because of the concern for syphilis, a modified Steiner stain was performed which demonstrated several spirochetes within the epidermis.

Plain radiography of the hands and feet revealed polyostotic cortical irregularities of the right foot and both hands, without joint involvement. Roentgenogram of the legs and forearms demonstrated cortical irregularities of the ulnar and radial diaphyses and of the tibial and fibular diaphyses, bilaterally (Figure 2). Roentgenogram of the skull was negative for bony lesions. Follow-up bone scintigraphy was impressive for bilateral, extensive polyostotic uptake within the hands, feet, forearms, and tibiae/fibulae (Figures 3(a)–3(e)).

Based on the positive serology and bone imaging findings, the patient was diagnosed with secondary syphilis osteitis and also now with acquired immunodeficiency syndrome (AIDS).

Given his penicillin allergy, the decision was made to treat the patient with an oral regimen: doxycycline 100 mg twice per day for a total of 6 weeks. He commenced receiving Atovaquone for *Pneumocystis jiroveci* prophylaxis. Prior to discharge (hospital course, day 8), a repeat RPR was performed, with a declining titer of 1 : 32.

The patient was subsequently referred to a HIV clinic where he commenced antiretroviral therapy with Darunavir/Cobicistat, Dolutegravir, and Tenofovir/Emtricitabine. He had one additional follow-up with the HIV clinic and was noted to be compliant with the medications and tolerating

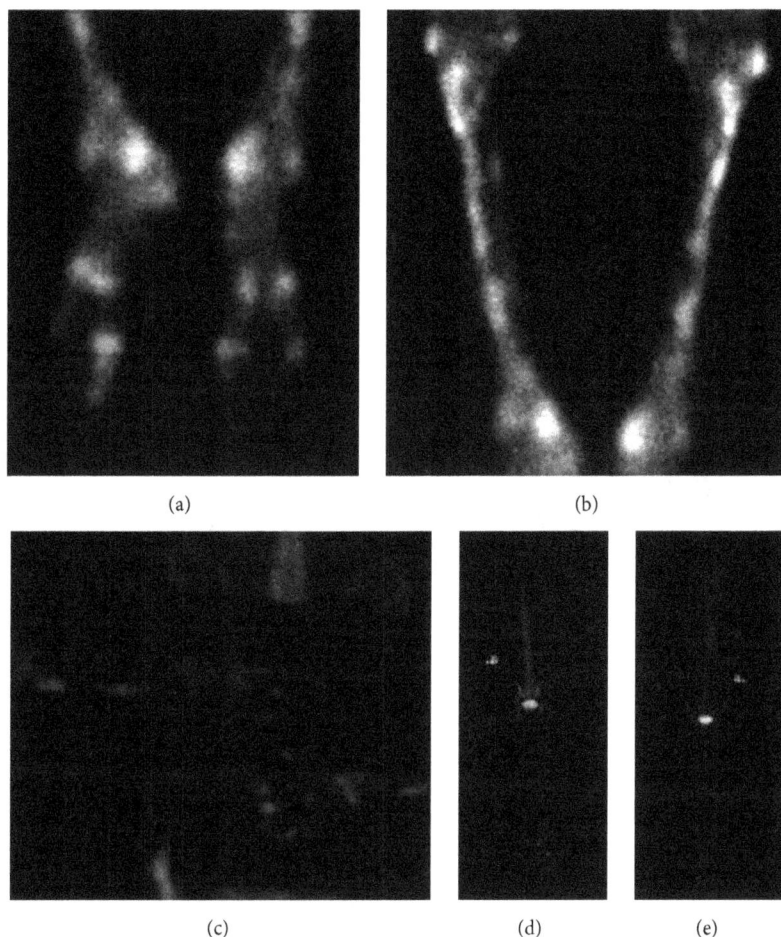

FIGURE 3: Nuclear medicine bone scan of the whole body showing extensive bilateral polyostotic patchy uptake within the distal appendicular skeleton, including the forearms, hands, tibias/fibulas, and feet. ((a) and (b)) Feet and tibiae, respectively. (c) Bilateral forearms and hands. ((d) and (e)) Whole body scans.

them well. He was followed up by his primary care provider at 2 and 6 weeks. During and upon completion of the course of doxycycline, the patient noted considerable improvement in bone pains and joint swelling, which was corroborated on physical examination. At this time, the skin eruption was completely resolved (Figure 4). A follow-up blood count revealed an improvement in the cytopenias. The patient was referred for repeat imaging and RPR titers but defaulted on additional follow-up. Multiple attempts at communication were unsuccessful, and the patient is yet to return to either the HIV clinic or his primary care provider.

3. Discussion

Syphilis osteitis remains an uncommon manifestation of secondary syphilis, with the largest quoted case series being performed by Reynolds, who identified 15 patients with destructive bone lesions in 10,000 cases of early syphilis over a 21-year period (1919 to 1940) [6]. Another study performed by Thompson and Preston investigated skull involvement among 80 patients with secondary syphilis via conventional skull radiography. Seven patients had osteolytic lesions, with

only 4 complaining of headaches [7]. Mindel et al. also performed a retrospective series spanning 20 years, with only 2 cases of syphilitic bone disease being diagnosed among 854 patients with secondary syphilis [8].

Secondary syphilis is associated with a disseminated stage and has varied clinical presentations, including mucocutaneous lesions, rash, and lymphadenopathy [9]. The skin rash in our patient was extensive and somewhat necrotic and has been described as "malignant" syphilis [5]. The presence of these clinical findings with concomitant bone pain or swelling prompted our investigation for syphilis osteitis. In syphilitic osteitis, examination may reveal tenderness over the involved bones, which is sharply localized and may be accompanied with local edema [10]. Additionally, pain has idiosyncratically been described to be exacerbated during the night and on exposure to heat [10, 11].

When spirochetemia occurs in syphilis, organisms can infect and involve the deeper vascular areas of the periosteum, with eventual extension into the Haversian canals and medullary spaces, resulting in periostitis, osteitis, or osteomyelitis [9]. Disease progression can develop into osteolytic or osteoblastic changes in the bones, often with

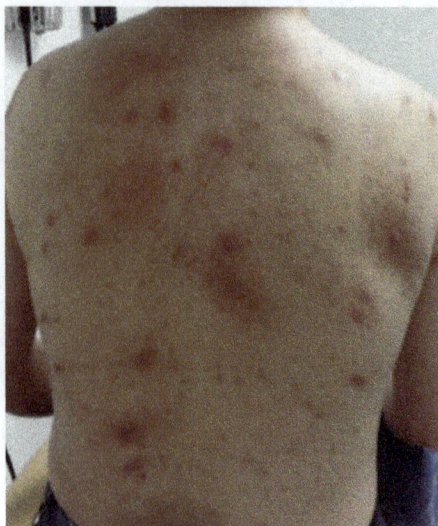

FIGURE 4: Photograph of the patient's back upon completion of treatment with doxycycline. Note dramatic improvement in lesions with few persistent areas of discoloration.

TABLE 1: Antibiotic treatment of 36 cases of secondary syphilis with bone involvement [4].

Antibiotic	Number (%) of patients
Penicillin	33
Benzathine penicillin G	19
Intravenous penicillin G	12
Procaine penicillin G	8
Other or unspecified penicillin regimens	4
Tetracycline	1
Doxycycline + azithromycin	1
Cephaloridine	1

predilection to the superficial bones [12, 13]. Orthodox radiography can occasionally demonstrate round areas with demineralization or sclerosis of the outer table and diploe, with less involvement of the inner table [7, 14]. Periosteal reactions are usually laminated or solid [15]. Generally, however, bone scintigraphy tends to be more sensitive than radiography in early detection of secondary syphilitic skeletal lesions and can be useful in ascertaining the extent of disease, guiding biopsy, and assessing response to therapy [16]. In a review performed by Park et al. of 37 patients with secondary syphilis and bone involvement, almost equal number of patients had disease affecting the limbs and skull, with multifocal lesions in 73% of cases. They also found that of the 13 bone lesions not detected by plain radiography 12 were detected by CT scan, MRI, and/or bone scintigraphy [4].

In addition to syphilis, multiple other etiologies should be considered in the HIV patient presenting with bone pain. Conditions more prone to the immunocompromised population include tuberculosis, pyogenic osteomyelitis, deep mycoses, and lymphoma, whereas non-HIV related conditions such as sarcoidosis or multiple myeloma are other possible differential diagnoses [17].

Identifying organisms on bone biopsy is inconsistent, with Halm reporting spirochete visualization by dark field microscopy in 50% of biopsied cases of bone involvement with early-stage syphilis [18]. Varied pathologic findings have been identified, including dense neutrophil infiltration without granuloma formation (Boone et al. [17]), perivascular infiltration with plasma cells and lymphocytes with some necrosis (Gurland et al. [19]), cortical and trabecular bone with attenuated inflammatory infiltrate composed largely of lymphocytes and plasma cells (Huang et al. [20]), bone necrosis with perivascular infiltration of plasma cells and lymphocytes and rare histiocytes (Kandelaki et al. [21]), and

acute and chronic osteomyelitis with numerous treponemes seen on silver stain (Kastner et al. [22]).

Documentation of syphilis osteitis has remained confined mainly to case reports and review articles. To date, there have been no formal clinical trials to ascertain choice of antibiotic or duration of therapy to guide treatment of syphilitic bone disease. By convention, the usual treatment of secondary syphilis is with intramuscular benzathine penicillin G [23]. Though some authors cite satisfactory results with this approach [9, 24, 25], other authors favor more prolonged duration of therapy, such as penicillin G intravenously for either 4 weeks or 6 weeks [20, 26]. Another regimen undertaken by Fabricius et al. was Ceftriaxone 2 grams intravenously daily for 5 weeks in a patient with vertebral syphilis osteitis, achieving resolution of pain after the first week of treatment, and stable lesions on follow-up MRI [13].

In the review by Park et al., they noted that of 36 patients with secondary syphilitic disease more than 90% received treatment with penicillin (see Table 1). The median duration of therapy was 3 weeks. Antibiotic regimens most often prescribed were intramuscular benzathine penicillin G 2.4 mU weekly for 2 to 4 weeks, intravenous aqueous penicillin G 12–24 mU daily for 2 to 6 weeks, and intramuscular procaine penicillin G 0.6–1.2 mU daily for 10 days. In terms of outcome, 33 (92%) of patients had uneventful improvement solely with antibiotic therapy [4].

The conundrum arises for those patients who are intolerant of penicillin or are allergic. Alternative therapies include doxycycline and azithromycin. Boix et al. are the only authors thus far who have used a regimen devoid of penicillin to treat syphilis osteitis [27]. In that particular case, the patient had a history of Stevens-Johnson syndrome induced by oral amoxicillin. As such, a regimen consisting of oral doxycycline 100 mg twice daily for 16 weeks with the addition of oral azithromycin 1 gram daily for the first 10 weeks was employed. Follow-up bone scan showed resolution of all foci of increased uptake and repeat serology 6 months later showed more than fourfold decline in RPR titers. Because of the penicillin allergy and a history of poor follow-up, we elected to treat our patient with oral doxycycline for 6 weeks.

Rapid symptomatic relief is common following therapy; however osseous lesions can persist for up to seven to eleven months [18, 28]. Nonetheless, reports have cited that once appropriate therapy is completed, radiographic resolution of the boney lesions can be expected [6, 19]. Park et al. described a review of 10 patients who had follow-up bone scintigraphy performed between 1 and 11 months after treatment completion. Eight patients had complete or partial resolution of bone lesions, while 2 patients had unaltered imaging [4]. Our patient did not return for follow-up serology and imaging.

It is recommended that for HIV patients coinfected with syphilis nontreponemal titers (RPR) be repeated at 3, 6, 9, 12, and 24 months after completion of treatment [29]. A fourfold decrease by 6 to 12 months is considered an appropriate response [30]. Retreatment should be considered in the following scenarios: (a) objective clinical features of persistent or recurrent syphilis or (b) persistent or increasing nontreponemal titers [29]. Additionally, all probable or confirmed cases of early syphilis and all reactive nontreponemal laboratory test results should be reported to the local health department within one working day by public and private providers and laboratories [30].

4. Closing Remarks

In the preantibiotic era, the protean manifestations of syphilis were well described, including uncommon clinical features such as bone involvement in early disease [31]. However, following the advent of penicillin therapy, these exceptional presentations have become a rarity. With the ever growing HIV burden, there seems to be reemergence of these esoteric manifestations. In fact, over the past years, more than two-thirds of the cases of syphilitic bone disease were described among HIV patients [29].

Our patient presented with both syphilitic osteitis and severe cutaneous manifestations of "malignant" syphilis and was treated with doxycycline because of a penicillin allergy. This case highlights that, for those patients with a significant penicillin allergy or intolerance, alternate regimens consisting of doxycycline with/without azithromycin for an extended course can be considered.

Competing Interests

The authors declare that there are no competing interests in publishing this paper.

References

[1] Centers for Disease Control and Prevention, *Sexually Transmitted Diseases Facts—Syphilis*, 2016.

[2] C. B. Hicks and P. F. Sparling, "Pathogenesis, clinical manifestations, and treatment of early syphilis," in *UpToDate*, T. W. Post, Ed., UpToDate, Waltham, Mass, USA, 2013.

[3] World Health Organization, *Sexually Transmitted Infections*, World Health Organization, Geneva, Switzerland, 2015.

[4] K.-H. Park, M. S. Lee, I. K. Hong et al., "Bone involvement in secondary syphilis: a case report and systematic review of the literature," *Sexually Transmitted Diseases*, vol. 41, no. 9, pp. 532–537, 2014.

[5] M. J. Romero-Jiménez, I. Suárez Lozano, J. M. Fajardo Picó, and B. Barón Franco, "Malignant syphilis in patient with human immunodeficiency virus (HIV): case report and literature review," *Anales de Medicina Interna*, vol. 20, no. 7, pp. 373–376, 2003.

[6] F. W. Reynolds, "Destructive osseous lesions in early syphilis," *Archives of Internal Medicine*, vol. 69, no. 2, pp. 263–276, 1942.

[7] R. G. Thompson and R. H. Preston, "Lesions of the skull in secondary syphilis," *American Journal of Syphilis, Gonorrhea, and Venereal Diseases*, vol. 36, no. 4, pp. 332–341, 1952.

[8] A. Mindel, S. J. Tovey, D. J. Timmins, and P. Williams, "Primary and secondary syphilis, 20 years' experience. 2. Clinical features," *Genitourinary Medicine*, vol. 65, no. 1, pp. 1–3, 1989.

[9] I. Ehrlich and M. E. Kricun, "Radiographic findings in early acquired syphilis: case report and critical review," *American Journal of Roentgenology*, vol. 127, no. 5, pp. 789–792, 1976.

[10] R. B. Roy and S. M. Laird, "Acute periostitis in early acquired syphilis," *British Journal of Venereal Diseases*, vol. 49, no. 6, article 555, 1973.

[11] S. Middleton, C. Rowntree, and S. Rudge, "Bone pain as the presenting manifestation of secondary syphilis," *Annals of the Rheumatic Diseases*, vol. 49, no. 8, pp. 641–642, 1990.

[12] G. L. Mandell, R. Doulin, and J. E. Bennett, *Principles and Practice of Infectious Diseases*, Churchill Livingstone, Philadelphia, Pa, USA, 2009.

[13] T. Fabricius, C. Winther, C. Ewertsen, M. Kemp, and S. D. Nielsen, "Osteitis in the dens of axis caused by Treponema pallidum," *BMC Infectious Diseases*, vol. 13, no. 1, article 347, 2013.

[14] C. L. Rumbaugh and R. T. Bergeron, "Infections involving the skull," in *Radiology of the Skull and Brain*, T. H. Newton and D. G. Potts, Eds., vol. 1, Book 2, pp. 716–742, CV Mosby, St. Louis, Canada, 1971.

[15] M. Samarkos, C. Giannopoulou, E. Karantoni, V. Papastamopoulos, I. Baraboutis, and A. Skoutelis, "Syphilitic periostitis of the skull and ribs in a HIV positive patient," *Sexually Transmitted Infections*, vol. 87, no. 1, pp. 44–45, 2011.

[16] K. Thakore, A. Viroslav, and J. Vansant, "Role of bone scintigraphy in the detection of periostitis in secondary syphilis," *Clinical Nuclear Medicine*, vol. 19, no. 6, pp. 536–541, 1994.

[17] P. M. Boone, V. Levy, and K. I. Relucio, "Early syphilis in an HIV-infected man presenting with bone lesions and orbital swelling," *Infections in Medicine*, vol. 26, no. 6, pp. 178–183, 2009.

[18] D. E. Halm, "Bone lesions in early syphilis: case report," *The Nebraska Medical Journal*, vol. 64, no. 10, pp. 310–312, 1979.

[19] I. A. Gurland, L. Korn, L. Edelman, and F. Wallach, "An unusual manifestation of acquired syphilis," *Clinical Infectious Diseases*, vol. 32, no. 4, pp. 667–669, 2001.

[20] I. Huang, J. L. Leach, C. J. Fichtenbaum, and R. K. Narayan, "Osteomyelitis of the skull in early-acquired syphilis: evaluation by MR imaging and CT," *American Journal of Neuroradiology*, vol. 28, no. 2, pp. 307–308, 2007.

[21] G. Kandelaki, R. Kapila, and H. Fernandes, "Destructive osteomyelitis associated with early secondary syphilis in an HIV-positive patient diagnosed by *Treponema pallidum* DNA polymerase chain reaction," *AIDS Patient Care and STDs*, vol. 21, no. 4, pp. 229–233, 2007.

[22] R. J. Kastner, J. L. Malone, and C. F. Decker, "Syphilitic osteitis in a patient with secondary syphilis and concurrent human immunodeficiency virus infection," *Clinical Infectious Diseases*, vol. 18, no. 2, pp. 250–252, 1994.

[23] K. A. Workowski and S. Berman, "Centers for Disease Control and Prevention (CDC). Sexually transmitted diseases treatment guidelines 2010," *MMWR Recommendations and Reports*, vol. 59, pp. 1–116, 2010.

[24] K. Coyne, R. Browne, C. Anagnostopoulos, and N. Nwokolo, "Syphilitic periostitis in a newly diagnosed HIV-positive man," *International Journal of STD and AIDS*, vol. 17, no. 6, pp. 421–423, 2006.

[25] S. H. Kang, S. W. Park, K. Y. Kwon, and W. J. Hong, "A solitary skull lesion of syphilitic osteomyelitis," *Journal of Korean Neurosurgical Society*, vol. 48, no. 1, pp. 85–87, 2010.

[26] Z.-Y. Liu, Y. Zhang, K.-F. Qiu, and S.-X. Du, "Osteomyelitis as the only manifestation of late latent syphilis: case report and literature review," *International Journal of STD & AIDS*, vol. 22, no. 6, pp. 353–355, 2011.

[27] V. Boix, E. Merino, S. Reus, D. Torrus, and J. Portilla, "Polyostotic osteitis in secondary syphilis in an HIV-infected patient," *Sexually Transmitted Diseases*, vol. 40, no. 8, pp. 645–646, 2013.

[28] W. E. Dismukes, D. G. Delgado, S. V. Mallernee, and T. C. Myers, "Destructive bone disease in early syphilis," *The Journal of the American Medical Association*, vol. 236, no. 23, pp. 2646–2648, 1976.

[29] S. T. Brown, A. Zaidi, S. A. Larsen, and G. H. Reynolds, "Serological response to syphilis treatment. A new analysis of old data," *The Journal of the American Medical Association*, vol. 253, no. 9, pp. 1296–1299, 1985.

[30] K. A. Workowski and S. M. Berman, "Sexually transmitted diseases treatment guidelines, 2006," *Morbidity and Mortality Weekly Report*, vol. 55, no. 11, pp. 1–94, 2006.

[31] U. J. Wile and F. E. Senear, "A study of the involvement of the bones and joints in early syphilis," *The American Journal of the Medical Sciences*, vol. 152, no. 5, pp. 689–746, 1916.

26

Detection of the Dimorphic Phases of *Mucor circinelloides* in Blood Cultures from an Immunosuppressed Female

Miguel A. Arroyo,[1,2] Bryan H. Schmitt,[1] Thomas E. Davis,[1] and Ryan F. Relich[1]

[1]*Department of Pathology and Laboratory Medicine, Indiana University School of Medicine, Indianapolis, IN 46202, USA*
[2]*U.S. Army Medical Department Center and School, Fort Sam Houston, TX 78234, USA*

Correspondence should be addressed to Ryan F. Relich; rrelich@iupui.edu

Academic Editor: Paul Horrocks

Mucormycosis fungemia is rarely documented since blood cultures are nearly always negative. We describe a case of *Mucor circinelloides* fungemia in a patient with a history of a sinus infection, sarcoidosis, and IgG deficiency. The identity of the isolate was supported by its microscopic morphology and its ability to convert into yeast forms under anaerobic conditions. The early detection, initiation of liposomal amphotericin B treatment, and reversal of underlying predisposing risk factors resulted in a good outcome.

1. Introduction

Mucormycoses are infectious diseases caused by filamentous fungi classified among the order Mucorales [1]. Infection occurs when a susceptible (e.g., immunocompromised) human is exposed to spores through inhalation, ingestion, or traumatic implantation. The resulting disease processes are characterized by an often rapid clinical progression and a high mortality rate [1, 2]. Mucorales rarely cause infection in immunocompetent persons but can cause fatal infection in immunocompromised patients. Risk factors include hematologic malignancies, bone marrow or solid organ transplantation, neutropenia, diabetes mellitus, corticosteroids, iron chelation therapy, broad spectrum antibiotics, antifungal prophylaxis, prolonged voriconazole use, cutaneous breakdown (from trauma, surgical wounds, needle-sticks, or burns), hyperalimentation, and severe malnutrition [1, 2]. Features of these organisms that contribute to their virulence include their rapid growth rate and their ability to invade blood vessels [1–3]. The latter characteristic permits their spread throughout the body, enabling access to numerous tissues and organs that may ultimately become infected [2]. However, documented mucormycosis fungemia is very rare, and blood cultures are usually negative. Demonstration of invasive disease by these organisms generally requires the identification of fungal elements directly in clinical specimens via histopathological examination or growth of these organisms from more than one specimen obtained from a normally sterile site [3].

Several *Mucor* spp., but not all, are known to be dimorphic. This distinct group of zygomycetes exhibits hyphal growth in aerobic conditions and multibudded yeast growth under anaerobic or high-CO_2 conditions [4]. *M. circinelloides* is one of these species, along with *M. racemosus*, *M. rouxii*, *M. genevensis*, *M. bacilliformis*, *M. subtilissimus*, and *M. amphibiorum*. *M. circinelloides* infections are well documented in the literature and have been associated with cutaneous, rhinocerebral, and pulmonary infections [5–9]. To our knowledge, only two cases of fungemia caused by this organism have been reported [10, 11]. In this report we describe a case of *M. circinelloides* fungemia in a female with a prior history of chronic sinus infection, sarcoidosis, and IgG deficiency.

2. Case Report

A 38-year-old female presented to the Emergency Department of a hospital in rural Indiana with shortness of breath and cough, sinus congestion, fevers as high as 39.4°C, nasal

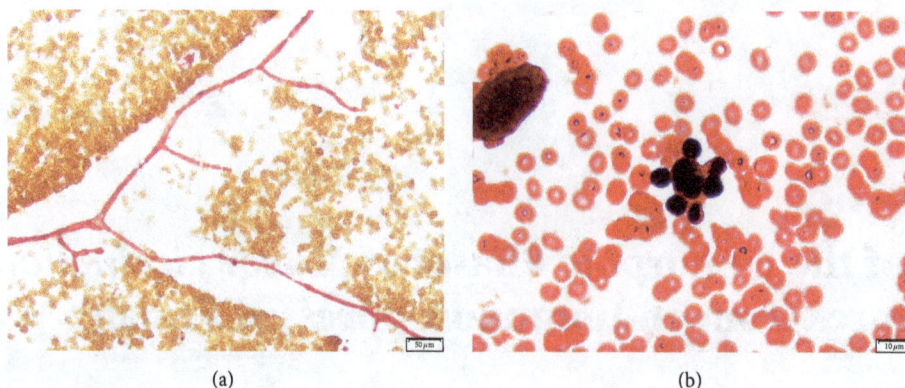

FIGURE 1: Gram stain of *M. circinelloides* dimorphic phases from a positive blood culture. (a) Pauciseptate wide hyphae with right-angle branching (100x magnification). (b) Circumferentially budding yeast resembling the yeast phase of *Paracoccidioides brasiliensis* (500x magnification).

TABLE 1: Clinical laboratory test results from blood specimens obtained at the time of patient presentation to the ED.

Test	Patient result	Reference range
WBC	13.7k/cumm	3.6–5.17k/cumm
Hgb	11.5 GM/dL	12.0–16.0 GM/dL
MCV	79 fL	81–99 fL
MCH	24.9 pg	27–34 pg
MCHC	31.5 GM/dL	32.0–36.0 GM/dL
RDW	15.8%	11.5–14.5%
Absolute neutrophil	8.2k/cumm	1.7–7.6k/cumm
Absolute lymphocyte	4.0k/cumm	1.0–3.2k/cumm
Absolute eosinophil	0.4k/cumm	0.0–0.3k/cumm
Potassium SerPl QN	2.8 mmol/L	3.5–5.5 mmol/L
Carbon dioxide SerPl QN	21 mmol/L	22–29 mmol/L
Glucose SerPl QN	138 mg/dL	70–99 mg/dL
Magnesium SerPl QN	1.3 mg/dL	1.6–2.9 mg/dL
AST SerPl QN	8 units/L	13–39 units/L
Total protein SerPl QN	6.0 GM/dL	6.4–8.0 GM/dL

drainage, sore throat, and yellow-green sputum production. The patient's medical history included sarcoidosis, IgG deficiency, and a sinus infection for which she completed treatment with cefdinir 1 week before admission. The patient stated improvement while on antibiotics but symptoms worsened after therapy completion. Upon physical examination, the patient had a temperature of 37.5°C and exhibited moderate respiratory distress with no wheezing, rales, or rhonchi. She was alert, awake, and oriented with no ear, nose, throat, cardiovascular, abdominal, back, extremities, skin, neurological, or psychiatric abnormalities. An X-ray of her chest was unremarkable. Peripheral blood specimens obtained at the time of initial presentation demonstrated leukocytosis, hyperglycemia and low potassium, CO_2, total protein, and magnesium (Table 1). The aerobic blood culture bottles (BD BACTEC™ Plus Aerobic/F) from two sets of blood cultures collected at the time of admission turned positive within 24 hours of incubation in a continuous-monitory blood culture system (BACTEC™ 9240, BD Diagnostics, Sparks, MD). Gram stains of the broth revealed pleomorphic yeast forms and wide, pauciseptate, hyphae with right-angle branching (Figure 1(a)). Yeast forms with single, bipolar, and circumferential buds were observed. Several of the yeast cells observed resembled the yeast phase of *Paracoccidioides brasiliensis* (Figure 1(b)). The Gram stain findings were reported as "fungal elements present" and were immediately phoned to the clinical care team.

The following day, mold growth was observed on the aerobic sheep blood agar and chocolate agar plates incubated at 35°C in 5% CO_2 and on potato dextrose and Sabouraud agars incubated at 30°C. Fast-growing, floccose colonies were initially pale gray to yellow, turning brown over time when incubated at 35°C. Microscopic examination of the mold colony by lactophenol cotton blue staining revealed broad, ribbon-like pauciseptate wide hyphae with right-angle branching. Sympodially branched and circinate sporangiophores were observed (Figures 2(a) and 2(b)). Globose sporangia measured within 25–80 μm and contained oval shaped sporangiospores (Figure 2(c)). Columellae were spherical, measuring up to 50 μm in diameter; collarettes were present (Figure 2(d)). Rhizoids and stolons were absent. The identity of the isolate as *M. circinelloides* was supported by its microscopic morphology, its ability to convert into yeast forms under anaerobic conditions, and its inability to grow at 42°C (Figure 3). Conclusive identification based on molecular and phenotypic methods was above the scope of this study. Following reporting of these findings, the patient was started on liposomal amphotericin B 500 mg IVPB every 24 hours; subsequent blood and sinus cultures were negative. In addition, sinus biopsy results and computerized tomography (CT scan) of the chest and sinuses did not show any clear evidence of fungal involvement. As a consequence, antifungal treatment was discontinued after 6 days and the patient was discharged home without further complications. The patient had no signs of *Mucor* infection 7 months after discharge.

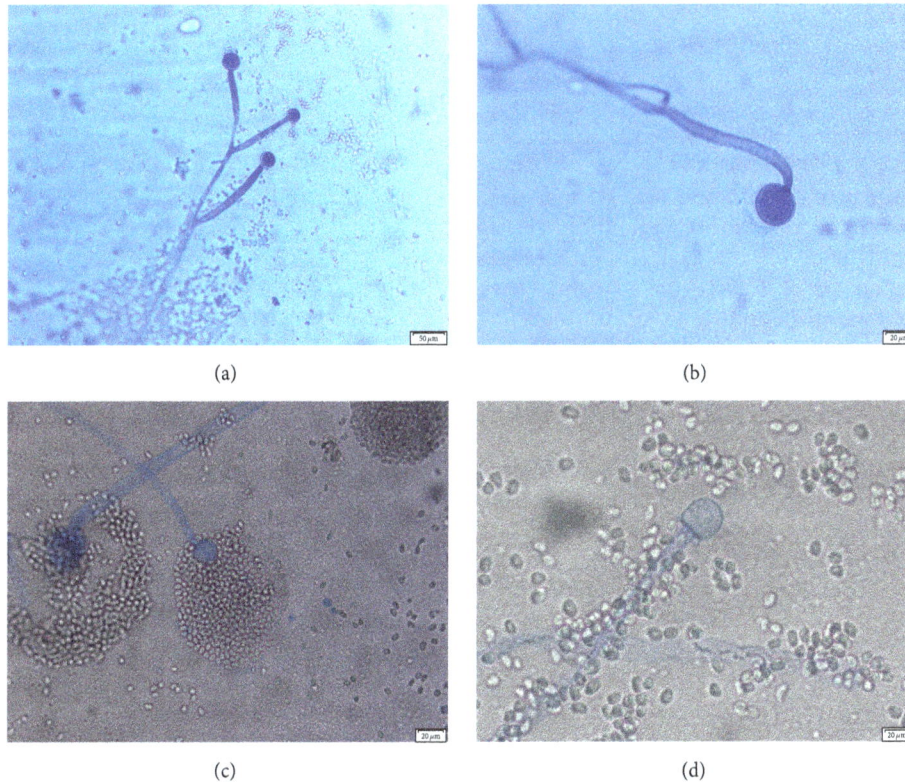

FIGURE 2: Microscopic examination of *Mucor circinelloides* on PDA by "tape prep" using lactophenol cotton blue stain. (a) Sympodially branched sporangiophores (100x magnification); (b) circinate sporangiophores (200x magnification); (c) deliquescent sporangia (100x magnification); (d) columella with collarette (200x magnification).

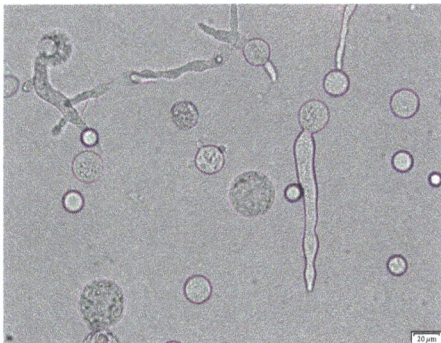

FIGURE 3: *Mucor circinelloides* yeast forms after cultivation of the isolate on Sabouraud dextrose agar incubated for 48 hrs under anaerobic conditions showing hyphae with single and multipolar buds (unstained, 200x)

3. Discussion

The saprophytic nature of the Mucorales makes the diagnosis of mucormycosis a challenging task when these organisms are isolated from nonsterile sites [1]. Because they are ubiquitous, the presence of these organisms can sometimes be dismissed, as, in many cases, they likely represent contamination of the clinical specimen or culture media. Therefore, it is essential that the physician and laboratory personnel work together to determine the clinical significance of the laboratory results. In most instances, the diagnosis of invasive mucormycosis is usually made when these organisms are identified directly from clinical specimens or isolated in culture from more than one specimen obtained from a normally sterile site. In the case presented, the diagnosis of mucormycosis was made by the isolation of *Mucor circinelloides* from two blood culture sets that were collected from two different sites. This finding was considered clinically significant since it represented multiple specimens obtained from a normally sterile site.

In this case, the source of infection is unknown, but we hypothesized that is likely related to her sinusitis. The successful treatment and optimal outcome were most likely attributed to the early detection and isolation of the organism from blood cultures, which prompted early implementation of antifungal therapy. In addition, the correction of her hypokalemia, hypomagnesemia, and hyperglycemia contributed to her recovery, as reversal of underlying physiological dyshomeostatic conditions has been reported to correlate with good patient outcomes [12]. Surgical debridement was not necessary since follow-up tests did not reveal foci of fungal infection. Based on the patient outcome, we can also hypothesize that this case might have represented a transient fungemia or that the causative organism is of low virulence [13].

To our knowledge, only two cases of fungemia associated with *M. circinelloides* have been previously described. The first reported cases occurred in a 48-year-old male with a history of short-gut syndrome secondary to multiple abdominal surgeries [10]. This patient had a central venous catheter (CVC) that was required for chronic total parenteral nutrition. Blood cultures obtained from the CVC on consecutive days grew both *Candida albicans* and *M. circinelloides*. Treatment with liposomal amphotericin B was started, and the CVC was removed. Similar to our case, the authors stated that early diagnosis of mucormycosis coupled with rapid therapeutic intervention led to a successful outcome. The second reported case was that of an 83-year-old diabetic woman who developed an acute left frontoparietal infarct while hospitalized in a neurological intensive care unit [11]. The initial isolation of a mold from a blood culture was considered to be a contaminant, but during the following days, the patient developed an erythematous and edematous lesion on her right hand. A skin biopsy culture grew a mold identical to that in the blood culture; both isolates were later identified as *M. circinelloides* by molecular methods. Despite treatment, the patient's clinical condition worsened and she later died.

4. Conclusion

This case represents the third documented case of fungemia cause by *M. circinelloides*. The most likely underlying factors were probably related to her chronic sinus infection, IgG deficiency, and chronic steroid use. The detection of this mold and reversal of the predisposing underlying conditions were vital in the successful treatment.

Disclosure

The views expressed are those of the authors and should not be construed to represent the positions of the U.S. Army or the Department of Defense.

Competing Interests

The authors declare that there is no conflict of interests regarding the publication of this paper.

References

[1] J. A. Ribes, C. L. Vanover-Sams, and D. J. Baker, "Zygomycetes in human disease," *Clinical Microbiology Reviews*, vol. 13, no. 2, pp. 236–301, 2000.

[2] G. Petrikkos, A. Skiada, O. Lortholary, E. Roilides, T. J. Walsh, and D. P. Kontoyiannis, "Epidemiology and clinical manifestations of mucormycosis," *Clinical Infectious Diseases*, vol. 54, supplement 1, pp. S23–S34, 2012.

[3] I. Weitzman, "Saprophytic molds as agents of cutaneous and subcutaneous infection in the immunocompromised host," *Archives of Dermatology*, vol. 122, no. 10, pp. 1161–1168, 1986.

[4] M. Orlowski, "Mucor dimorphism," *Microbiological Reviews*, vol. 55, no. 2, pp. 234–258, 1991.

[5] S. P. Lazar, J. M. Lukaszewicz, K. A. Persad, and J. F. Reinhardt, "Rhinocerebral *Mucor circinelloides* infection in immunocompromised patient following yogurt ingestion," *Delaware Medical Journal*, vol. 86, no. 8, pp. 245–248, 2014.

[6] Z. U. Khan, S. Ahmad, A. Brazda, and R. Chandy, "*Mucor circinelloides* as a cause of invasive maxillofacial zygomycosis: an emerging dimorphic pathogen with reduced susceptibility to posaconazole," *Journal of Clinical Microbiology*, vol. 47, no. 4, pp. 1244–1248, 2009.

[7] M. Dodémont, M. Hites, B. Bailly et al., "When you can't see the wood for the trees. *Mucor circinelloides*: a rare case of primary cutaneous zygomycosis," *Journal de Mycologie Médicale*, vol. 25, no. 2, pp. 151–154, 2015.

[8] P. C. Iwen, L. Sigler, R. K. Noel, and A. G. Freifeld, "*Mucor circinelloides* was identified by molecular methods as a cause of primary cutaneous zygomycosis," *Journal of Clinical Microbiology*, vol. 45, no. 2, pp. 636–640, 2007.

[9] M. Shindo, K. Sato, J. Jimbo et al., "Breakthrough pulmonary mucormycosis during voriconazole treatment after reduced-intensity cord blood transplantation for a patient with acute myeloid leukemia," *Rinsho Ketsueki*, vol. 48, no. 5, pp. 412–417, 2007.

[10] K. M. Chan-Tack, L. L. Nemoy, and E. N. Perencevich, "Central venous catheter-associated fungemia secondary to mucormycosis," *Scandinavian Journal of Infectious Diseases*, vol. 37, no. 11-12, pp. 925–927, 2005.

[11] M. Dizbay, E. Adisen, S. Kustimur et al., "Fungemia and cutaneous zygomycosis due to *Mucor circinelloides* in an intensive care unit patient: case report and review of literature," *Japanese Journal of Infectious Diseases*, vol. 62, no. 2, pp. 146–148, 2009.

[12] B. Spellberg, J. Edwards Jr., and A. Ibrahim, "Novel perspectives on mucormycosis: pathophysiology, presentation, and management," *Clinical Microbiology Reviews*, vol. 18, no. 3, pp. 556–569, 2005.

[13] S. C. Lee, A. Li, S. Calo et al., "Calcineurin orchestrates dimorphic transitions, antifungal drug responses and host-pathogen interactions of the pathogenic mucoralean fungus *Mucor circinelloides*," *Molecular Microbiology*, vol. 97, no. 5, pp. 844–865, 2015.

27

Voriconazole-Induced Periostitis Mimicking Chronic Graft-versus-Host Disease after Allogeneic Stem Cell Transplantation

Karen Sweiss,[1,2] **Annie Oh,**[3] **Damiano Rondelli,**[2,3] **and Pritesh Patel**[2,3]

[1]*Department of Pharmacy Practice, University of Illinois at Chicago, Chicago, IL 60612, USA*
[2]*Cancer Center, University of Illinois, Chicago, IL 60612, USA*
[3]*Division of Hematology/Oncology, University of Illinois at Chicago, Chicago, IL 60612, USA*

Correspondence should be addressed to Karen Sweiss; ksweis2@uic.edu

Academic Editor: Pere Domingo

Voriconazole is an established first-line agent for treatment of invasive fungal infections in patients undergoing allogeneic stem cell transplantation (ASCT). It is associated with the uncommon complication of periostitis. We report this complication in a 58-year-old female undergoing HSCT. She was treated with corticosteroids with minimal improvement. The symptoms related to periostitis can mimic chronic graft-versus-host disease in patients undergoing HSCT and clinicians should differentiate this from other diagnoses and promptly discontinue therapy.

1. Introduction

Invasive fungal infections lead to significant morbidity and mortality in patients who are undergoing allogeneic stem cell transplantation (ASCT) [1–3]. Treatment is typically prolonged and continues until complete clinical and radiographic resolution. Voriconazole is an established first-line treatment for invasive aspergillosis [2]. Although mostly well tolerated, it is associated with the uncommon yet clinically relevant complication of periostitis [1]. Here we report this underrecognized complication of voriconazole and its unique implications in the setting of ASCT.

2. Case Report

A 58-year-old woman with intermediate risk acute myeloid leukemia in first complete remission underwent ASCT from an HLA-matched sibling. Her initial induction was complicated by hypoxia, pulmonary infiltrates, and fevers despite broad-spectrum antibiotics. She was treated with voriconazole with clinical improvement and was presumed to have invasive fungal infection. Voriconazole was continued throughout her transplant course given persistent chest CT abnormalities.

At day 79 after ASCT, the patient complained of swelling in her left middle finger. Physical examination revealed discrete tender swelling of the middle phalanx on the third finger. This continued to worsen and one month later she was complaining of further swelling involving the fourth finger (Figure 1(a)). In addition, she reported fatigue and proximal muscle myalgia especially in her lower extremities. An X-ray of her hand (Figure 1(b)) reported multifocal periosteal reaction involving multiple bones of the right hand with associated soft tissue swelling. Laboratory testing showed elevated alkaline phosphatase (ALP) of 341 u/L (normal 40–125 u/L). Her liver function tests and kidney function were within normal limits. Erythrocyte sedimentation rate was mildly elevated at 31 mm/hr (normal 0–10 mm/hr). C reactive protein (CRP) and creatine kinase (CK) levels were normal. At that time, she was prescribed 1 milligram per kilogram per day of prednisone for musculoskeletal complaints associated with a presumed diagnosis of chronic graft-versus-host disease (cGVHD). However, she had only minor improvement in her symptoms after one week of treatment. An MRI of the hand was performed and showed exuberant disorganized periostitis involving the second, third, and fourth digits. It was suspected that the patient had

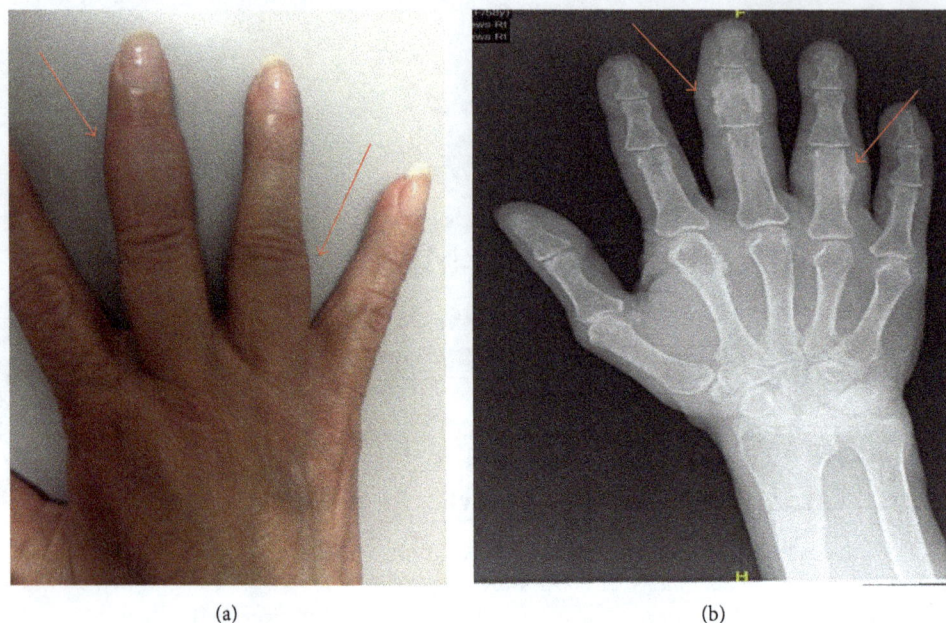

(a)   (b)

FIGURE 1: Examination findings and radiograph illustrating periostitis of the right hand. (a) Examination revealed swelling with tenderness of the third middle phalange as well as the less marked swelling of the fourth proximal phalange. (b) Radiograph showed multifocal periosteal reaction with associated soft tissue swelling.

voriconazole-induced periostitis. Of note, she had received voriconazole for 6 months with trough concentrations within therapeutic range. Voriconazole was discontinued and one week later the patient's symptoms began improving. Her ALP level improved from 341 u/L to 179 u/L and continued to improve over the next couple weeks. At day 175 after transplant, her symptoms had completely resolved.

3. Discussion

Voriconazole is a triazole antifungal that is indicated for the treatment of invasive aspergillosis. Common adverse effects include visual disturbances, hallucinations, QT prolongation, and hepatotoxicity. With prolonged use however, newly described adverse effects, including periostitis, alopecia, and development of skin cancers, have been noted [1]. Painful periostitis is a well-recognized, albeit uncommon, complication of prolonged voriconazole therapy [4–7]. The clinical features of voriconazole-induced periostitis are similar to skeletal fluorosis. As opposed to other azole antifungals, voriconazole is trifluorinated [8]. Therefore it is theorized that periostitis occurs due to high circulating levels of fluoride released during hepatic metabolism. The calculated daily fluoride intake at a standard dose of voriconazole may be as high as 62.6 mg which exceeds the fluoride toxicity threshold as defined by the World Health Organization 10-fold [8–10].

Most cases of voriconazole-induced periostitis have been reported in patients who have undergone solid organ transplantation [4–7]. Few cases in ASCT patients have been published [8, 11, 12]. Barajas et al. [12] have retrospectively analyzed 242 ASCT patients who received prolonged voriconazole treatment. Twenty-nine of 31 patients who experienced pain had elevated fluoride levels. These patients, however,

did not have confirmed radiologic diagnosis of periostitis. Commonly described locations of involvement among both solid organ and ASCT patients are the clavicles, ribs, scapula, acetabulum, and hands [8–10, 12]. Patients typically complain of bone pain that is not alleviated by analgesics. Symptoms can occur within days of starting treatment but typically are seen after 3 to 6 months of therapy. Prompt discontinuation of the drug results in resolution of symptoms within a few weeks [10].

The clinical presentation and radiologic findings of patients who develop voriconazole-induced periostitis are nonspecific and insidious and may be confused with rheumatologic or endocrinologic disorders. In the setting of ASCT, symptoms may mimic cGVHD. Prior cases reported in the ASCT setting were also treated with corticosteroids for cGVHD, resulting in temporary symptom relief and a delay in discontinuing voriconazole [9–11]. In our case, there was a 3-month delay from time of symptom onset to voriconazole discontinuation due to a presumed diagnosis of cGVHD. Laboratory tests that help differentiate cGVHD from periostitis include ALP level, CRP, CK, and rheumatologic testing. Alkaline phosphatase levels are often elevated in periostitis but normalize within 1 to 2 months after discontinuation [4–7].

Given that long-term voriconazole therapy is increasingly common, clinicians managing ASCT patients should be aware of this complication. We recommend periodic measurement of ALP and fluoride levels in patients on prolonged voriconazole therapy. In patients on voriconazole who report nonspecific musculoskeletal complaints following ASCT, drug-induced periostitis should be included in the differential diagnosis along with cGVHD.

Competing Interests

The authors declare no competing interests.

Authors' Contributions

All authors contributed to the clinical care of the patient as well as the writing of the paper. All authors approved the final version of the paper for submission.

References

[1] L. K. Scott and D. Simpson, "Voriconazole: a review of its use in the management of invasive fungal infections," *Drugs*, vol. 67, no. 2, pp. 269–298, 2007.

[2] J. R. Wingard, "Fungal infections after bone marrow transplant," *Biology of Blood and Marrow Transplantation*, vol. 5, no. 2, pp. 55–68, 1999.

[3] A. B. Halpern, G. H. Lyman, T. J. Walsh, D. P. Kontoyiannis, and R. B. Walter, "Primary antifungal prophylaxis during curative-intent therapy for acute myeloid leukemia," *Blood*, vol. 126, no. 26, pp. 2790–2797, 2015.

[4] T. F. Wang, T. Wang, R. Altman et al., "Periostitis secondary to prolonged voriconazole therapy in lung transplant recipients," *American Journal of Transplantation*, vol. 9, no. 12, pp. 2845–2850, 2009.

[5] L. Chen and M. E. Mulligan, "Medication-induced periostitis in lung transplant patients: periostitis deformans revisited," *Skeletal Radiology*, vol. 40, no. 2, pp. 143–148, 2011.

[6] A. Ayub, C. V. Kenney, and F. E. Mckiernan, "Multifocal nodular periostitis associated with prolonged voriconazole therapy in a lung transplant recipient," *Journal of Clinical Rheumatology*, vol. 17, no. 2, pp. 73–75, 2011.

[7] M. D. Bucknor, A. J. Gross, and T. M. Link, "Voriconazole-induced periostitis in two post-transplant patients," *Journal of Radiology Case Reports*, vol. 7, no. 8, pp. 10–17, 2013.

[8] R. A. Wermers, K. Cooper, R. R. Razonable et al., "Fluoride excess and periostitis in transplant patients receiving long-term voriconazole therapy," *Clinical Infectious Diseases*, vol. 52, no. 5, pp. 604–611, 2011.

[9] J. L. Skiles, E. A. Imel, J. C. Christenson, J. E. Bell, and M. L. Hulbert, "Fluorosis because of prolonged voriconazole therapy in a teenager with acute myelogenous leukemia," *Journal of Clinical Oncology*, vol. 29, no. 32, pp. e779–e782, 2011.

[10] G. R. Thompson III, D. Bays, S. H. Cohen, and D. Pappagianis, "Fluoride excess in coccidioidomycosis patients receiving long-term antifungal therapy: an assessment of currently available triazoles," *Antimicrobial Agents and Chemotherapy*, vol. 56, no. 1, pp. 563–564, 2012.

[11] B. Gerber, R. Guggenberger, D. Fasler et al., "Reversible skeletal disease and high fluoride serum levels in hematologic patients receiving voriconazole," *Blood*, vol. 120, no. 12, pp. 2390–2394, 2012.

[12] M. R. Barajas, K. B. McCullough, J. A. Merten et al., "Correlation of pain and fluoride concentration in allogeneic hematopoietic stem cell transplant recipients on voriconazole," *Biology of Blood and Marrow Transplantation*, vol. 22, no. 3, pp. 579–583, 2016.

28

Immune Reconstitution Inflammatory Syndrome: Opening Pandora's Box

Mariana Meireles,[1] Conceição Souto Moura,[2] and Margarida França[3]

[1]*Internal Medicine Department, Porto Hospital Centre, Porto, Portugal*
[2]*Pathological Anatomy Department, São João Hospital Centre, Porto, Portugal*
[3]*Clinical Immunology Unit, Porto Hospital Centre, Porto, Portugal*

Correspondence should be addressed to Mariana Meireles; mra.meireles@gmail.com

Academic Editor: Sinésio Talhari

One of the purposes of antiretroviral therapy (ART) is to restore the immune system. However, it can sometimes lead to an aberrant inflammatory response and paradoxical clinical worsening known as the immune reconstitution inflammatory syndrome (IRIS). We describe a 23-year-old male, HIV1 infected with a rapid progression phenotype, who started ART with TCD4+ of 53 cells/mm^3 (3,3%) and HIV RNA $= 890000$ copies/mL (6 log). Four weeks later he was admitted to the intensive care unit with severe sepsis. The diagnostic pathway identified progressive multifocal leukoencephalopathy, digestive Kaposi sarcoma, and *P. aeruginosa* bacteraemia. Five weeks after starting ART, TCD4+ cell count was 259 cells/mm^3 (15%) and HIV RNA $= 3500$ copies/mL (4 log). He developed respiratory failure and progressed to septic shock and death. Those complications might justify the outcome but its autopsy opened *Pandora*'s box: cerebral and cardiac toxoplasmosis was identified, as well as hemophagocytic syndrome, systemic candidiasis, and *Mycobacterium avium complex* infection. IRIS remains a concern and eventually a barrier to ART. Male gender, young age, low TCD4 cell count, and high viral load are risk factors. The high prevalence of subclinical opportunistic diseases highlights the need for new strategies to reduce IRIS incidence.

1. Background

Antiretroviral therapy (ART) led to a dramatic change in the clinical picture and prognosis of the Human Immunodeficiency Virus (HIV) infection. However, some patients develop a paradoxical worsening of their clinical status after starting therapy. HIV-associated immune reconstitution inflammatory syndrome (IRIS) has emerged as an important early complication of ART introduction, particularly in patients with severe immunosuppression. The diagnosis is based on an unexpected clinical worsening, days to months after the ART introduction, an abrupt rise of TCD4+ cell count, and a decrease >1 log in HIV RNA load in the presence of pathological antigens [1]. Mortality rate is around 5.4% [2] reaching up to 45% if concomitant opportunistic diseases occur. Early diagnosis and therapy are crucial to a favorable outcome but diagnosis of the leading opportunistic antigen can be challenging.

2. Case Presentation

A 23-year-old male was diagnosed with HIV infection in July 2011, having a negative HIV serology 6 months earlier. By September 2011, his TCD4+ cell count was 563 cells/mm^3 (15%) with a HIV RNA of 88500 copies/mL. HBV, HCV, syphilis, *Mycobacterium tuberculosis*, CMV, and *Toxoplasma* screenings were negative and chest X-ray, abdominal ultrasound, and colonoscopy were unremarkable. During the follow-up, although presenting with a stable TCD4+ cell count, he kept high viral load and a serodiscordant sexual partner, those being reasons for initiating ART, which he refused. In February 2012 secondary syphilis was diagnosed with a TCD4+ count of 264 cells/mm^3 (7,5%) and a HIV RNA load of 339000 copies/mL (5,5 log). Three months later, with 53 TCD4+ cells/mm^3 (3.3%) and a viral load of 890000 copies/mm^3 (6 log) he was started on TDF + FTC + EFV.

Four weeks later he was admitted to the emergency department with fever, oral candidiasis, diarrhea, hypotension, and pancytopenia. Gastrointestinal sepsis was suspected and he was started on ciprofloxacin and fluconazole. He developed shock and respiratory failure in the next 48 h and was admitted to the intensive care unit. Antibiotic regimen was changed to imipenem, metronidazole, and fluconazole. Faeces microbiological and parasitological tests were negative, blood and urine cultures were sterile, and CMV plasma antigen was negative. Five weeks after starting ART there was an increase in TCD4+ cell count [259 cells/mm^3 (15%)] and a 2 log drop in the HIV viral load [3500 copies/mm^3 (4 log)]. Initial thoracic, abdominal, and pelvic CT scan were unremarkable. Bronchial aspirate and bronchoalveolar lavage (BAL) were sterile for fungi and fast growing bacteria. PCR assays to identify *Chlamydophila*, *Legionella*, *Mycoplasma*, CMV, HSV, and *Mycobacterium tuberculosis* were negative. The patient remained febrile, and due to severe pancytopenia, hepatosplenomegaly, and an elevated ferritin, hemophagocytic syndrome was suspected, not being confirmed on the bone marrow aspirate though. By the 9th hospitalization day he presented with seizures and the MRI scan showed bilateral and multifocal white matter with high signal intensity on T2-weighted and FLAIR images. This, associated with the presence of JC virus in CSF, led to the diagnosis of progressive multifocal leukoencephalopathy (PML). Diarrhea persisted but due to clinical instability and severe anemia and thrombocytopenia, endoscopic studies were only performed on the 24th hospitalization day. Upper and lower endoscopy revealed multiple polypoid lesions with a cherry-red appearance in the stomach and colon, compatible with Kaposi sarcoma (Figure 1(a)). He was started on doxorubicin. Three days later, along with *Pseudomonas aeruginosa* bacteraemia, the clinical state deteriorated and the patient died.

The clinical course and the documented complications, some of them defining AIDS, would be sufficient to explain the poor outcome but the autopsy opened an unexpected underworld: Kaposi sarcoma was confirmed in the stomach and colon but also in the esophagus and mediastinal lymph nodes (Figure 1(b)); *Candida* species was found in the anal canal, colon (Figure 1(c)), and lung, where hyaline membranes compatible with an acute respiratory distress syndrome were also seen (Figure 1(d)). As previously suspected, prominent phagocytosis of blood cells in the bone marrow confirmed hemophagocytic syndrome (Figure 1(e)); brain histology showed enlarged oligodendroglial cells nucleus with ground glass inclusions consistent with PML (Figure 1(f)); multiple basophilic dot-like parasites in cysts were documented in cerebral (Figure 1(g)) and heart tissues (Figure 1(h)) configuring cerebral and myocardial toxoplasmosis. *Mycobacterium avium complex* culture from the bronchial aspirate became positive after death. *A. baumannii* grew from the right atrium blood culture and aspects of anal condyloma and intraepithelial low-grade neoplasm were also identified, as well as several aspects consistent with systemic shock.

3. Discussion/Conclusion

Chronic HIV infection is a disease of coinfections with immunosuppression allowing reactivation of dormant pathogens or increasing susceptibility to exogenous ones. The vast majority of HIV-infected patients have one or more coinfections at some point during the disease course, which play an important role in chronic immune activation. The higher the antigen burden, the higher the risk for IRIS. This case presents multiple unmasking-IRIS with systemic Kaposi sarcoma, systemic candidiasis, and PML, coupled with several more or less quiescent defining AIDS diseases.

A meta-analysis with 13103 HIV-infected patients showed that IRIS occurred in 16.1% of the cases after starting ART [2]. This number can significantly increase in the presence of coinfections, reaching 45%. Male gender, young age, low TCD4+ cell count, and high viral load are all IRIS risk factors. It has been showed that low TCD4+ cell count and high plasma HIV RNA levels at the time of diagnosis are associated with a faster progression to AIDS [3]. At least 1 value of CD4+ <100 cells/mm^3 in the first year of seroconversion seems to identify a rare group of individuals at high risk for faster disease progression [4]. The patient in this report had a decrease of almost 80% in TCD4+ cell count in 3 months. This subset of patients has the ability to collect several opportunistic infections (OI) in few months, before the risk for specific OI be identified and effective prophylaxis started.

Several factors are independently associated with occurrence of OI such as African American/Black race or Hispanic/Latino ethnicity, intravenous drug users, heterosexual HIV transmission, lower TCD4+ cell count, and higher viral load [5]. Sixteen large cohorts of HIV-infected patients were recently evaluated and reported a decrease in the incidence rates of first OIs, from 2.96 events/100 person-years in 2000–2003 to 1.45 events/100 person-years in 2008–2010 [5]. The improvements in viral suppression and immune status associated with newer ART regimens played a major role in the picture of OI. Levels of TCD4+ cell count below which specific OIs tend to occur were never absolute. Patients that started ART during 2008–2010 had a 7% probability of developing a new OI within 2 years when the initial TCD4+ cell count was <200 cell/mm^3 but only 1% when the initial TCD4+ cell count was ≥500 cells/mm^3 [5]. The median TCD4+ cell count is usually above or close to 200 cells/mm^3 for tuberculosis and isosporiasis infections and less than 100 cells/mm^3 for candidiasis, PCP, CMV infection, and MAC infection [5]. On the other hand, OIs also have an impact on TCD4+ cell count as the latter decrease at a rate of 24.1 cells/mL per three months in the presence of OI, compared to an increase of 21.3 cells/mL per three months in its absence [6]. In this report, the patient had a rapid decline in TCD4+ cells to 53 cells/mm^3 leading to a profound immunosuppressed state, which dramatically increased the risk for several OI in a short period of time.

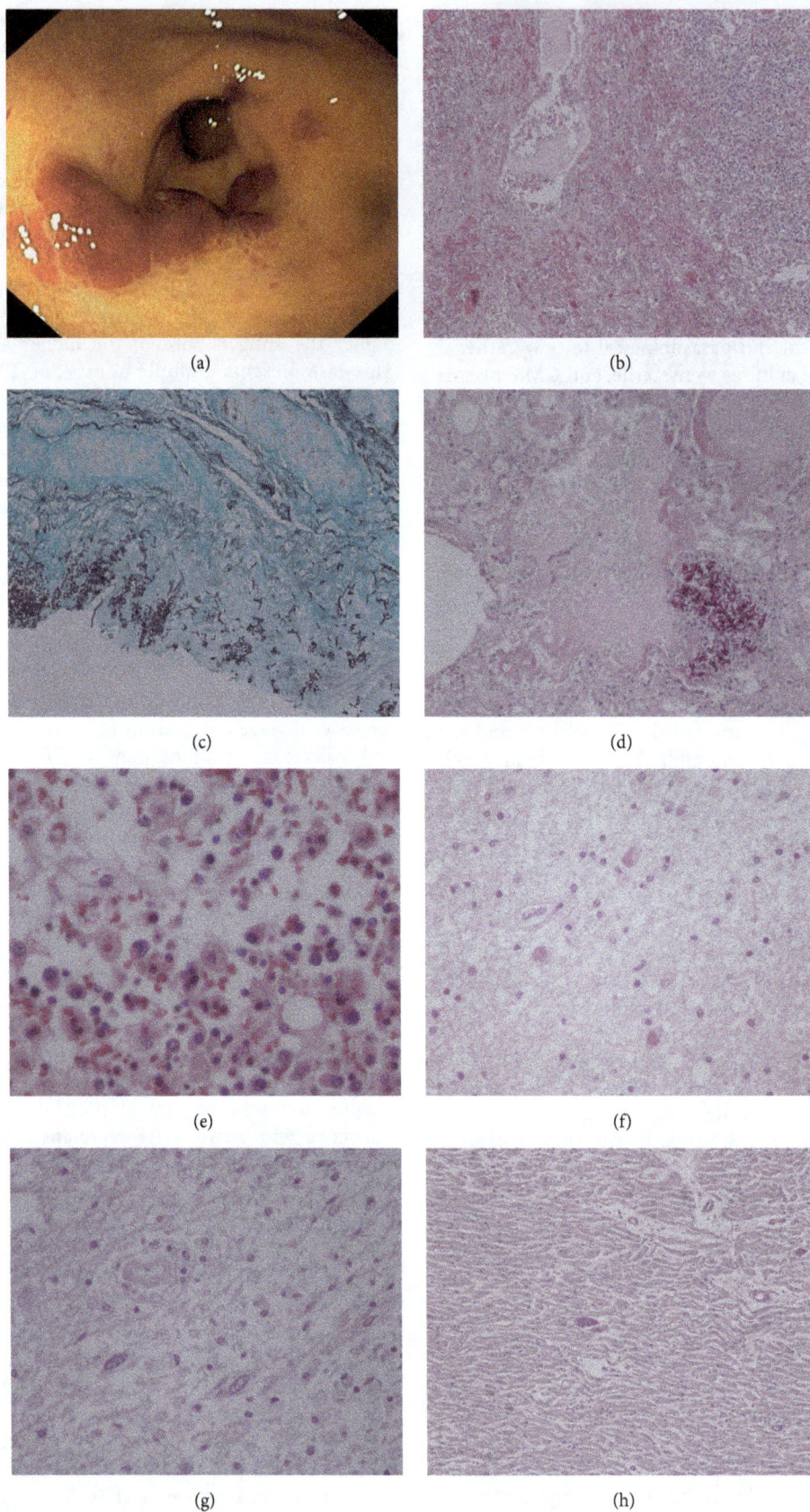

FIGURE 1: (a) Gastric Kaposi sarcoma: scarlet slightly elevated lesions of the antral gastric mucosal surface (upper gastrointestinal endoscopy). (b) Mediastinal ganglia Kaposi sarcoma: submucosal vascular spindle-shaped cells (H&E-stain, 100x). (c) *Candida* spp. in colon (Grocott methenamine silver-stain, 100x). (d) *Candida* spp. in lung and hyaline membranes suggesting acute respiratory distress syndrome (H&E-stain, 100x). (e) Bone marrow hemophagocytosis (H&E-stain, 400x). (f) Progressive multifocal leukoencephalopathy: enlarged homogeneous oligodendrocyte nucleus with inclusion (H&E-stain, 100x). (g) Cerebral toxoplasmosis: *Toxoplasma* cyst (H&E-stain, 100x). (h) Cardiac toxoplasmosis: *Toxoplasma* cyst (H&E-stain, 100x).

Along with depression of immune system, OI presentation becomes blurred and the diagnosis is difficult. Our patient, despite his profound immunosuppression, was asymptomatic until the start of ART. KS is the most common HIV-associated malignancy and disease exacerbation or presentation after starting ART can be as high as 29% [7]. Central nervous system IRIS contributes to the bulk of IRIS mortality: JC virus infection is the third cause after *Mycobacterium* tuberculosis and *Cryptococcus neoformans*; cerebral toxoplasmosis is rare. Twelve to 22% of AIDS patients had endomyocardial involvement by *T. gondii* at autopsy; in the highly active ART era the prevalence of cardiac toxoplasmosis confirmed *postmortem* has been reported to be less than 10% [8]. The incidence of *M. avium complex* infection related to IRIS, in the presence of TCD4+ <100 cells/mm^3, is 3.5% [9].

Early HIV infection detection and treatment are crucial to a better prognosis. Recent changes in the treatment guidelines are expected to reduce IRIS incidence, particularly by reducing the duration and degree of immunosuppression. Nevertheless, systematic screening for OI before starting ART is still a key element to prevent this phenomenon. The risk of paradoxical IRIS could also be substantially altered by deferral of ART initiation, particularly in central nervous system IRIS. This approach is postulated to ensure adequate treatment of OI, reduce the antigen burden before starting ART in HIV-infected patients with severe immune deficiency, and promote immune recovery.

Despite the lack of standardized treatment protocol for IRIS, ART should not be interrupted and there may be a need for corticosteroid therapy. As such, treatment of these patients is a huge challenge and further research regarding the immunopathogenesis, diagnosis, and its management should be pursued.

Competing Interests

The authors have no conflict of interests to declare.

References

[1] N. F. Walker, J. Scriven, G. Meintjes, and R. J. Wilkinson, "Immune reconstitution inflammatory syndrome in HIV-infected patients," *HIV/AIDS—Research and Palliative Care*, vol. 7, pp. 49–64, 2015.

[2] M. Müller, S. Wandel, R. Colebunders, B. A. Suzanna Attia, M. D. Hansjakob Furrer, and M. Egger, "Immune reconstitution inflammatory syndrome in patients starting antiretroviral therapy for HIV infection: a systematic review and meta-analysis," *The Lancet Infectious Diseases*, vol. 10, no. 4, pp. 251–261, 2010.

[3] C. Goujard, M. Bonarek, L. Meyer et al., "CD4 cell count and HIV DNA level are independent predictors of disease progression after primary HIV type 1 infection in untreated patients," *Clinical Infectious Diseases*, vol. 42, no. 5, pp. 709–715, 2006.

[4] A. D. Olson, M. Guiguet, R. Zangerle et al., "Evaluation of rapid progressors in HIV infection as an extreme phenotype," *Journal of Acquired Immune Deficiency Syndromes*, vol. 67, no. 1, pp. 15–21, 2014.

[5] K. Buchacz, B. Lau, Y. Jing et al., "Incidence of AIDS-defining opportunistic infections in a multicohort analysis of HIV-infected persons in the United States and Canada, 2000–2010," *The Journal of Infectious Diseases*, vol. 214, no. 6, pp. 862–872, 2016.

[6] J. P. Ekwaru, J. Campbell, S. Malamba, D. M. Moore, W. Were, and J. Mermin, "The effect of opportunistic illness on HIV RNA viral load and CD4+ T cell count among HIV-positive adults taking antiretroviral therapy," *Journal of the International AIDS Society*, vol. 16, Article ID 17355, 2013.

[7] L. Shahani and R. J. Hamill, "Therapeutics targeting inflammation in the immune reconstitution inflammatory syndrome," *Translational Research*, vol. 167, no. 1, pp. 88–103, 2016.

[8] A. Hidron, N. Vogenthaler, J. I. Santos-Preciado, A. J. Rodriguez-Morales, C. Franco-Paredes, and A. Rassi Jr., "Cardiac involvement with parasitic infections," *Clinical Microbiology Reviews*, vol. 23, no. 2, pp. 324–349, 2010.

[9] P. Phillips, S. Bonner, N. Gataric et al., "Nontuberculous mycobacterial immune reconstitution syndrome in HIV-infected patients: spectrum of disease and long-term folow-up," *Clinical Infectious Diseases*, vol. 41, no. 10, pp. 1483–1497, 2005.

29

Nocardia transvalensis Disseminated Infection in an Immunocompromised Patient with Idiopathic Thrombocytopenic Purpura

Jorge García-Méndez,[1,2] **Erika M. Carrillo-Casas,**[3]
Andrea Rangel-Cordero,[4] **Margarita Leyva-Leyva,**[3] **Juan Xicohtencatl-Cortes,**[5]
Roberto Arenas,[6] **and Rigoberto Hernández-Castro**[7]

[1]*Departamento de Posgrado y Educación Médica Continua, Instituto Nacional de Cancerología, Mexico*
[2]*Departamento de Microbiología, Facultad de Medicina, UNAM, 04510 Coyoacán, MEX, Mexico*
[3]*Departamento de Biología Molecular e Histocompatibilidad, Dirección de Investigación,*
 Hospital General "Dr. Manuel Gea González", 14080 Tlalpan, MEX, Mexico
[4]*Laboratorio de Microbiología Clínica, Instituto Nacional de Ciencias Médicas y Nutrición "Salvador Zubirán",*
 14080 Tlalpan, MEX, Mexico
[5]*Departamento de Infectología, Hospital Infantil de México "Federico Gómez", Dr. Márquez 162, Cuauhtémoc,*
 06720 Ciudad de México, DF, Mexico
[6]*Servicio de Micología, Hospital General "Dr. Manuel Gea González", 14080 Tlalpan, MEX, Mexico*
[7]*Departamento de Ecología de Agentes Patógenos, Hospital General "Dr. Manuel Gea González", 14080 Tlalpan, MEX, Mexico*

Correspondence should be addressed to Rigoberto Hernández-Castro; rigo37@gmail.com

Academic Editor: Larry M. Bush

Nocardia transvalensis complex includes a wide range of microorganisms with specific antimicrobial resistance patterns. *N. transvalensis* is an unusual *Nocardia* species. However, it must be differentiated due to its natural resistance to aminoglycosides while other *Nocardia* species are susceptible. The present report describes a *Nocardia* species involved in an uncommon clinical case of a patient with idiopathic thrombocytopenic purpura and pulmonary nocardiosis. Microbiological and molecular techniques based on the sequencing of the 16S rRNA gene allowed diagnosis of *Nocardia transvalensis* sensu stricto. The successful treatment was based on trimethoprim-sulfamethoxazole and other drugs. We conclude that molecular identification of *Nocardia* species is a valuable technique to guide good treatment and prognosis and recommend its use for daily bases diagnosis.

1. Introduction

Nocardia species are Gram-positive ubiquitous, aerobic actinomycetes, saprophytic of soil, water, and organic matter. *Nocardia* genus is an opportunistic pathogen which may cause disease in immunocompromised or immunocompetent patients [1, 2]. The primary source of infection is through inhalation. However, more than 90% patients have underlying conditions compromising their cellular or humoral immunity. *N. transvalensis* must be differentiated due to its natural resistance to aminoglycosides, while other *Nocardia*

species are typically susceptible such as *N. blacklockiae* and *N. wallacei* [3, 4].

N. transvalensis was first described by Pijper and Pullinger in 1927 as the causative agent of mycetoma of the foot in a South African patient [5]; since then, it has turned to be a cause of life threatening infections and other non-threatening infections [4]. *N. asteroides* and *N. brasiliensis* are common species recognized in clinical cases, while *N. transvalensis* sensu stricto is one of the least frequent *Nocardia* species. It has restricted susceptibility to cotrimoxazole, third-generation cephalosporin, imipenem, and linezolid. *N.*

transvalensis is a pathogen rarely reported, particularly in a case of cystic fibrosis with chronic pulmonary infections [5], brain abscess [3], keratitis [4], ocular infections, HIV patients [6], mycetoma [1, 7], and pulmonary infections [8].

Here we present an uncommon report of pulmonary nocardiosis with haematological and neurological involvement caused by *N. transvalensis* in a patient with idiopathic thrombocytopenic purpura.

2. Case Description

A 59-year-old male from Guerrero, Mexico, was referred to the National Cancer Institute at Mexico City, diagnosed with prostate adenocarcinoma (Gleason 8), and treated with flutamide (Androgen Receptor Inhibitor) plus goserelin (gonadotropin releasing hormone superagonist (GnRH agonist)). After exhaustive physical examination and thrombocytopenia ($51/mm^3$), presumptive drug-induced idiopathic thrombocytopenic purpura was recognized. This condition was managed with prednisone 100 mg/day plus 6-mercaptopurine 50 mg/day, for 7 weeks. After 12 weeks at his hometown, the patient developed progressive respiratory insufficiency, diagnosed with right pneumonia and treated with oral levofloxacin (500 mg/daily). He was readmitted to the Cancer Institute with hyperglycaemia because of steroid use, and no bacterial isolation was obtained from the first sputum. One week later, the patient was received at the Emergency Room complaining of fever (39°C), dyspnea, cachexia, and haemoptysis. Clinically with right basal hypoventilation, the imaging studies (chest X-ray, followed by a thoracic computed tomography scan) revealed cavitated right middle lobe pneumonia, as well as lesions in other lung segments (Figures 1 and 2). The antimicrobial regimen was changed to ceftriaxone and clindamycin. In spite of mild improvement, the patient was submitted to a CT-guided lung biopsy. Gram and Ziehl-Neelsen stains were negative and until the fourth day waxy colonies were detected in blood agar and Sabouraud plates under incubation at 37°C and 5% CO_2 atmosphere. Microscopically, weak Gram-positive, branched filamentous bacilli were observed. Trimethoprim-sulfamethoxazole (15 mg/kg/day) was the successful treatment. Almost immediately to diagnosis, the patient referred to right arm weakness, which reversed on the third day of treatment with trimethoprim-sulfamethoxazole. A Magnetic Resonance of the brain reported minimum changes in the meningeal layers, and the lumbar puncture showed moderate pleocytosis without recovering any microorganisms. A follow-up thoracic CT scan showed the resolution of more than half of lung involvement and trimethoprim-sulfamethoxazole was continued at home. The resolution of the idiopathic thrombocytopenic purpura was followed by tapering prednisone and 6-mercaptopurine (25 mg/48 h) for the next 6 and 12 months until discontinuation. One year after the episode and maintenance treatment with amoxicillin-clavulanate (40 mg/10 mg/kg/day) plus trimethoprim-sulfamethoxazole (15 mg/kg/day) for the *Nocardia* infection, the imaging studies confirmed the complete resolution of the lung pathology. Since then, the patient has not relapsed and the cancer treatment continued.

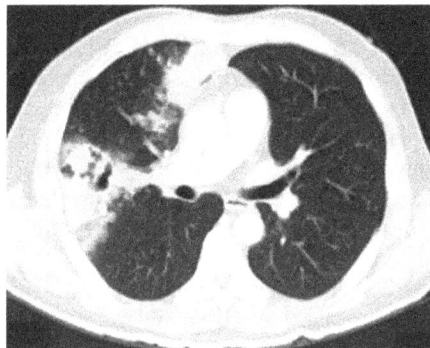

FIGURE 1: Axial computed tomography showing middle right lobe involvement.

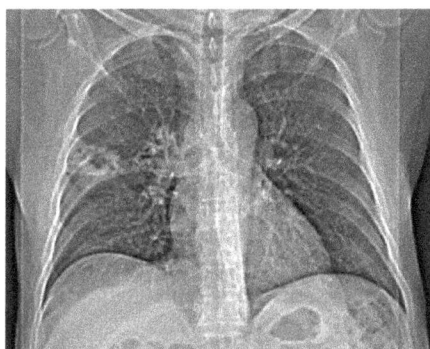

FIGURE 2: Chest computed tomographic scan at ER admission.

3. Materials and Methods

The genus identification was based on the Gram-positive stain of branching and filamentous bacilli, positive modified acid-fast stain, colonial morphology, and conventional biochemical reactions. Further species identification was based on sequencing of the 16S rRNA gene, using the primers Noc1 (5′-GCTTAACACATGCAAGTCG-3′) and Noc2 (5′-GAATTCCAGTCTCCCCTG-3′) [9]. The PCR product was purified with the QIAquick purification kit (Qiagen, Ventura, CA, USA), according to the manufacturer, and DNA sequences were determined with Taq FS Dye Terminator Cycle Sequencing Fluorescence-Based Sequencing and analysed on an Applied Biosystems 3730 DNA sequencing system (Foster City, CA, USA). The sequence of the 16S showed 100% homology with *N. transvalensis* accession number FJ516749.

4. Discussion

A marked increased number of human *Nocardia* infections have been reported worldwide since the decade of 1960. However, *N. transvalensis* is an infrequent pathogen and probably misdiagnosed. Pulmonary nocardiosis is a mayor clinical manifestation of *Nocardia* species infection and may pose a challenge when distinguishing it from tuberculosis. To the best of our knowledge, only few cases had been related involving *N. transvalensis* as the primary cause of acute or chronic infections. Predisposing factors of human nocardiosis are chronic obstructive pulmonary disease, bronchiectasis, pulmonary fibrosis, emphysema, asthma, neoplastic disease (thoracic or induced by potent immunosuppressant drugs), organ transplant (bone marrow or solid transplantation), or immunosuppressive therapy used in autoimmune diseases, cancer, diabetes mellitus, previous or concurrent tuberculosis, and advanced HIV infection (acquired immunodeficiency syndrome) [8].

The geographical differences among continents should be taken into account. *N. transvalensis* sensu stricto is common in Africa and absent in Asia. *N. wallacei* is the most frequent species isolated in the United States, whereas scarce information is available in the rest of America, maybe due to misdiagnosis or underestimation of human cases and difficulties in clinical and laboratory diagnosis.

The routine diagnosis has been microbiological culture and morphological features. However, the phenotypic identification has 37% misidentification of *Nocardia* species based on the 16S rRNA gene which discern among the *N. transvalensis* cluster and other species by two base insertions. Few reports have used molecular techniques to identify the involvement of *N. transvalensis* in clinical cases [4, 10]; nonetheless, its molecular identification is of great value as guidance for treatment choice [4]. The delay in the *Nocardia* species identification has clinical implications because these bacteria have been classified according to their antibiotic resistance patterns but share similar clinical manifestations; therefore, the treatment election may be hindered. In the current case, the use of trimethoprim-sulfamethoxazole (an antimicrobial of choice for nocardiosis) was the right choice in combination with other antimicrobials, which may include imipenem, amikacin, ceftriaxone, and amoxicillin-clavulanate.

5. Conclusion

The present report describes an uncommon *N. transvalensis* infection in an immunocompromised patient with idiopathic thrombocytopenic purpura. This work underlines the value of early diagnosis by microbiological culture combined with accurate molecular identification of the *Nocardia* species; in addition, sulfonamide extended use and the reduction in immunosuppression are key factors for good prognosis. We encourage the use of molecular identification at the species level for further understanding of the epidemiology, taxonomy, antimicrobial susceptibility, and clinical and epidemiological aspects of nocardiosis.

Competing Interests

The authors declare that there are no competing interests regarding the publication of this paper.

References

[1] S. H. Mirza and C. Campbell, "Mycetoma caused by Nocardia transvalensis," *Journal of Clinical Pathology*, vol. 47, no. 1, pp. 85–86, 1994.

[2] M. M. McNeil, J. M. Brown, P. R. Georghiou, A. M. Allworth, and Z. M. Blacklock, "Infections due to *Nocardia transvalensis*: clinical spectrum and antimicrobial therapy," *Clinical Infectious Diseases*, vol. 15, no. 3, pp. 453–463, 1992.

[3] R. F. Yorke and E. Rouah, "Nocardiosis with brain abscess due to an unusual species, Nocardia transvalensis," *Archives of Pathology and Laboratory Medicine*, vol. 127, no. 2, pp. 224–226, 2003.

[4] E. Trichet, S. Cohen-Bacrie, J. Conrath, M. Drancourt, and L. Hoffart, "Nocardia transvalensis keratitis: an emerging pathology among travelers returning from Asia," *BMC Infectious Diseases*, vol. 11, article 296, 2011.

[5] A. Aravantagi, K. Patra, M. Broussard, and K. Jones, "A case of Nocardia transvalensis pneumonia in a 19-year-old cystic fibrosis patient," *Lung India*, vol. 29, no. 3, pp. 283–285, 2012.

[6] N. Poonwan, M. Kusum, Y. Mikami et al., "Pathogenic Nocardia isolated from clinical specimens including those of AIDS patients in Thailand," *European Journal of Epidemiology*, vol. 11, no. 5, pp. 507–512, 1995.

[7] H. C. Gugnani, J. O. Ojukwu, and A. V. Suseelan, "Mycetoma of thumb caused by Nocardia transvalensis," *Mycopathologia*, vol. 80, no. 1, pp. 55–60, 1982.

[8] A. Kageyama, K. Yazawa, J. Ishikawa, K. Hotta, K. Nishimura, and Y. Mikami, "Nocardial infections in Japan from 1992 to 2001, including the first report of infection by *Nocardia transvalensis*," *European Journal of Epidemiology*, vol. 19, no. 4, pp. 383–389, 2004.

[9] C.-K. Tan, C.-C. Lai, S.-H. Lin et al., "Clinical and microbiological characteristics of Nocardiosis including those caused by emerging Nocardia species in Taiwan, 1998–2008," *Clinical Microbiology and Infection*, vol. 16, no. 7, pp. 966–972, 2010.

[10] W. L. Liu, C. C. Lai, W. C. Ko et al., "Clinical and microbiological characteristics of infections caused by various Nocardia species in Taiwan: A multicenter study from 1998 to 2010," *European Journal of Clinical Microbiology and Infectious Diseases*, vol. 30, no. 11, pp. 1341–1347, 2011.

30

Acute and Fatal Isoniazid-Induced Hepatotoxicity: A Case Report and Review of the Literature

Wissam K. Kabbara,[1] **Aline T. Sarkis,**[2] **and Paola G. Saroufim**[2]

[1]*Department of Pharmacy Practice, School of Pharmacy, Lebanese American University (LAU), P.O. Box 36/F-37, Byblos, Lebanon*
[2]*School of Pharmacy, Lebanese American University (LAU), Byblos, Lebanon*

Correspondence should be addressed to Wissam K. Kabbara; wissam.kabbara@lau.edu.lb

Academic Editor: Daniela M. Cirillo

This paper describes a case of an acute and fatal isoniazid-induced hepatotoxicity and provides a review of the literature. A 65-year-old female diagnosed with latent *Mycobacterium tuberculosis* infection was receiving oral isoniazid 300 mg daily. She was admitted to the hospital for epigastric and right sided flank pain of one-week duration. Laboratory results and imaging confirmed hepatitis. After ruling out all other possible causes, she was diagnosed with isoniazid-induced acute hepatitis (probable association by the Naranjo scale). After discharge, the patient was readmitted and suffered from severe coagulopathy, metabolic acidosis, acute kidney injury, hepatic encephalopathy, and cardiorespiratory arrest necessitating two rounds of cardiopulmonary resuscitation. Despite maximal hemodynamic support, the patient did not survive. A review of the literature, from several European countries and the United States of America, revealed a low incidence of mortality due to isoniazid-induced hepatotoxicity when used as a single agent for latent *Mycobacterium tuberculosis* infection. As for the management, the first step consists of withdrawing isoniazid and rechallenge is usually discouraged. Few treatment modalities have been proposed; however there is no robust evidence to support any of them. Routine monitoring for hepatotoxicity in patients receiving isoniazid is warranted to prevent morbidity and mortality.

1. Introduction

Isoniazid (INH) is an antituberculosis agent that is commonly used for the treatment and prophylaxis of tuberculosis (TB). It inhibits bacterial cell wall synthesis, thus killing *Mycobacterium tuberculosis* organisms. Due to its significant potential in reducing morbidity, the use of INH in treating latent *Mycobacterium tuberculosis* infection (LTBI) is recommended as a first-line option since the 1965 American Thoracic Society guidelines especially in high risk individuals [1].

Since its introduction in 1952, several cases of INH-induced hepatotoxicity were reported [2–11]. Drug-induced liver injury guidelines caused by INH appears to be due to metabolic idiosyncratic reactions. INH is metabolized mostly by the liver, primarily by acetylation by N-acetyl transferase 2 (NAT-2) to acetyl-isoniazid. Acetyl-isoniazid is metabolized mainly to monoacetyl hydrazine (MAH) and to the non-toxic diacetyl hydrazine, as well as other minor metabolites.

The influence of acetylation rate on INH hepatotoxicity is controversial; however, the involvement of INH's metabolites has been proposed: first by free radical generation from reactive metabolites of MAH and second by the covalent bond of acetyl hydrazine to liver macromolecules. Patients with enhanced cytochrome P450 2E1 activity carrying the homozygous cytochrome P450 2E1 c1/c1 host gene polymorphism showed an increased risk of developing hepatotoxicity particularly if known to be slow acetylators [12].

Multiple risk factors may contribute to INH-related hepatotoxicity. Some of them have conflicting evidence such as racial difference [13–15] and female gender [16, 17]. Other risk factors are well-confirmed including age [13, 18, 19], alcohol consumption [14, 15], and the concomitant administration of other hepatotoxic drugs such as acetaminophen [20], methotrexate [21], sulfasalazine [21], or carbamazepine [22].

Reports of severe and fatal hepatitis associated with INH emerged after the 1970 TB outbreak in Capitol Hill in Washington, DC, among workers who were receiving it for prophylaxis. Nineteen patients developed signs and symptoms of liver damage; and two of them died [23].

Accordingly, the guidelines published in 1971 were updated to include pretreatment screening and monitoring to reduce the risk of such complications [24]. In 1979, the USPHS trial showed a rate of death due to INH of 0.06% [15]. The IUAT study, a large eastern European clinical trial, estimated the rates of fatal INH hepatitis as 14 per 100,000 person-years [25]. Again, the 1983 guidelines were further reviewed to recommend routine clinical and laboratory monitoring for patients who are older than 35 years and for those with additional risk factors for hepatotoxicity [26]. Another report published in 1992 revealed rates of INH fatal hepatitis of around 0.02% which is lower than the incidence stated in the USPHS trial [17]. Salpeter evaluated articles published from 1966 to 1992 on INH use (with or without other antituberculosis drugs) in chemoprophylaxis. All patients were appropriately monitored according to the guidelines. Results showed 2 hepatotoxic deaths in 202,497 patients (an adjusted fatality rate of 0.003%). Both patients were taking INH monotherapy but had additional risk factors for hepatotoxicity [27]. In 1996, Millard et al. estimated rates of fatal INH hepatitis to be around 4.2 per 100,000 persons newly starting therapy and around 7 per 100,000 while completing therapy [28].

The most recent American Thoracic Society guidelines (2003) recommends INH 300 mg monotherapy daily for 9 months for human immunodeficiency virus (HIV) negative and positive individuals. Routine baseline and follow-up laboratory monitoring is only recommended for those who are HIV positive, have chronic liver disease, and are regular alcohol consumers or pregnant [29]. A recent case report (2015) was published presenting the case of a 53-year-old Japanese male diagnosed with INH-induced acute liver failure during a course of preventive therapy for LTBI [30]. Liver transplant was refused by the patient and his family leading to his death 4 months after admission.

Here, we present a probable case, as determined by the Naranjo adverse drug reaction probability scale score [31], of INH-induced fulminant hepatic failure in a 65-year-old woman who was receiving INH for LTBI.

2. Case Presentation

We present the case of a 65-year-old (weight, 80 Kg, height, 150 cm) Sri Lankan black woman, known to have LTBI treated with INH and dyslipidemia. She was diagnosed with LTBI based on a positive purified protein derivative test. The patient's main indication for LTBI treatment was recent arrival (within 5 years) from a high prevalence country. She presented to the emergency department with epigastric and right sided flank pain of one-week duration. The history goes back to one week prior to admission when the patient started to experience pain along with one episode of vomiting and dark (tea-colored) urine without any other urinary symptoms. She reported a severe pain of 8/10, relieved by sitting and lying forward and worsened by lying backwards. The patient denied any nausea, diarrhea, constipation, or fever prior to the presentation.

TABLE 1: Laboratory data upon admission.

Laboratory test	Result	Normal range
Biochemistry		
Total bilirubin	*11.4 mg/dL	<1 mg/dL
Direct bilirubin	*9.9 mg/dL	0–0.2 mg/dL
Indirect bilirubin	*1.5 mg/dL	0–1 mg/dL
γ-GTP	*202 U/L	<40 U/L
ALP	*316 U/L	35–105 U/L
AST (SGOT)	*2099 U/L	<33 U/L
ALT (SGPT)	*1096 U/L	<34 U/L
CRP	*1.54 mg/dL	<0.5 mg/dL
Amylase	*115 U/L	28–100 U/L
Lipase	*97 U/L	13–60 U/L
Total proteins	*5.2 g/dL	6.6–8.7 g/dL
Albumin	*2.9 g/dL	3.5–5.2 g/dL
Hematology		
WBC	*4.8 × 10^3/μL	5.2–12.4 × 10^3/μL
RBC	4.5 × 10^6/μL	4.2–5.4 × 10^6/μL
Hb	13.7 g/dL	12–16 g/dL
PLT	237 × 10^3/μL	130–400 × 10^3/μL
Coagulation		
INR	*1.58	1–1.3

*Abnormal value.
γ-GTP: Gamma-Glutamyl Transpeptidase; ALP: Alkaline Phosphatase; AST: Aspartate Aminotransferase; SGOT: Serum Glutamic Oxaloacetic Transaminase; ALT: Alanine Aminotransferase; SGPT: Serum Glutamic Pyruvic Transaminase; CRP: C-Reactive Protein; WBC: White Blood Cell Count; RBC: Red Blood Cell; Hb: Hemoglobin; PLT: Platelet; INR: International Normalized Ratio.

Her past medical history includes LTBI (6 months prior to the presentation with no laboratory and clinical monitoring for the isoniazid treatment) and dyslipidemia without any known liver disease. Her medications are Rimifon® (INH) 150 mg two tablets by mouth once daily and Panadol® (Acetaminophen) 500 mg two tablets by mouth as needed for headache. The patient was previously on Liponorm® (Atorvastatin) 10 mg one tablet by mouth once daily and Neurobion® (Vitamin B12, 200 mcg, Vitamin B6, 200 mg, and Vitamin B1, 100 mg) both of which were discontinued when INH was initiated (6 months prior to the presentation). The patient works as a housekeeper; she denied any known drug or food allergies, the use of recreational drugs, tobacco smoke, or alcohol.

Her vital signs were as follows: blood pressure of 120/78 mmHg, heart rate of 83 beats per minute, respiratory rate of 15 breaths per minute, and a body temperature of 36.2°C. Her review of systems was normal except for icteric sclera, pale conjunctiva, and epigastric tenderness. Pending laboratory results, she was given Perfalgan® (acetaminophen) 1 g IV STAT for pain and normal saline 0.9% 1 L every 24 hours. The patient's laboratory data upon admission are shown in Table 1.

The patient was admitted to the internal medicine service for further investigation. INH was discontinued and medication orders were the following: Profenid® (ketoprofen)

100 mg IV every 8 hours as needed for pain, Nexium® (Esomeprazole) 40 mg IV once daily, and Buscopan® (Scopolamine Butylbromide) 1 ampoule of 20 mg IV every 8 hours as needed for abdominal pain. Based on negative infectious serology, hepatitis A, hepatitis B, hepatitis C, cytomegalovirus (CMV), and Epstein-Barr virus were all ruled out. The patient had a positive CMV IgG Ab (160 AU/mL) suggesting a previous infection. Hepatic autoimmune disease was ruled out as well based on negative immunology markers. An abdominal ultrasound showed a normal liver size of 11 cm, perihepatic fluid effusion, and pericholecystic edema that are most probably related to hepatitis rather than cholecystitis. CT scan of the abdomen and pelvis showed a diffusely thickened gallbladder wall with neither the evidence of obstructive process nor portal vein thrombosis. After ruling out all the possible causes of acute hepatitis in our patient, the final diagnosis was made as INH-induced acute hepatitis.

Throughout the hospital stay, there was a slight reduction (around 15% from baseline) in liver function tests (LFTs); however INR and bilirubin remained elevated. The patient was clinically improving and her laboratory values were slightly better. Upon physician's order, the patient was discharged on Nexium 40 mg one tablet by mouth daily for one week. The patient did not resume the isoniazid treatment upon discharge after the initial hospital admission.

Six days later, the patient was readmitted to the hospital for abdominal distention and increased upper right quadrant pain that radiated to the flanks and increases with food intake and exertion. She also reported decreased appetite, fatigue, and dyspnea with exertion. Upon readmission, she presented with jaundice, icteric sclera, dark urine, and prominent ascites confirmed by wave fluid test. In the ER, she received Nexium 40 mg IV, Profenid 100 mg IV STAT, and NS 0.9% 500 mL every 24 hours which was increased to 1 L every 24 hours when her blood pressure dropped to 85/55 mmHg. Laboratory values were the following: total bilirubin 27.8 mg/dL, γ-GTP 95 U/L, ALP 283 U/L, ALT (SGPT) 873 U/L, AST (SGOT) 1582 U/L, amylase 164 U/L, lipase 65 U/L, Cr 0.66 mg/dL, and INR 2.28. Bilirubin was also detected in urine. Accordingly, the patient was admitted to the internal medicine floor for fulminant hepatic failure due to INH.

In an attempt to normalize INR, multiple administrations of Konakion® (Phytomenadione) were given. Profenid was discontinued due to the increased risk of bleeding and Buscopan 20 mg IV every 8 hours as needed for abdominal pain was ordered. Furthermore, Primperan® (Metoclopramide) 10 mg IV STAT, one vial of Albumin (20%) IV STAT, and morphine sulfate 2 mg SC STAT twice for pain were given. The patient had several episodes of hypotension responsive to fluid resuscitation with NS. The ultrasound showed diffused and clear moderate ascites as well as marked edematous thickening of the gallbladder wall with clear content related to intra-abdominal fluid effusion. The patient developed hypoglycemia (32–37 mg/dL) and oxygen saturation dropped to 86%. Due to deterioration, reduced level of consciousness, and poor response to oxygen, she was intubated and transferred to the intensive care unit.

On physical exam she was unresponsive, her pupils were middilated, and nonreactive, her lungs had few scattered rhonchi, and she had abdominal distention and ascites. She had metabolic acidosis (pH 6.8) and multiple doses of sodium bicarbonate were administered. The patient was consistently hypoglycemic and hypotensive despite fluid resuscitation and vasopressor administration. Serum creatinine increased from 0.66 mg/dL to 2.34 mg/dL in two days confirming acute kidney injury. She was also suffering from severe coagulopathy and hepatic encephalopathy. Additionally, blood cultures revealed a sensitive *Escherichia coli* and sputum cultures showed α-*Streptococcus* and *Neisseria* species. The patient had cardiorespiratory failure necessitating cardiopulmonary resuscitation (CPR). Spontaneous circulation was achieved after 15 minutes of CPR. Unfortunately, this was followed by a second cardiac arrest and despite maximal hemodynamic support, the patient passed away.

3. Discussion

The American College of Gastroenterology (ACG) clinical guidelines recommend the use of a specific formula (R = ALT/ULN ÷ ALP/ULN) to differentiate between three different types of drug-induced liver injury (DILI): acute hepatocellular ($R \geq 5$), mixed (R 2–5), or cholestatic ($R \leq 2$) [32]. The most common presentation of DILI is acute hepatocellular injury or cholestatic injury [33]. The former is more life-threatening (may lead to coagulopathy and encephalopathy) and is characterized by severe elevation of LFTs but mild elevation of ALP [34–36]. In cholestatic disease, there is a marked elevation of ALP, minimal elevation of LFTs, and it is accompanied by jaundice and pruritus [33]. Finally, the mixed type is somewhere in-between where the elevation of LFTs and ALP are both intermediate, resembling atypical hepatitis and granulomatous hepatitis [36]. INH fits the acute hepatocellular injury profile that is similar to acute viral hepatitis with a moderate to long latency period of 30 to more than 90 days [32, 33]. The reported patient's R score was 10 confirming the acute hepatocellular injury as expected. Other reports show latency period of approximately one week to three months; in most cases, however, the INH-induced hepatotoxicity can occur up to one year later or more [14]. An acute DILI may proceed to a chronic DILI in 15–20% of the cases. A chronic DILI is confirmed if the condition (clinical and laboratory) does not resolve 6 months after its onset. Usually, patients with cholestatic liver injury are at higher risk compared to those with acute liver injury [32].

We presented the case of a 65-year-old female with acute INH-induced hepatic failure that progressed dramatically in a short period of time leading to death. As mentioned earlier, hepatic involvement is a common side effect of INH. The patient's Naranjo adverse drug reaction probability score was 7, indicating a probable association [31]. Similarly, both the Yale Algorithm [37] and the WHO-UMC system for standardized case causality assessment [38] showed a probable association. It is also important to note that the patient received other potentially hepatotoxic medications: acetaminophen, by mouth and by intravenous injection, ketoprofen and esomeprazole, by intravenous injection and then by mouth, and metoclopramide. These medications could have contributed to the ultimate deterioration of the liver.

A recent case report presents a 53-year-old Japanese male receiving INH for LTBI [30]. Similar to our case, there was no routine laboratory monitoring. Our patient had a longer latency period (180 days versus 70 days) but a similar time from INH initiation until death (around 190 days). Both patients had a slight improvement in LFTs upon discontinuation of INH but remained extremely elevated. As for disease progression, hepatic encephalopathy and coagulopathy were noted in both cases. The Japanese patient developed sepsis and liver atrophy and died of liver failure, while our patient had acute kidney injury and metabolic acidosis and died of cardiorespiratory arrest. Liver transplant was an appropriate treatment option for both but was not feasible for different reasons.

The Center for Disease Control and Prevention published a report that quantified the frequency of severe adverse effects in patient receiving isoniazid for LTBI treatment during 2004–2008 [39]. Severe liver injury due to isoniazid was reported in 17 patients, 5 of whom underwent liver transplantation. Five patients died, including one patient who had a liver transplantation. The report emphasized the need for monthly clinical monitoring and counselling of patients receiving isoniazid for LTBI, including those with no evident additive risk factors for liver injury, to identify any treatment-associated adverse event.

According to The Diagnosis and Management of Idiosyncratic Drug-Induced Liver Injury published by the ACG, it is strongly discouraged to rechallenge a patient with a drug that was considered to be a causative agent for hepatotoxicity especially when the injury is severe (LFTs > 5x ULN). However, exceptions do occur in life-threatening situations when no other alternative is available [32]. As for the appropriate management, the first step would be withdrawing the offending agent and, if possible, other hepatotoxic agents as well [32]. Corticosteroids and ursodeoxycholic acid have been proposed as a treatment for DILI associated with acute liver failure (ALF) [40]; however, no robust evidence supports these treatment modalities [32]. The use of intravenous N-acetylcysteine (NAC) in non-acetaminophen acute liver failure (DILI in one subgroup) was tested in a prospective, double blind trial. Intravenous NAC did not enhance overall survival; however, it improved transplant-free survival in patients with early coma grade. Patients with advanced coma grades do not benefit from NAC and typically require emergency liver transplantation [41]. Another prospective double blind trial was conducted to determine the association between clinical benefit seen with IV NAC and improvement in hepatic function. In early grade coma patients with non-acetaminophen acute liver failure, the reduction in transplantation or death or of transplantation alone was associated with an improvement in ALT and bilirubin (parameters reflecting hepatocyte necrosis and bile excretion) but not in INR, creatinine, or AST [42]. Findings suggest an accelerated hepatic recovery with the use of IV NAC in such patients [42]. However, NAC use in pediatric non-acetaminophen related ALF showed conflicting results [43, 44].

A 4-month regimen of rifampin can be considered for persons who cannot tolerate INH, who have been exposed to INH-resistant tuberculosis, or who require a shortened duration of therapy for better completion rates [45]. It should not be used to treat HIV-infected persons taking some combinations of antiretroviral therapy [45]. In a pooled data from 3586 patients, a 4-month rifampin regimen was associated with a significant reduction in the risk of hepatotoxicity as compared to 9-month isoniazid therapy [46].

4. Conclusion

We reported a case of acute, fulminant, and fatal hepatotoxicity due to INH in a 65-year-old female with LTBI. Although hepatotoxicity is a well-known side effect of INH, mortality rates remain low as reported in the literature. It is important for clinicians and pharmacists to appropriately follow up patients, counsel them on the signs and symptoms of hepatotoxicity, and encourage them to report it.

Ethical Approval

The institutional review board of the Lebanese American University approved this study.

Competing Interests

The authors of this paper report no competing interests and no financial support.

Authors' Contributions

All authors participated in the conception and design of the study, contributed to the analysis of data and to the drafting and critical revision of the article, and approved the final manuscript.

References

[1] American Thoracic Society, "Preventive treatment in tuberculosis: a statement by the committee on therapy," The American Review of Respiratory Disease, vol. 91, pp. 297–298, 1965.

[2] H. Randolph and S. Joseph, "Toxic hepatitis with jaundice occurring in a patient treated with Isoniazid," Journal of the American Medical Association, vol. 152, no. 1, pp. 38–40, 1953.

[3] S. N. Gellis and R. V. Murphy, "Hepatitis following isoniazid," Diseases of the Chest, vol. 28, no. 4, pp. 462–464, 1955.

[4] A. D. Merritt, "Toxic hepatic necrosis (hepatitis) due to isoniazid: report of a case with cirrhosis and death due to hemorrhage from esophageal varices," Annals of Internal Medicine, vol. 50, no. 3, pp. 804–801, 1959.

[5] E. Haber and R. K. Osborne, "Icterus and febrile reactions in response to isonicotinic acid hydrazine; Report of two cases and review of the literature," The New England Journal of Medicine, vol. 260, no. 9, pp. 417–420, 1959.

[6] S. Gillis and K. Texler, "Unusual reactions to anti-tuberculous chemotherapy," The Medical Journal of Australia, vol. 47, no. 2, pp. 99–101, 1960.

[7] R. Cohen, M. H. Kalser, and R. V. Thomson, "Fatal hepatic necrosis secondary to isoniazid therapy," *The Journal of the American Medical Association*, vol. 176, no. 10, pp. 877–879, 1961.

[8] D. Davies and J. J. Glowinski, "Jaundice due to isoniazid," *Tubercle*, vol. 42, pp. 504–506, 1961.

[9] E. S. Assem, N. Ndoping, H. Nicholson, and J. R. Wade, "Liver damage and isoniazid allergy," *Clinical and Experimental Immunology*, vol. 5, no. 4, pp. 439–442, 1969.

[10] L. Scharer and J. P. Smith, "Serum transaminase elevations and other hepatic abnormalities in patients receiving isoniazid," *Annals of Internal Medicine*, vol. 71, no. 6, pp. 1113–1120, 1969.

[11] C. E. Martin and J. B. Arthaud, "Hepatitis after isoniazid administration," *The New England Journal of Medicine*, vol. 282, no. 8, pp. 433–434, 1970.

[12] J. J. Saukkonen, D. L. Cohn, R. M. Jasmer et al., "An official ATS statement: hepatotoxicity of antituberculosis therapy," *American Journal of Respiratory and Critical Care Medicine*, vol. 174, no. 8, pp. 935–952, 2006.

[13] C. M. Nolan, S. V. Goldberg, and S. E. Buskin, "Hepatotoxicity associated with isoniazid preventive therapy: a 7-year survey from a public health tuberculosis clinic," *The Journal of the American Medical Association*, vol. 281, no. 11, pp. 1014–1018, 1999.

[14] Isoniazid, September 2015, http://livertox.nlm.nih.gov/Isoniazid.htm.

[15] D. E. Kopanoff, D. E. Snider Jr., and G. J. Caras, "Isoniazid-related hepatitis: a U.S. Public Health Service cooperative surveillance study," *The American Review of Respiratory Disease*, vol. 117, no. 6, pp. 991–1001, 1978.

[16] T. S. Moulding, A. G. Redeker, and G. C. Kanel, "Twenty isoniazid-associated deaths in one state," *American Review of Respiratory Disease*, vol. 140, no. 3, pp. 700–705, 1989.

[17] D. E. Snider Jr. and G. J. Caras, "Isoniazid-associated hepatitis deaths: a review of available information," *American Review of Respiratory Disease*, vol. 145, no. 2, pp. 494–497, 1992.

[18] P. A. LoBue and K. S. Moser, "Isoniazid- and rifampin-resistant tuberculosis in San Diego County, California, United States, 1993–2002," *International Journal of Tuberculosis and Lung Disease*, vol. 9, no. 5, pp. 501–506, 2005.

[19] F. F. Fountain, E. Tolley, C. R. Chrisman, and T. H. Self, "Isoniazid hepatotoxicity associated with treatment of latent tuberculosis infection: a 7-year evaluation from a public health tuberculosis clinic," *Chest*, vol. 128, no. 1, pp. 116–123, 2005.

[20] J. S. Crippin, "Acetaminophen hepatotoxicity: potentiation by isoniazid," *The American Journal of Gastroenterology*, vol. 88, no. 4, pp. 590–592, 1993.

[21] J. Vanhoof, S. Landewe, E. Van Wijngaerden, and P. Geusens, "High incidence of hepatotoxicity of isoniazid treatment for tuberculosis chemoprophylaxis in patients with rheumatoid arthritis treated with methotrexate or sulfasalazine and antitumour necrosis factor inhibitors," *Annals of the Rheumatic Diseases*, vol. 62, no. 12, pp. 1241–1242, 2003.

[22] F. E. Berkowitz, S. L. Henderson, N. Fajman, B. Schoen, and M. Naughton, "Acute liver failure caused by isoniazid in a child receiving carbamazepine," *International Journal of Tuberculosis and Lung Disease*, vol. 2, no. 7, pp. 603–606, 1998.

[23] R. A. Garibaldi, R. E. Drusin, S. H. Ferebee, and M. B. Gregg, "Isoniazid-associated hepatitis. Report of an outbreak," *American Review of Respiratory Disease*, vol. 106, no. 3, pp. 357–365, 1972.

[24] "Preventive treatment of tuberculosis. A joint statement of the American Thoracic Society, National Tuberculosis and Respiratory Disease Association, and the Center for Disease Control," *The American Review of Respiratory Disease*, vol. 104, no. 3, pp. 460–463, 1971.

[25] "Efficacy of various durations of isoniazid preventive therapy for tuberculosis: five years of follow-up in the IUAT trial. International Union Against Tuberculosis Committee on Prophylaxis," *Bulletin of the World Health Organization*, vol. 60, no. 4, pp. 555–564, 1982.

[26] W. C. Bailey, R. K. Albert, P. T. Davidson et al., "Treatment of tuberculosis and other mycobacterial diseases," *American Review of Respiratory Disease*, vol. 127, no. 6, pp. 790–796, 1983.

[27] S. R. Salpeter, "Fatal isoniazid-induced hepatitis. Its risk during chemoprophylaxis," *Western Journal of Medicine*, vol. 159, no. 5, pp. 560–564, 1993.

[28] P. S. Millard, T. C. Wilcosky, S. J. Reade-Christopher, and D. J. Weber, "Isoniazid-related fatal hepatitis," *Western Journal of Medicine*, vol. 164, no. 6, pp. 486–491, 1996.

[29] "Targeted tuberculin testing and treatment of latent tuberculosis infection," *American Journal of Respiratory and Critical Care Medicine*, vol. 161, no. 4, part 2, pp. S221–S247, 2000.

[30] S. Miyazawa, S. Matsuoka, S. Hamana et al., "Isoniazid-induced acute liver failure during preventive therapy for latent tuberculosis infection," *Internal Medicine*, vol. 54, no. 6, pp. 591–595, 2015.

[31] C. A. Naranjo, U. Busto, E. M. Sellers et al., "A method for estimating the probability of adverse drug reactions," *Clinical Pharmacology & Therapeutics*, vol. 30, no. 2, pp. 239–245, 1981.

[32] N. P. Chalasani, P. H. Hayashi, H. L. Bonkovsky, V. J. Navarro, W. M. Lee, and R. J. Fontana, "ACG clinical guideline: the diagnosis and management of idiosyncratic drug-induced liver injury," *The American Journal of Gastroenterology*, vol. 109, no. 7, pp. 950–966, 2014.

[33] N. Kaplowitz, "Drug-induced liver injury," *Clinical Infectious Diseases*, vol. 38, supplement 2, pp. S44–S48, 2004.

[34] N. Kaplowitz, "Drug-induced liver disorders: implications for drug development and regulation," *Drug Safety*, vol. 24, no. 7, pp. 483–490, 2001.

[35] H. Zimmerman, *Hepatotoxicity: The Adverse Effects of Drugs and Other Chemicals on the Liver*, Lippincott Williams & Wilkins, Philadelphia, Pa, USA, 2nd edition, 1999.

[36] N. Kaplowitz, "Drug-induced liver disorders: introduction and overview," in *Drug-Induced Liver Disease*, N. Kaplowitz and L. D. DeLeve, Eds., pp. 1–13, Marcel Dekker, New York, NY, USA, 2002.

[37] M. S. Kramer and T. A. Hutchinson, "The Yale algorithm. Special workshop—clinical," *Drug Information Journal*, vol. 18, no. 3-4, pp. 283–291, 1984.

[38] The use of the WHO-UMC system for standardized case causality assessment, http://www.who.int/medicines/areas/quality_safety/safety_efficacy/WHOcausality_assessment.pdf.

[39] CDC, "Severe isoniazid-associated liver injuries among persons being treated for latent tuberculosis infection—United States, 2004–2008," *Morbidity and Mortality Weekly Report*, vol. 59, no. 8, pp. 224–229, 2010.

[40] A. Wree, A. Dechêne, K. Herzer et al., "Steroid and ursodesoxycholic acid combination therapy in severe drug-induced liver injury," *Digestion*, vol. 84, no. 1, pp. 54–59, 2011.

[41] W. M. Lee, L. S. Hynan, L. Rossaro et al., "Intravenous N-acetylcysteine improves transplant-free survival in early stage

non-acetaminophen acute liver failure," *Gastroenterology*, vol. 137, pp. 856–864, 2009.

[42] S. Singh, L. S. Hynan, and W. M. Lee, "Improvements in hepatic serological biomarkers are associated with clinical benefit of intravenous *N*-acetylcysteine in early stage non-acetaminophen acute liver failure," *Digestive Diseases and Sciences*, vol. 58, no. 5, pp. 1397–1402, 2013.

[43] C. Kortsalioudaki, R. M. Taylor, P. Cheeseman, S. Bansal, G. Mieli-Vergani, and A. Dhawan, "Safety and efficacy of N-acetylcysteine in children with non-acetaminophen-induced acute liver failure," *Liver Transplantation*, vol. 14, no. 1, pp. 25–30, 2008.

[44] R. H. Squires, A. Dhawan, E. Alonso et al., "Intravenous N-acetylcysteine in pediatric patients with nonacetaminophen acute liver failure: a placebo-controlled clinical trial," *Hepatology*, vol. 57, no. 4, pp. 1542–1549, 2013.

[45] J. T. Denholm and E. S. McBryde, "The use of anti-tuberculosis therapy for latent TB infection," *Infection and Drug Resistance*, vol. 3, pp. 63–72, 2010.

[46] P. D. Ziakas and E. Mylonakis, "4 Months of rifampin compared with 9 months of isoniazid for the management of latent tuberculosis infection: a meta-analysis and cost-effectiveness study that focuses on compliance and liver toxicity," *Clinical Infectious Diseases*, vol. 49, no. 12, pp. 1883–1889, 2009.

31

Neisseria meningitidis Infecting a Prosthetic Knee Joint:
A New Case of an Unusual Disease

Berta Becerril Carral,[1] **Elvira Alarcón Manoja,**[2] **Salvador López Cárdenas,**[1]
and Jesús Canueto Quintero[1]

[1]*Unidad Clínica de Gestión de Enfermedades Infecciosas y Microbiología del Área Sanitaria del Campo de Gibraltar, Cádiz, Spain*
[2]*Unidad Clínica de Gestión de Medicina Interna del Área Sanitaria del Campo de Gibraltar, Cádiz, Spain*

Correspondence should be addressed to Elvira Alarcón Manoja; elviraalarconmanoja@hotmail.com

Academic Editor: Oguz R. Sipahi

Primary meningococcal meningitis is an infrequent but known disease. However, the infection of a prosthetic joint with *Neisseria meningitidis* is rare. We hereby describe the second case of an arthroplasty infected with *Neisseria meningitidis* that responded favourably to prosthesis retention with surgical debridement, in combination with antibiotics treatment.

1. Introduction

Neisseria meningitidis is a Gram-negative, facultative, aerobic, or anaerobic diplococcus. It was isolated for the first time by Anton Weischselbaum in 1887 in the cerebrospinal fluid of a meningitis patient [1]. It is a strict human pathogen with a wide variety of clinical manifestations. *N. meningitidis* can cause extremely severe diseases, such as meningitis and life-threatening sepsis, as well as the asymptomatic colonization of the nasopharynx in approximately 10% of the population during endemic periods of infection [2]. It rarely provokes localized forms, such as septic arthritis, pneumonia, pericarditis, otitis, sinusitis, and urethritis [3]. Primary purulent arthritis caused by *N. meningitidis* is a rare but known disease. However, as far as we know, there is only one published case report of an arthroplasty infected with *Neisseria meningitidis* [4]. We hereby present a new case of this exceptional infection.

The duration and form of administration of antibiotic agents in these infections are based on expert opinions. The traditional recommendation duration of total postdebridement antibiotic treatment of 6 to maximal 12 weeks or the duration of its initial parental part (2–4 weeks) is discussed in favour of an oral antibiotic treatment from the start [5].

2. Case Presentation

A 78-year-old Caucasian female patient with dislipemia, stable ischemic cardiopathology, degenerative aortic and mitral valves, and generalized osteoarthritis arrived at the Emergency Department of Hospital Punta de Europa, Algeciras, Spain, a 328-bed general hospital, with a chief complaint of pain in her left knee. The patient had undergone a total left knee arthroplasty 7 months before due to a severe functional limitation secondary to osteoarthritis. Seven days before admission and while experiencing symptoms of pharyngitis, she had an accident at home and suffered a sprain in her left ankle. The patient complained of pain and swelling in the above joint that radiated towards her left knee. Within days of the accident, the patient reported a gradual reduction in the symptoms in her ankle but an increase of pain in her knee. She started complaining of intense pain, functional impairment, redness, and increase of local temperature but without evidence of skin rash. The presence of intra-articular fluid was confirmed in the operated knee. There were no other affected joints or presence of skin lesions. Main analytical data were as follows: leukocytes: 13.6×10^9/L with 80% granulocytes; haemoglobin: 11.8 g/dL; platelets: 486×10^9/L; immunoglobulin levels in serum were normal. An arthrocentesis was performed and it yielded an amber-coloured fluid with 9.9 × 109/L (67% polymorphonuclear), glucose: 97 mg/dL, proteins: 4.2 g/dL, and LDH: 1866 U/L. No crystals were observed. The joint fluid culture was positive for *N. meningitidis* serogroup B (latex agglutination (Difco™ Neisseria Meningitidis Antiserum, Becton, Dickinson and Company®, Sparks, MD)), with an intermediate sensitivity to penicillin (minimum inhibitory concentration (MIC): 0,25 microg/ml by *E*-test (BioMerieux® Inc, Marcy L'Etoil, France)) and sensitivity to cefotaxime (0,01 microg/ml by *E*-test (BioMerieux Inc, Marcy L'Etoil, France)) and ciprofloxacin (by disk diffusion (Sensi-Disc™, Becton, Dickinson and Company, Sparks, MD) according to the CLSI guidelines [6, 7]. *N. meningitidis* was identified by growth on chocolate agar and blood agar, and by utilization of enriched media (API NH biochemical testing (BioMerieux Inc, Marcy L'Etoil, France)). Blood cultures were negatives (BacT/ALERT® 3D system (BioMerieux Inc, Mercy L'Etoil, France)). The procedure included arthroscopic debridement with implant retention because of individual patient circumstances and acute onset of symptoms in the setting of a well-fixed prosthesis without a sinus tract and antibiotics and 2 grams ceftriaxone administered intravenously every 24 hours over a 3-week period, followed by oral administration of 750 mg ciprofloxacin every 12 hours over the total 12-week study period. No recurrence has been observed during a two-year follow-up. The Department of Preventive Medicine and Public Health was notified of the case and the recommendations on prophylaxis and treatment of possible carriers were followed, and the patient was vaccinated with meningococcal vaccines following this episode [8].

3. Discussion

Infection is the most feared complication after an arthroplasty and has proven to be the cause for a notable rate of morbidity and a nonnegligible rate of mortality [9]. There are two ways of how microorganisms can infect a prosthetic joint, and the most frequent is direct inoculation during surgery. The second one is haematogenous dissemination, responsible for 10% of the cases.

In his article, Aslam et al. [10] include nonsurgical trauma to the implant as a risk factor for the acquisition of a haematogenous prosthetic infection. In the case described, a traumatic event that had happened in the past and that had affected the left ankle and knee could have created an environment allowing the bacteria, which just happened to be in the blood at the time due to a concomitant pharyngitis, to seed the prosthetic joint.

The most frequently isolated bacteria in prosthetic joint infections are: *Staphylococcus aureus*, *Streptococcus* spp., and Gram-negative bacilli, although the proportions vary depending on the series [11].

Three clinical syndromes have been described in association to the bloodstream infection with *Neisseria meningitidis*. The first one, acute meningococcemia, is a severe condition that occurs within the context of a sepsis, a septic shock, or meningitis. Although rarer, bacteraemia adopts a less aggressive clinical course, such as chronic meningococcemia, indistinguishable from chronic gonococcemia, which is a rare infection characterized by intermittent fever episodes, maculopapular rash, and arthralgia; it can also adopt the form of transient meningococcemia, characterized by fever and unspecified rash over a 2–5-day evolution period where presence of *N. meningitidis* in the blood usually comes as an unexpected finding [12].

Besides, the ability of *N. meningitidis* to infect prosthetic joints shall depend upon the affinity for the osteoarticular tissue, the type of prosthesis employed, and the residual joint tissue. The frequency of arthritis complicating acute meningococcal disease in adults ranges from 4 to 50%. Schaad [13] describes the following three clinical types of arthritis in meningococcal disease. (1) The most common type is arthritis complicating acute meningococcal disease. Its mechanism is of an immunologic basis and affects larger joints, mainly knees, and, less frequently, the direct invasion of the joint by the bacteria. (2) Chronic meningococcemia is accompanied more often by arthralgia. (3) Primary meningococcal arthritis, which is a rare form of acute septic arthritis, affects large joints almost exclusively and is monoarticular in two-thirds of the cases.

Both the case described by Vikram et al. [4] and the present description should be classified in the third category, where the germ's route of entry is supposedly haematogenous.

Biofilm formation plays a crucial role in the ability of germs to colonize nonbiological surfaces. Both encapsulated and nonencapsulated forms of *N. meningitidis* are capable of producing biofilm. This favours its persistence in the nasopharynx and seems to play an important role in the process of colonization and the carrier status (in this case the pharyngitis seven days before admission was the probable entry site but was not confirmed). Nonetheless, the role of biofilm-forming strains in the different clinical syndromes associated with the meningococcal disease is still to be determined.

To our knowledge, this is the second reported case of primary meningococcal arthritis in a prosthetic joint. The previous case, published in 2001, described the infection of a total knee prosthesis by *N. meningitidis* serogroup Y in an 80-year-old female patient. This patient's prosthesis had been placed 3 years before and, as in the case hereby presented, it did not have any distinctive clinical feature. The management included prosthesis retention and a 6-week course of i.v. ceftriaxone.

In both cases, the most likely route of entry for the germ into the joint was the haematogenous route, although the presence of this germ in blood could never be confirmed. The case presented was probably favoured by a minor local trauma. Besides, the infection of other types of nonarticular prosthetic grafts with *N. meningitidis* is very rare and limited to a very reduced number of endocarditis on prosthetic valves [14, 15]. Therefore, *N. meningitidis* is a germ that has low affinity for the joint tissue and, although capable of producing biofilm in order to survive in the surface secretions of the nasopharynx, it has very limited capacity to cause infections in abiotic surfaces, and here lies the exceptional significance of the case hereby presented.

Competing Interests

The authors declare that there is no conflict of interests regarding the publication of this paper.

Authors' Contributions

Berta Becerril Carral and Elvira Alarcón Manoja contributed equally to this case report.

References

[1] A. Weichselbaum, "Über die aetiologie der akuten meningitis cerebro-spinalis," *Fortschritte der Medizin*, vol. 5, pp. 573–583, 1887.

[2] S. P. Yazdankhah and D. A. Caugant, "*Neisseria meningitidis*: an overview of the carriage state," *Journal of Medical Microbiology*, vol. 53, no. 9, pp. 821–832, 2004.

[3] A. P. Yung and M. I. McDonald, "Early clinical clues to meningococcaemia," *Medical Journal of Australia*, vol. 178, no. 3, pp. 134–137, 2003.

[4] H. R. Vikram, R. B. Buencamino, and S. I. Aronin, "Primary meningococcal arthritis in a prosthetic knee joint," *Journal of Infection*, vol. 42, no. 4, pp. 279–281, 2001.

[5] L. Deabate, P. Leonardo, and U. İlker, "Modern antibiotic treatment of chronic long bone infections in adults-theory, evidence and practice," *Mediterranean Journal of Infection, Microbes and Antimicrobials*, vol. 3, article 9, 2014.

[6] Clinical and Laboratory Standards Institute, *Methods for Dilution Antimicrobial Susceptibility Tests for Bacteria That Grow Aerobically*, Approved Standard M07-A8, CLSI, Wayne, Pa, USA, 8th edition, 2009.

[7] Clinical and Laboratory Standards Institute, *Performance Standards for Antimicrobial Susceptibility Testing: Twentieth Informational Supplement*, CLSI Document M100-S22, CLSI, Wayne, Pa, USA, 2012.

[8] D. van de Beek, C. Cabellos, O. Dzupova et al., "ESCMID guideline: diagnosis and treatment of acute bacterial meningitis," *Clinical Microbiology and Infection*, vol. 22, pp. S37–S62, 2016.

[9] D. Rodríguez, C. Pigrau, G. Euba et al., "Acute haematogenous prosthetic joint infection: prospective evaluation of medical and surgical management," *Clinical Microbiology and Infection*, vol. 16, no. 12, pp. 1789–1795, 2010.

[10] S. Aslam, C. Reitman, and R. O. Darouiche, "Risk factors for subsequent diagnosis of prosthetic joint infection," *Infection Control and Hospital Epidemiology*, vol. 31, no. 3, pp. 298–301, 2010.

[11] C. J. E. Kaandorp, H. J. Dinant, M. A. F. J. Van De Laar, H. J. Bernelot Moens, A. P. A. Prins, and B. A. C. Dijkmans, "Incidence and sources of native and prosthetic joint infection: a community based prospective survey," *Annals of the Rheumatic Diseases*, vol. 56, no. 8, pp. 470–475, 1997.

[12] D. S. Stephens, B. Greenwood, and P. Brandtzaeg, "Epidemic meningitis, meningococcaemia, and *Neisseria meningitidis*," *Lancet*, vol. 369, no. 9580, pp. 2196–2210, 2007.

[13] U. B. Schaad, "Arthritis in disease due to *Neisseria meningitidis*," *Reviews of Infectious Diseases*, vol. 2, no. 6, pp. 880–888, 1980.

[14] J. Dennis, L. D. Edwards, T. N. Fisher, and L. Makeever, "Endocarditis on a Bjork-Shiley mitral prosthesis due to Neisseria meningitidis," *Scandinavian Journal of Thoracic and Cardiovascular Surgery*, vol. 11, no. 3, pp. 205–209, 1977.

[15] A. E. Jephcott and C. A. Hardisty, "Meningococcal septicaemia in a patient with a prosthetic valve—a sucessfully treated case," *The British Journal of Clinical Practice*, vol. 30, no. 9, pp. 180–185, 1976.

32

Lemierre's Syndrome Associated with Mechanical Ventilation and Profound Deafness

Lukas Birkner

Department of Internal Medicine, Ev. Krankenhaus Witten gGmbH, University of Witten/Herdecke, Pferdebachstr 27, 58455 Witten, Germany

Correspondence should be addressed to Lukas Birkner; lukasbirkner@freenet.de

Academic Editor: Tomoyuki Shibata

Lemierre's syndrome is a rare disorder that is characterized by anaerobic organisms inducing a thrombophlebitis of the internal jugular vein (IJV) following a course of oropharyngeal infection. It often occurs in young and healthy patients. Clinicians continuously misinterpret early symptoms until infection disseminates systematically and life-threatening sepsis transpires. We report the case of a 58-year-old female developing Lemierre's syndrome accompanied by invasive ventilation support and a profound deafness requiring the implementation of a cochlear implant. This is one of two reported cases of Lemierre's syndrome associated with mechanical ventilation support and the only case associated with a cochlear implant.

1. Introduction

Lemierre's syndrome is a condition caused by primarily anaerobic organisms that induce thrombophlebitis of the internal jugular vein (IJV) and bacteraemia, following a course of oropharyngeal infection [1]. Firstly described in 1936, its incidence and mortality rate decreased drastically after the introduction of antibiotics [2, 3]. Although it is often called "forgotten disease" its occurrence increases since the 1990s [4]. Still Lemierre's syndrome is a rare disease with 0.6–2.3 cases per 1000000 population and a mortality rate of 4–18%. Clinicians frequently misinterpret early symptoms until infection disseminates systematically and life-threatening sepsis transpires [1]. Often the disease occurs in young, healthy patients that show prolonged symptoms of pharyngitis later accompanied by symptoms of septicaemia and pneumonia. Identification of IJV thrombophlebitis as well as cultivation of anaerobic bacteria, mostly *Fusobacterium necrophorum*, confirms the diagnosis [5].

2. Case Report

We report a 58-year-old female patient with a previously fractured elbow. Pain continued throughout the physiotherapy. Swelling of the left arm prolonged over the course of three weeks. Additionally, the patient developed a sore throat, shivering attacks, and fever accompanied by growing nausea. Thereafter she was admitted to the hospital due to a poor general condition, increasing fever, and a developing pharyngitis. On general examination patient was lethargic and disoriented with over 39-degree fever. The patients respiratory condition worsened considerably causing multiorgan failure and a resulting severe pneumonia transpired. Thus, invasive ventilation and administration of catecholamines were started. Ventilator-associated pneumonia could be excluded, because of the sequence of events.

Subsequently computed tomography (CT) revealed thrombosis of right and left internal jugular vein (Figures 1 and 2). Furthermore, a bilateral mastoiditis and a chronic sinusitis were discovered (Figures 3 and 4). It must be noted that this could be a coincidental radiological finding. The following magnetic resonance tomography (MRT) displayed multiple sources of infection, likely to be septic emboli, located in the brain (Figure 5). Blood tests revealed a positive anaerobic blood culture bottle. To identify a possible bacterial infection the blood was subcultured. Susceptible testing recognized *Fusobacterium necrophorum* as the responsible agent. The organism was susceptible to penicillin. Antibiotic therapy was reorganized and the patient received metronidazole and penicillin. Based on

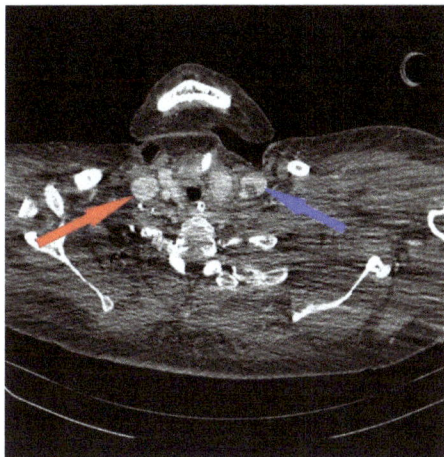

FIGURE 1: CT scan (axial image) of the thorax with a contrast enhancing agent. Results with thrombus adhering to the wall in both internal jugular veins (left IJV, blue arrow, and right IJV, red arrow).

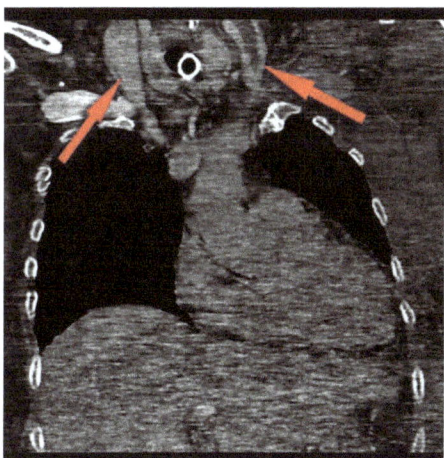

FIGURE 2: CT scan (coronal image) of the thorax with thrombus adhering to the wall in both internal jugular veins (red arrow).

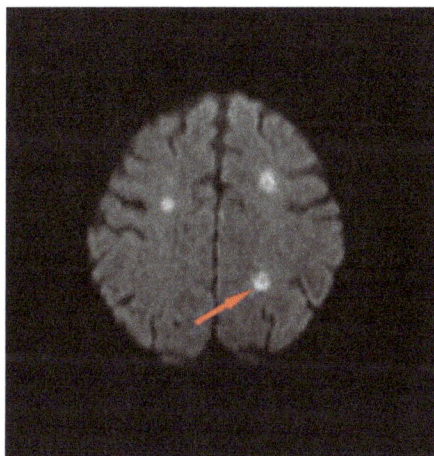

FIGURE 3: MR imaging of the cranium with bilateral mastoiditis (blue arrow) and sphenoidal sinus with air-fluid level (red arrow). In addition, polypoid swelling of mucous in both ethmoid sinuses.

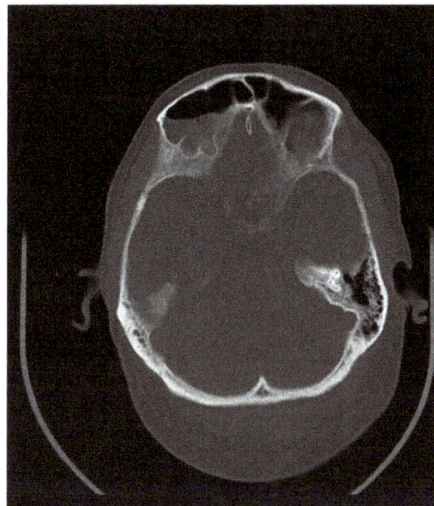

FIGURE 4: MR imaging of the cranium with air-fluid level in both frontal sinuses.

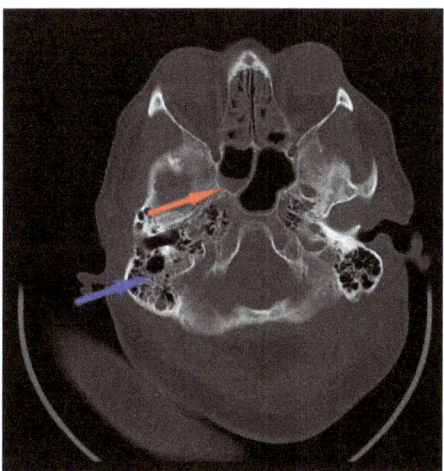

FIGURE 5: MR imaging of the cranium with multiple small rotund lesions in the sense of septic emboli (red arrow).

those findings Lemierre's syndrome was diagnosed. In time the patient's general condition improved and invasive ventilation was stopped. A temporary tracheostomy was performed. Severe dysphagia was discovered and the patient required a PEG (percutaneous endoscopic gastrostomy) feeding tube. Additionally, a profound deafness, which presumably started during the septic shock, complicated communication with the patient. As a result, a cochlear implant was agreed upon and the patient was transferred to a specialized hospital. Intensive physiotherapy enabled the patient to walk for very short distances again.

3. Discussion

Lemierre's syndrome is a thrombophlebitis of the IJV originated from an initial oropharyngeal infection. It most commonly occurs in the 2nd decade of life (51%), followed by the 3rd decade (20%), and is least common in the 1st decade (8%) [6]. Clinically the disease presents not unlike pharyngitis and pneumonia. The most common symptom is a sore throat as in our patient. It typically outdates other symptoms by 4-5 days although the time period may extend in some cases. Other symptoms frequently associated with Lemierre's syndrome are neck mass and pain often mistaken for enlarged lymph nodes, ear pain, dental pain, pleuritic chest pain often indicating metastatic infection, dyspnea, hemoptysis, bone and joint pain, and abdominal pain [7]. Discovering the thrombus within the IJV is the first crucial step towards diagnosing Lemierre's syndrome. For visualisation of the IJV ultrasonography, contrast enhanced CT or less frequently MR imagining is used. As cheapest, but most inexact, ultrasonography may miss thrombi with a low echogenicity [8]. Since CT is more effective it is often used for a specific diagnosis as in our case [9]. The second step in diagnosing Lemierre's syndrome is the growth of characteristic anaerobic bacteria from blood culture [7]. In conclusion Karkos et al. suggest that the concurrent presentation of a recent history of oropharyngeal infection, pharyngitis in our case, clinical or radiological evidence of IJV thrombosis, and the isolation of anaerobic pathogens, mainly *Fusobacterium necrophorum*, pose the main diagnostic criteria for Lemierre's syndrome [6]. Although most cases have been associated with *Fusobacterium necrophorum* there have been reports of other cases associated with other bacteria of the genus *Fusobacterium* [10]. Several antibiotics have been proven to be effective against *Fusobacterium*, such as penicillin, lincomycin, clindamycin, and carbenicillin [11, 12]. Of interest, there have been a few strains of *F. necrophorum* that have reported resistance to penicillin due to beta-lactamase production [13].

Mechanical ventilation support has been reported only in one other case associated with Lemierre's syndrome [14]. The sequence of events suggests that the severe respiratory exhaustion and resulting multiorgan failure the patient displayed may be a consequence of the transpiring sepsis most likely due to the *Fusobacterium*. Sepsis is a common condition accompanying Lemierre's syndrome [2, 6]. Furthermore, Lemierre's syndrome has never been accompanied by profound deafness. This could be a rare effect of the disease possibly caused by damage to auditory pathways due to the septic emboli in the brain or by expansion of the mastoiditis resulting in damage of the inner ear. Mastoiditis has been associated with Lemierre's syndrome before, but our case illustrates that it poses a severe side effect clinicians need to be aware of [6].

4. Conclusion

Generally, this case proves that the clinical presentation of Lemierre's syndrome can be diverse. Clinicians need to be aware of severe and possibly lethal side effects Lemierre's syndrome can have and be able to distinguish and interpret the few telltale signs correctly. Ongoing oropharyngeal infections should be investigated at once to prevent critical progression of the disease. Possibly lethal complications such as sepsis and multiorgan failure should not be neglected.

Competing Interests

The author declares no conflict of interests in this work.

References

[1] M. D. Williams, C. A. Kerber, and H. F. Tergin, "Unusual presentation of lemierre's syndrome due to Fusobacterium nucleatum," *Journal of Clinical Microbiology*, vol. 41, no. 7, pp. 3445–3448, 2003.

[2] A. Lemierre, "On certain septicæmias due to anaerobic organisms," *The Lancet*, vol. 227, no. 5874, pp. 701–703, 1936.

[3] C. L. Weesner and J. E. Cisek, "Lemierre syndrome: the forgotten disease," *Annals of Emergency Medicine*, vol. 22, no. 2, pp. 256–258, 1993.

[4] S. Ramirez, T. G. Hild, C. N. Rudolph et al., "Increased diagnosis of Lemierre syndrome and other Fusobacterium necrophorum infections at a Children's Hospital," *Pediatrics*, vol. 112, no. 5, article no. e380, 2003.

[5] A. V. Hadjinicolaou and Y. Philippou, "Lemierre's syndrome: a neglected disease with classical features," *Case Reports in Medicine*, vol. 2015, Article ID 846715, 4 pages, 2015.

[6] P. D. Karkos, S. Asrani, C. D. Karkos et al., "Lemierre's syndrome: a systematic review," *The Laryngoscope*, vol. 119, no. 8, pp. 1552–1559, 2009.

[7] W. Eilbert and N. Singla, "Lemierre's syndrome," *International Journal of Emergency Medicine*, vol. 6, no. 1, article 40, 2013.

[8] R. Golpe, B. Marín, and M. Alonso, "Lemierre's syndrome (necrobacillosis)," *Postgraduate Medical Journal*, vol. 75, no. 881, pp. 141–144, 1999.

[9] A. Kushawaha, M. Popalzai, E. El-Charabaty, and N. Mobarakai, "Lemierre's syndrome, reemergence of a forgotten disease: a case report," *Cases Journal*, vol. 2, no. 3, 2009.

[10] T. Riordan and M. Wilson, "Lemierre's syndrome: more than a historical curiosa," *Postgraduate Medical Journal*, vol. 80, no. 944, pp. 328–334, 2004.

[11] B. F. Langworth, "Fusobacterium necrophorum: its characteristics and role as an animal pathogen," *Bacteriological Reviews*, vol. 41, no. 2, pp. 373–390, 1977.

[12] P. Bondy and T. Grant, "Lemierre's syndrome: what are the roles for anticoagulation and long-term antibiotic therapy?" *Annals of Otology, Rhinology and Laryngology*, vol. 117, no. 9, pp. 679–683, 2008.

[13] A. S. Hackman and T. D. Wilkins, "In vivo protection of Fusobacterium necrophorum from penicillin by Bacteroides fragilis," *Antimicrobial Agents and Chemotherapy*, vol. 7, no. 5, pp. 698–703, 1975.

[14] A. Chuncharunee and T. Khawcharoenporn, "Lemierre's syndrome caused by Klebsiella pneumoniae in diabetic patient: a case report and review of the literature," *Hawai'i Journal of Medicine & Public Health*, vol. 74, no. 8, pp. 260–266, 2015.

33

Acute Acalculous Cholecystitis: A Rare Presentation of Primary Epstein-Barr Virus Infection in Adults—Case Report and Review of the Literature

Zuhal Yesilbag,[1] Asli Karadeniz,[2] and Fatih Oner Kaya[3]

[1]*Department of Infectious Diseases and Clinical Microbiology, Bakirkoy Dr. Sadi Konuk Education and Research Hospital, Istanbul, Turkey*
[2]*Department of Infectious Diseases and Clinical Microbiology, Maltepe University Faculty of Medicine, Istanbul, Turkey*
[3]*Department of Internal Medicine, Maltepe University Faculty of Medicine, Istanbul, Turkey*

Correspondence should be addressed to Zuhal Yesilbag; zuhalyes@gmail.com

Academic Editor: Tomoyuki Shibata

Primary Epstein-Barr virus (EBV) infection is almost always a self-limited disease characterized by sore throat, fever, and lymphadenopathy. Hepatic involvement is usually characterized by mild elevations of aminotransferases and resolves spontaneously. Although isolated gallbladder wall thickness has been reported in these patients, acute acalculous cholecystitis is an atypical presentation of primary EBV infection. We presented a young women admitted with a 10-day history of fever, nausea, malaise who had jaundice and right upper quadrant tenderness on the physical examination. Based on diagnostic laboratory tests and abdominal ultrasonographic findings, cholestasis and acute acalculous cholecystitis were diagnosed. Serology performed for EBV revealed the acute EBV infection. Symptoms and clinical course gradually improved with the conservative therapy, and at the 1-month follow-up laboratory findings were normal. We reviewed 16 adult cases with EBV-associated AAC in the literature. Classic symptoms of EBV infection were not predominant and all cases experienced gastrointestinal symptoms. Only one patient underwent surgery and all other patients recovered with conservative therapy. The development of AAC should be kept in mind in patients with cholestatic hepatitis due to EBV infection to avoid unnecessary surgical therapy and overuse of antibiotics.

1. Introduction

Epstein-Barr virus (EBV) is a member of Herpesviridae family and causes infectious mononucleosis (IM) characterized by sore throat, fever, and lymphadenopathy. IM is common worldwide and is almost always a self-limited disease most commonly seen in young adults. Hepatic involvement is usually characterized by mild elevations of aminotransferases seen in 80–90% of the cases and resolves spontaneously; severe cholestasis and jaundice are rare [1–6]. Acute acalculous cholecystitis (AAC), an inflammatory process of gallbladder in the absence of gallstones, usually occurs in critically ill patients with severe infections or injuries and antibiotic treatment and surgery may be needed [7]. Although isolated gallbladder wall thickness (GWT) or hydrops have been reported in the patients with IM, AAC is an atypical presentation of primary EBV infection [8, 9]. We described a

patient with AAC due to acute EBV infection presented with jaundice and successfully treated with conservative therapy and reviewed similar adult cases reported in the literature.

2. Case Presentation

A 30-year-old woman was admitted to our hospital with a 10-day history of fever, nausea, and malaise. She had a recent upper respiratory tract infection with sore throat and nonproductive cough and took a beta-lactam antibiotic and paracetamol. She noted that 3 days prior to admission she had realised the jaundice of her sclera. Her past medical history was unremarkable. She had no drug allergies and she had no history of alcohol consumption, blood transfusion, injection drug use, and recent travel. She had no family history of liver disease. On admission she had a body temperature of 39.2°C, pulse rate of 112/min, and respiratory rate of 16/min.

Blood pressure was 110/70 mmHg and jaundice of sclera and skin was observed. Tonsil and pharynx were normal. On examination of the abdomen, the right upper quadrant was tender and painful, hepatomegaly was not present, and the spleen was enlarged two fingers below the costal margin. Initial laboratory tests revealed aspartate aminotransferase (AST): 233 (8–37) U/L, alanine aminotransferase (ALT): 220 (15–65) U/L, gamma glutamyl transferase (GGT): 471 (5–55) U/L, alkaline phosphatase (ALP): 376 (50–136) U/L, lactate dehydrogenase (LDH): 909 (81–234) U/L, C-reactive protein (CRP): 13.6 (0–0.5) mg/dL, erythrocyte sedimentation rate (ESR): 34 (0–15) mm/h, total bilirubin: 15.4 (0.0–1.0) mg/dL and direct bilirubin: 14.5 (0.0–0.3) mg/dL, white blood cell (WBC) count: 8.7×10^3 $(4.5–11 \times 10^3)$/mm^3 with 66.4% neutrophils, 27.1% lymphocytes, and 5.6% monocytes, hemoglobin (Hb): 10.4 (11.7–15.5) g/dL, hematocrit: 30.6 (35–45)%, and platelets: 121×10^3 $(150–450 \times 10^3)$/mm^3. Bacterial cultures of urine and blood were negative. Chest X-ray did not show any pathologic changes. Serological markers for hepatitis A, B, and C viruses, anti-HIV, CMV IgM, toxoplasma IgM, anti-nuclear antibody, anti-mitochondrial antibody, smooth muscle antibody, anti-dsDNA, and ANCA tests were negative. Brucella agglutination and Gruber Widal tests were negative. Serology performed for EBV revealed the acute EBV infection: IgM and IgG antibodies against viral capsid antigen (VCA) were positive whereas IgG antibodies against Epstein-Barr nuclear antigen (EBNA) were negative. An ultrasound scan of the upper abdomen showed a thickened and oedematous gallbladder wall (7.4 mm) with pericholecystic and perihepatic fluid and absence of cholelithiasis or dilatation of the biliary tract, suggesting an acute acalculous cholecystitis. On the 4th day of hospital stay, AST, ALT, total bilirubin, and direct bilirubin increased to 469 U/L, 361 U/L, 19.1 mg/dL, and 17.7 mg/dL, respectively, and ALP and GGT decreased to 289 U/L and 308 U/L, respectively. During admission hemolysis developed with a drop in Hb from 10.4 to 8.6 g/dL. After the 5th day of hospital stay, aminotransferase and bilirubin levels began to decrease; ALP and GGT levels continued to fall which were already decreasing since the first day of admission. Platelets were low on the day of admission (121×10^3/mm^3) and rose to normal level on the 4th day. We did not use antibiotic and because symptoms and clinical course gradually improved with the conservative therapy, percutaneous drainage was thought to be unnecessary. Abdominal pain and fever resolved, and the patient was discharged on the 7th day of admission. At the 1-month follow-up, the patient was asymptomatic, jaundice had resolved, and laboratory findings were normal.

3. Discussion

AAC is defined as acute inflammatory process of the gallbladder without evidence of gallstones and it contributes to 5–10% of overall cholecystitis in adults. It is usually described in patients with abdominal trauma, extensive burns, long term total parenteral nutrition, and systemic diseases including systemic lupus erythematosus and Kawasaki disease [24, 25]. It has also been reported during several infections such as viral hepatitis A, cytomegalovirus, *Salmonella* spp., malaria

infections [26]. Although hepatitis with mild elevations in serum aminotransferases is a common characteristic of EBV infection, AAC is rare in the course of primary EBV infection.

Reviewing the literature, we found 16 adult cases (including the present case) of AAC due to primary EBV infection published between 2007 and 2016 (Table 1) [10–23]. It has been noticed that almost all cases were seen in females (15 out of 16). Eicosanoid proinflammatory mediators also play a role in AAC and eicosanoid synthesis depends on estrogen levels, suggesting a probable relationship between estrogen and the development of disease [27]. AAC can be seen at any age of people, but it is most commonly seen in the fourth or eighth decades of life [28]. Although AAC represents 30–50% of all cases of acute cholecystitis in pediatric population, it is rare in childhood compared with the adults. Most of the cases we reviewed were younger than 25 years. This can be explained by the fact that EBV infections are most commonly seen in young adults. Most of the reported cases occurred in Europe, and 2 of the cases were from our country.

Cholestasis, increased bile viscosity, ischemia, and secondary infections were described in the pathogenesis of AAC [22]. The mechanism of EBV-associated AAC is not clear. Most of the authors hypothesized that EBV-induced hepatitis is a cause of cholestasis, inducing gallbladder inflammation and AAC [20]. We had documented elevations in cholestatic markers in 14 of 16 cases (Table 1). Our patient had cholestatic hepatitis with jaundice and markedly elevations in gamaglutamyltransferase, alkaline phosphatase and bilirubin levels without biliary obstruction. Therefore, it could be postulated that EBV-associated cholestasis induced gallbladder inflammation and the development of AAC in these patients. In hepatitis A infection, direct viral invasion of the gallbladder has been documented by detection of viral antigen in most epithelial cells of the gallbladder [13]. However EBV is known to infect oral epithelial cells, but direct invasion of the gallbladder wall has not been described [22]. The presence of Gilbert's syndrome in children with EBV-associated cholestasis could also play a role in the development of AAC [29].

The main clinical symptoms of AAC are represented by fever, vomiting, and right upper quadrant pain. In our case, the patient was admitted with fever, nausea, malaise, and jaundice, and also the right upper quadrant was tender and painful. The classical symptoms of EBV infection such as sore throat, pharyngitis, and lymphadenopathy have been reported in only three patients (9 with missing information), six patients (4 with missing information), and eight patients (2 with missing information), respectively. However all of the patients had abdominal symptoms and almost all cases had positive Murphy's sign (1 with missing information).

14 of the patients had ALT elevations (2 with missing information), 13 patients had markedly elevated bilirubin levels and 14 patients had high ALP or GGT levels (2 with missing information). In a retrospective study Vine et al. recently showed that EBV was the causative agent in only 0.85% of 1995 adult patients with jaundice and hepatitis and the increase of liver enzymes did not exceed 1400 IU/L, and more profound impairment of liver enzymes usually suggests other causes [30]. In our review the mean ALT level was 281 IU/L, mean AST level was 253 IU/L, and the highest increase in

TABLE 1: Characteristics of reported cases of AAC due to primary EBV infection in adults.

Authors	Age, sex	Country	Sore throat	Pharyngitis	Lymph-adeno-pathy	Murphy's sign positive	Hepato-spleno-megaly	AST (IU/l)	ALT (IU/l)	Total bilirubin	ALP (IU/l)	GGT (IU/L)	GWT	Antibiotics
Koch et al. (2007) [10]	53, F	Netherlands	—	—	—	—	—	—	339	120 μmol/L (0–17)	1081 (40–120)	—	10 mm	No
Iaria et al. (2008) [11]	18, F	Italy	Yes	Yes	Yes	Yes	Yes	220 (5–45)	328 (5–45)	7 mg/dL (0–1.9)	312 (38–148)	142 (7–32)	9 mm	Yes
Cholongitas et al. (2009) [12]	19, F	Greece	Yes	Yes	Yes	Yes	—	426 (<40)	584 (<40)	6.5 mg/dL	710 (<280)	156 (<50)	8 mm	No
Yang et al. (2010) [13]	20, F	Korea	Yes	Yes	Yes	Yes	Yes	171	299	0.7 mg/dL	727	202		Yes
Chalupa et al. (2009) [14]	22, F	Czech Republic	—	Yes	Yes	Yes	Yes	6.87 μkat/L (0–0.65)	12.79 μkat/L (0–0.8)	143 μmol/L (0–20)	2.2 μkat/L (0.5–2)	3.06 μkat/L (0–0.6)	6 mm	Yes
Hagel et al. (2009) [15]	22, F	Germany	—	—	—	Yes	Spleno-megaly	—	—	254 μmol/L	—	—	7 mm	Yes
Beltrame et al. (2012) [16]	29, F	Italy	—	Yes	Yes	Yes	—	121 (10–35)	166 (10–35)	23.2 μmol/L (1.7–17)	161 (53–151)	145 (3–45)	15 mm	Yes
Nagdev and Ward (2011) [17]	18, F	California	No	No	No	Yes	—	118	—	1.2 mg/dL	146	—	>10 mm	Yes
Dylewski (2012) [18]	22, F	Canada	—	No	No	Yes	Spleno-megaly	—	89	Normal	—	—	5 mm	Yes
Carrascosa et al. (2012) [19]	22, F	Spain	—	—	No	Yes	Yes	329	464	43 μmol/L	239	—	14 mm	No
Gagneux-Brunon et al. (2014) [20]	18, F	France	—	No	Yes	Yes	No	321	214	20 μmol/L	165	64	12 mm	Yes
Gagneux-Brunon et al. (2014) [20]	20, F	France	—	No	Yes	Yes	No	453	494	38 μmol/L	133	286	16 mm	Yes
Celik et al. (2014) [21]	48, F	Turkey	—	—	Yes	Yes	—	221 (5–35)	165 (5–40)	14.43 mg/dL (0.1–1)	516 (90–260)	224 (7–32)	Marked thickened	Yes
Agergaard and Larsen (2015) [22]	34, F	Denmark	No	Yes	No	Yes	No	—	61 (10–45)	42 μmol/L (5–25)	429 (35–105)	—	11.3 mm	Yes
Koufakis and Gabranis (2016) [23]	21, M	Greece	No	No	No	Yes	—	172 (<40)	232 (<40)	6.31 mg/dL (0–1)	179 (<140)	350 (<30)	4.5 mm	No
Present Case	30, F	Turkey	No	No	Yes	Yes	Spleno-megaly	233 (8–37)	220 (15–65)	15.4 mg/dL (0–1)	376 (50–136)	471 (5–55)	7.4 mm	No

ALT: alanine aminotransferase, AST: aspartate aminotransferase, ALP: Alkaline phosphatase, GGT: gamma-glutamyl transferase, GWT: gallbladder wall thickness, (): normal values only noted when described in the study, and —:missing values.

ALT was in Cholongitas's study (584 IU/L). Severe liver injury during EBV infection is very rare and is mostly reported in the posttransplant and immunodeficiency settings [30]. Markers of severe involvement such as hyperammonemia or prolonged prothrombin time were not documented in any of the cases we reviewed.

The diagnosis of AAC is based on clinical symptoms, laboratory tests, and ultrasonographic image. Abdominal ultrasonography is the main diagnostic method. Criteria such as GWT of over 3.5 mm, distention of the gallbladder, localized tenderness (sonographic Murphy's sign), and pericholecystic fluid and sludge have been used for the diagnosis of AAC. The combination of two or more of the above-mentioned findings, in the appropriate clinical setting, is considered to be diagnostic [7, 31]. Deitch and Engel reported a specificity of 90% with a 3 mm GWT and 98,5% with a 3.5 mm GWT, whereas sensitivity was 100% at 3 mm but only 80% at 3.5 mm [32, 33]. According to this, a GWT of 3.5 mm or more is generally accepted to be diagnostic for AAC. In our case the GWT was 7.4 mm with a pericholecystic fluid and GWT of other cases we reviewed were between 4.5 and 16 mm. Isolated GWT is a well-known feature during IM and has been been proposed as a sign of severity of the illness [8, 34]. However we consider that the wall thickening of our patient's gallbladder was a consequence of the developed AAC.

The treatment of AAC involves serial examinations, gallbladder ultrasonography, and cholecystectomy when indicated by deteriorating clinical or ultrasonographic findings. AAC due to bacterial infections should be severe and treated with antibiotics, and gallbladder percutaneous drainage should be performed [7]. In our case percutaneous drainage was thought to be unnecessary, because her symptoms and clinical course were gradually improved with conservative therapy. The treatment of EBV-associated AAC is usually supportive and antibiotics are not indicated and most cases resolve spontaneously. All the cases we reviewed had favourable outcomes. In most of the cases, antibiotics were discontinued after the diagnosis of EBV infection was performed. There was no difference in clinical course of the patients treated with antibiotics compared with patients not receiving antibiotics in the cases we reviewed. We did not use antibiotics in our case. The patient was admitted to our hospital with a history of beta-lactam antibiotic usage for the last 7 days, but her symptoms gradually increased despite antibiotic usage. Therefore we wanted to see the results of viral markers and the 3rd day of hospital stay primary EBV infection was investigated. While AAC is considered as a surgical emergency in critically ill patients, in the course of EBV-associated AAC surgical intervention is rarely necessary. In our review, only one patient, receiving azathioprine for an inflammatory bowel disease, reported by Hagel et al. underwent cholecystectomy [15]. Although EBV infections are rarely severe, AAC may cause gallbladder perforation [20]. Thus, a 22-year-old woman with severe EBV-associated AAC with suspected gallbladder perforation was described by Chalupa et al. and was treated without surgery [14].

In summary we reviewed sixteen adult cases with AAC associated with primary EBV infection reported in the

literature since 2007. All but one case were females and most of them were young adults. In general all patients had similar gastrointestinal symptoms (classic symptoms of EBV infection were not predominant), and markedly elevations in cholestatic markers and moderate transaminase level elevations were the most common laboratory findings. GWT in the ultrasound scanning were between 4.5 and 16 mm. Only one patient required surgical intervention and all other patients recovered with conservative therapy even though one was suspected to have perforation of the gallbladder.

4. Conclusion

Acute acalculous cholecystitis may develop during the course of primary EBV infection, especially in young women with cholestatic hepatitis. Abdominal ultrasonography should be performed when a patient is admitted with right upper quadrant pain or jaundice during the course of IM, to avoid unnecessary surgical therapy and overuse of antibiotic.

Competing Interests

The authors declare that they have no competing interests.

References

[1] Y. Edoute, Y. Baruch, J. Lachter, E. Furman, L. Bassan, and N. Assy, "Case report: Severe cholestatic jaundice induced by Epstein-Barr virus infection in the elderly," *Journal of Gastroenterology and Hepatology*, vol. 13, no. 8, pp. 821–824, 1998.

[2] M. Barreales, M. Pérez-Carreras, T. Meizoso et al., "Epstein-Barr virus infection and acute cholestatic hepatitis," *Anales de Medicina Interna*, vol. 23, no. 10, pp. 483–486, 2006.

[3] D. P. Kofteridis, M. Koulentaki, A. Valachis et al., "Epstein Barr virus hepatitis," *European Journal of Internal Medicine*, vol. 22, no. 1, pp. 73–76, 2011.

[4] T. B. Hinedi and R. S. Koff, "Cholestatic hepatitis induced by Epstein-Barr virus infection in an adult," *Digestive Diseases and Sciences*, vol. 48, no. 3, pp. 539–541, 2003.

[5] G. Barlow, R. Kilding, and S. T. Green, "Epstein-Barr virus infection mimicking extrahepatic biliary obstruction," *Journal of the Royal Society of Medicine*, vol. 93, no. 6, pp. 316–318, 2000.

[6] E. C. Johannsen, R. T. Schooley, and K. M. Kaye, "Epstein-Barr virüs (infectious mononucleosis)," in *Principles and Practice of Infectious Diseases*, G. L. Mandell, J. E. Bennett, and R. Dolin, Eds., pp. 1801–1820, Churchill Livingstone, Philadelphia, Pa, USA, 6th edition, 2005.

[7] P. S. Barie and S. R. Eachempati, "Acute acalculous cholecystitis," *Gastroenterology Clinics of North America*, vol. 39, no. 2, pp. 343–357, 2010.

[8] N. O'Donovan and E. Fitzgerald, "Gallbladder wall thickening in infectious mononucleosis: an ominous sign," *Postgraduate Medical Journal*, vol. 72, no. 847, pp. 299–300, 1996.

[9] E. Lagona, F. Sharifi, A. Voutsioti, A. Mavri, M. Markouri, and A. Attilakos, "Epstein-barr virus infectious mononucleosis associated with acute acalculous cholecystitis," *Infection*, vol. 35, no. 2, pp. 118–119, 2007.

[10] A. D. Koch, H. C. M. Van Den Bosch, and B. Bravenboer, "Epstein-Barr virus-associated cholecystitis," *Annals of Internal Medicine*, vol. 146, no. 11, pp. 826–827, 2007.

[11] C. Iaria, L. Arena, G. Di Maio et al., "Acute acalculous cholecystitis during the course of primary Epstein-Barr virus infection: a new case and a review of the literature," *International Journal of Infectious Diseases*, vol. 12, no. 4, pp. 391–395, 2008.

[12] E. Cholongitas, K. Katsogridakis, and M. Dasenaki, "Acalculous cholecystitis during the course of acute Epstein-Barr virus infection," *International Journal of Infectious Diseases*, vol. 13, no. 3, pp. e129–e130, 2009.

[13] H. N. Yang, K. W. Hong, J. S. Lee, and J. S. Eom, "A case of acute cholecystitis without cholestasis caused by Epstein-Barr virus in a healthy young woman," *International Journal of Infectious Diseases*, vol. 14, no. 5, pp. e448–e449, 2010.

[14] P. Chalupa, M. Kaspar, and M. Holub, "Acute acalculous cholecystitis with pericholecystitis in a patient with Epstein-Barr Virus infectious mononucleosis," *Medical Science Monitor*, vol. 15, no. 2, pp. CS30–CS33, 2009.

[15] S. Hagel, T. Bruns, M. Kantowski, P. Fix, T. Seidel, and A. Stallmach, "Cholestatic hepatitis, acute acalculous cholecystitis, and hemolytic anemia: primary Epstein-Barr virus infection under azathioprine," *Inflammatory Bowel Diseases*, vol. 15, no. 11, pp. 1613–1616, 2009.

[16] V. Beltrame, A. Andres, F. Tona, and C. Sperti, "Epstein-barr virus—associated acute acalculous cholecystitis in an adult," *American Journal of Case Reports*, vol. 13, pp. 153–156, 2012.

[17] A. Nagdev and J. Ward, "Bedside ultrasound diagnosis of acalculous cholecystitis from Epstein-Barr virus," *Western Journal of Emergency Medicine*, vol. 12, no. 4, pp. 481–483, 2011.

[18] J. Dylewski, "Acute acalculous cholecystitis caused by Epstein-Barr virus infection," *Clinical Microbiology Newsletter*, vol. 34, no. 1, pp. 7–8, 2012.

[19] M. F. Carrascosa, J.-R. S. Caviedes, G. Soler-Dorda, and C. Saiz-Pérez, "Epstein-Barr virus acute cholecystitis," *BMJ Case Reports*, vol. 2012, 2012.

[20] A. Gagneux-Brunon, F. Suy, A. Pouvaret et al., "Acute acalculous cholecystitis, a rare complication of Epstein-Barr virus primary infection: report of two cases and review," *Journal of Clinical Virology*, vol. 61, no. 1, pp. 173–175, 2014.

[21] F. Çelik, F. Tekin, T. Yamazhan, and F. Gunsar, "Epstein-barr virüs associated acute acalculous cholecystitis," *Journal of Gastroenterology and Hepatology Research*, vol. 3, no. 7, pp. 1179–1180, 2014.

[22] J. Agergaard and C. S. Larsen, "Acute acalculous cholecystitis in a patient with primary Epstein-Barr virus infection: a case report and literature review," *International Journal of Infectious Diseases*, vol. 35, pp. 67–72, 2015.

[23] T. Koufakis and I. Gabranis, "Another report of acalculous cholecystitis in a greek patient with infectious mononucleosis: a matter of luck or genetic predisposition?" *Case Reports in Hepatology*, vol. 2016, Article ID 6080832, 3 pages, 2016.

[24] J. A. Mendonça, J. F. Marques-Neto, P. Prando, and S. Appenzeller, "Acute acalculous cholecystitis in juvenile systemic lupus erythematosus," *Lupus*, vol. 18, no. 6, pp. 561–563, 2009.

[25] C.-J. Chen, F.-C. Huang, M.-M. Tiao et al., "Sonographic gallbladder abnormality is associated with intravenous immunoglobulin resistance in Kawasaki disease," *The Scientific World Journal*, vol. 2012, Article ID 485758, 5 pages, 2012.

[26] P. S. Barie and S. R. Eachempati, "Acute acalculous cholecystitis," *Current Gastroenterology Reports*, vol. 5, no. 4, pp. 302–309, 2003.

[27] S. I. Myers, "The role of eicosanoids in experimental and clinical gallbladder disease," *Prostaglandins, Leukotrienes and Essential Fatty Acids*, vol. 45, no. 3, pp. 167–180, 1992.

[28] R. R. Babb, "Acute acalculous cholecystitis. A review," *Journal of Clinical Gastroenterology*, vol. 15, no. 3, pp. 238–241, 1992.

[29] A. Attilakos, A. Prassouli, G. Hadjigeorgiou et al., "Acute acalculous cholecystitis in children with Epstein-Barr virus infection: a role for Gilbert's syndrome?" *International Journal of Infectious Diseases*, vol. 13, no. 4, pp. e161–e164, 2009.

[30] L. J. Vine, K. Shepherd, J. G. Hunter et al., "Characteristics of Epstein-Barr virus hepatitis among patients with jaundice or acute hepatitis," *Alimentary Pharmacology & Therapeutics*, vol. 36, no. 1, pp. 16–21, 2012.

[31] F. Alkhoury, D. Diaz, and J. Hidalgo, "Acute acalculous cholecystitis (AAC) in the pediatric population associated with Epstein-Barr Virus (EBV) infection. Case report and review of the literature," *International Journal of Surgery Case Reports*, vol. 11, pp. 50–52, 2015.

[32] E. A. Deitch and J. M. Engel, "Ultrasound in elective biliary tract surgery," *The American Journal of Surgery*, vol. 140, no. 2, pp. 277–283, 1980.

[33] E. A. Deitch and J. M. Engel, "Acute acalculous cholecystitis. Ultrasonic diagnosis," *The American Journal of Surgery*, vol. 142, no. 2, pp. 290–292, 1981.

[34] K. Yamada and H. Yamada, "Gallbladder wall thickening in mononucleosis syndromes," *Journal of Clinical Ultrasound*, vol. 29, no. 6, pp. 322–325, 2001.

34

Rapidly Progressive Spontaneous Spinal Epidural Abscess

Abdurrahman Aycan,[1] **Ozgür Yusuf Aktas,**[2] **Feyza Karagoz Guzey,**[2]
Azmi Tufan,[2] **Cihan Isler,**[2] **Nur Aycan,**[3] **İsmail Gulsen,**[1] **and Harun Arslan**[1]

[1]*Neurosurgery Department, Yuzuncu Yıl University Faculty of Medicine, 65040 Van, Turkey*
[2]*Neurosurgery Department, Bagcilar Training and Research Hospital, Istanbul, Turkey*
[3]*Pediatric Department, Private İstanbul Hospital, Van, Turkey*

Correspondence should be addressed to Abdurrahman Aycan; abdurrahmanaycan07@gmail.com

Academic Editor: Paola Di Carlo

Spinal epidural abscess (SEA) is a rare disease which is often rapidly progressive. Delayed diagnosis of SEA may lead to serious complications and the clinical findings of SEA are generally nonspecific. Paraspinal abscess should be considered in the presence of local low back tenderness, redness, and pain with fever, particularly in children. In case of delayed diagnosis and treatment, SEA may spread to the epidural space and may cause neurological deficits. Magnetic resonance imaging (MRI) remains the method of choice in the diagnosis of SEA. Treatment of SEA often consists of both medical and surgical therapy including drainage with percutaneous entry, corpectomy, and instrumentation.

1. Case

A 13-year-old girl presented to our clinic with a 10-day history of low back pain, muscle tenderness, fever, and skin rash. Lumbar MRI showed abscess formation in the paravertebral area at the level of L4-L5 (Figures 1(a) and 1(b)). Initially, the patient refused treatment but after three days, she was readmitted to our clinic due to the increasing complaints including paraparesis in the lower extremities, loss of sensation, and sphincter dysfunction. Systemic examination was normal. Neurological examination revealed a positive Lasègue sign at an angle of 30 degrees, bilateral hypoesthesia at the L3, L4, L5, and S1 dermatomes, paraparesis in the proximal and distal muscle groups of both lower extremities (3/5 and 1/5, resp.), and hypoactive reflex at the lower extremities.

Laboratory parameters were as follows: WBC: 18,500, HB: 5.13, HCI: 34, sedimentation: 80/h, CRP 95/2 h: 115 mg/L, RF: negative, *Salmonella* tests: negative *Brucella* tests: negative and ASO: N. Blood biochemistry and urine analysis were normal. The second thoracic and lumbar MRI scans demonstrated that the paravertebral abscess had spread to the epidural space extending between the levels of S1 and T12.

The patient was operated on under emergency conditions. Abscess drainage was achieved via the L-1, L-2, L-3, L-4, and L-5 hemilaminectomies and the epidural space was flushed with physiological serum. No bacterial growth was detected in the blood culture. Following the consultation with the Department of Infectious Diseases, an empirical antibiotic therapy including imipenem, aminoglycoside, and Metronidazole was started. Methicillin-resistant *Staphylococcus aureus* (MRSA) was detected in the pus culture of the patient. Depending on the culture-antibiogram results and the consultation with the Department of Infectious Diseases, imipenem was stopped and the antibiotic therapy was restarted with Vancomycin 4 × 500 mg (2 weeks), Penicillin 4 × 1 g, third-generation ceftriaxone 1 g/flk 2 × 1 (14 days), Metronidazole 500 mg flk 2 × 1 (5 days), and Paracetamol suspension (60 days). Rapid clinical improvement was observed within the first days after surgery. In the control lumbar MRI, no abscess was detected in the epidural and paravertebral areas and several scar tissues were seen in the paravertebral area (Figures 2(a) and 2(b)). Pathological examination revealed intensive active chronic nonspecific pus turning to abscess formation in the irregular bones,

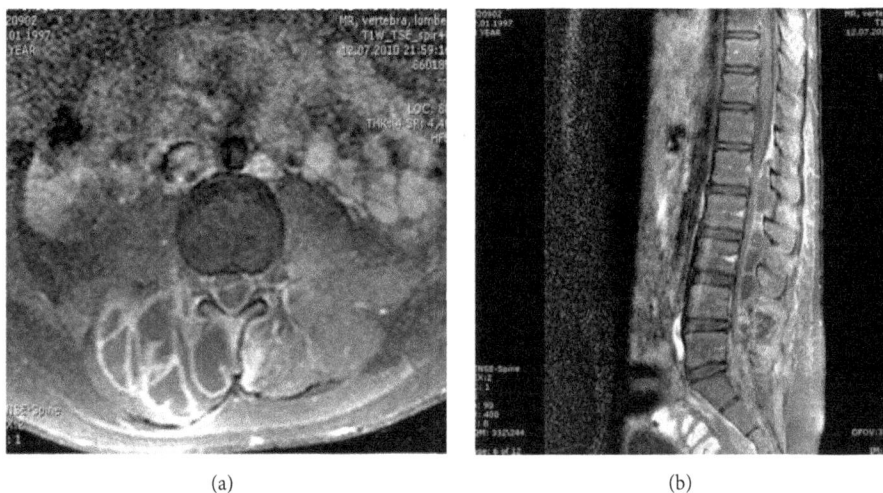

(a)   (b)

FIGURE 1: (a) Preoperative axial lumbar MRI. (b) Preoperative sagittal MRI.

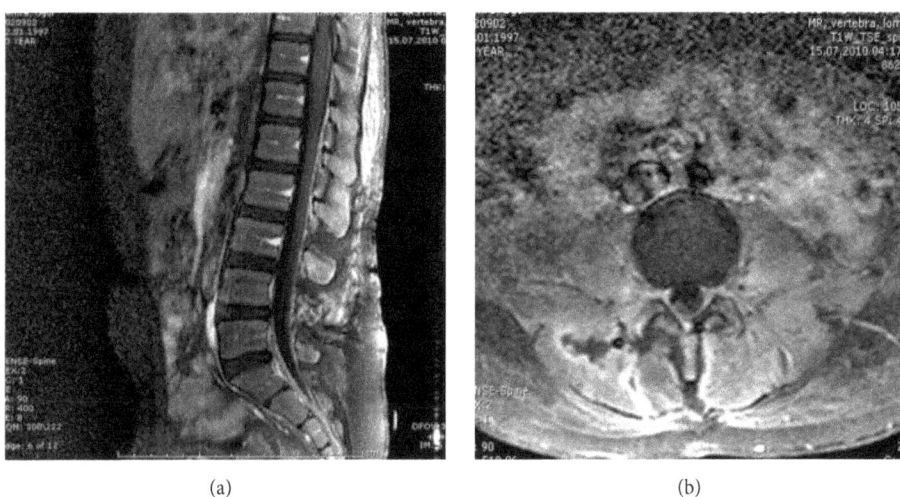

(a)   (b)

FIGURE 2: (a) Postoperative sagittal MRI. (b) Postoperative axial MRI with contrast.

cartilage, striated muscles, and fat tissue fragments, abundant lipogranuloma formation caused by the macrophages in the fat tissues, and an increase in connective tissues.

The patient was followed up for 3 years. At annual follow-up visits, no low back pain or sign of infection was detected. No kyphotic increase was observed. The present lumbar MRI images were obtained at follow-up year 3 (Figures 3(a) and 3(b)).

2. Discussion

Spontaneous spinal epidural abscess (SEA) is not common in neurosurgical practice. The incidence of SEA is reported to be 1/100,000 individuals, whereas some other studies have reported higher rates [1, 2]. SEA was first reported by Morgagni in 1796 [3, 4] and is usually known as a complication caused by spinal surgery. Epidural abscess may occur with hematogenously spreading infections in another part of the body or through the relation of contamination

during surgery, lumbar drainage, and spinal anesthesia or after discography. Most of the SEA patients present with an immunosuppressive disease such as AIDS, diabetes mellitus (DM), chronic renal failure, and tumor. Of these, DM is the most common comorbidity [5]. About 10–20% of the SEA patients present no predisposing factors [6, 7]. Similarly, no predisposing factor was detected in our patient.

SEA is mostly characterized by the fluid collection and inflammatory process on the surrounding dura mater and adipose tissue [8]. The most common strain isolated in SEA patients is *S. aureus*, followed by Streptococci, anaerobic bacteria, and Gram-negative bacilli [9]. Similarly, *S. aureus* was the most common bacterium detected in our patient.

SEA presents three clinical manifestations: acute, subacute, and chronic [10]. The acute symptoms of SEA may be manifested in a few hours or days and are characterized by significant fluid collection. The chronic symptoms of SEA, characterized by inflammatory granular tissue, are relatively slower and may be manifested within weeks or months.

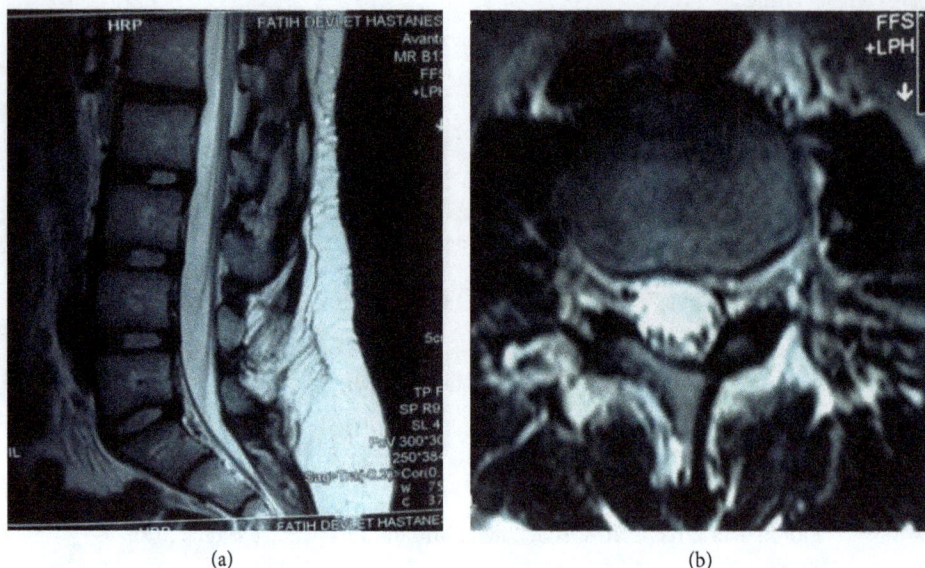

(a)   (b)

FIGURE 3: The 3rd year after the operation.

SEA is mostly seen at the thoracic area, followed by lumbar and cervical areas. Common clinical findings of SEA include pain, inflammation, radicular symptoms, spinal cord compression, and the symptoms of cauda equina syndrome [8]. SEA may be mislocalized by the clinical findings and thus the diagnosis of SEA is difficult.

In 1986, three different pathogenic mechanisms were described for paraparesis regarding bacterial infections: (I) with nonspecific polyarthritis, (II) with mass effect of epidural abscess or vertebral collapse related to spondylitis, and (III) with ischemic spinal cord lesion as a result of the abdominal aorta septic thromboembolism [11]. In our patient, depending on their mechanisms of paraparesis, the abscess was considered to be with mass effect.

Magnetic resonance imaging (MRI) remains the method of choice in the diagnosis of SEA [9, 12]. When compared to other methods, MRI provides better outcomes particularly in the early stages of SEA [13, 14].

The primary aims in the treatment of SEA are to identify microorganisms, ensure the drainage of abscess, perform the debridement of granulation tissue, and, if needed, perform spinal stabilization. Treatment of SEA often consists of both medical and surgical therapy including drainage with percutaneous entry, corpectomy, and instrumentation [15]. SEA often is posterior spinal settled. So with hemilaminectomy or laminectomy, it is adequate drainage and debridement. If vertebral osteomyelitis is present, discectomy, corpectomy, or debridement should be performed with stabilization [16].

SEA is a rapidly progressive disease resulting in severe morbidity and mortality in children. Therefore, SEA should be considered in the children presenting with tenderness in the spinal area and pain with or without fever. As in our case, empirical antibiotic therapy is required in SEA patients. In the patients presenting with paravertebral abscess, blood sample should be obtained via abscess drainage and the patient should be strictly monitored during the antibiotic therapy.

If neurological deficits or a worsening clinical status appears, radiological imaging should be immediately performed (particularly, MRI) and if neural compression is detected, surgical procedure should be promptly performed. Otherwise, SEA may progress rapidly and may consequently lead to sequela. Paraparesis should be kept in mind in the patients presenting with lumbosacral SEA.

Competing Interests

The authors declare that they have no competing interests.

References

[1] O. V. Batson, "The vertebral vein system," *The American Journal of Roentgenology, Radium Therapy and Nuclear Medicine*, vol. 78, pp. 195–212, 1957.

[2] D. Rigamonti, L. Liem, P. Sampath et al., "Spinal epidural abscess: contemporary trends in etiology, evaluation, and management," *Surgical Neurology*, vol. 52, no. 2, pp. 189–197, 1999.

[3] R. K. Khanna, G. M. Malik, J. P. Rock, and M. L. Rosenblum, "Spinal epidural abscess: evaluation of factors influencing outcome," *Neurosurgery*, vol. 39, no. 5, pp. 958–964, 1996.

[4] G. L. Rea, J. M. McGregor, C. A. Miller, and M. E. Miner, "Surgical treatment of the spontaneous spinal epidural abscess," *Surgical Neurology*, vol. 37, no. 4, pp. 274–279, 1992.

[5] M. L. Hlavin, H. J. Kaminski, J. S. Ross, and E. Ganz, "Spinal epidural abscess; a ten-year perspective," *Neurosurgery*, vol. 27, no. 2, pp. 177–184, 1990.

[6] G. M. Vilke and E. A. Honingford, "Cervical spine epidural abscess in a patient with no predisposing risk factors," *Annals of Emergency Medicine*, vol. 27, no. 6, pp. 777–780, 1996.

[7] H.-J. Tang, H.-J. Lin, Y.-C. Liu, and C.-M. Li, "Spinal epidural abscess-experience with 46 patients and evaluation of prognostic factors," *Journal of Infection*, vol. 45, no. 2, pp. 76–81, 2002.

[8] P. Sampath and D. Rigamonti, "Spinal epidural abscess: a review of epidemiology, diagnosis, and treatment," *Journal of Spinal Disorders*, vol. 12, no. 2, pp. 89–93, 1999.

[9] J. A. Shulman and H. M. Blumberg, "Paraspinal andspinal infections," in *Infections of the Central Nervous System*, H. P. Lambert, Ed., pp. 374–391, BC Decker, Philadelphia, Pa, USA, 1991.

[10] S.-N. H. Khan, M. S. Hussain, R. W. Griebel, and S. Hattingh, "Title comparison of primary and secondary spinal epidural abscesses: a retrospective analysis of 29 cases," *Surgical Neurology*, vol. 59, no. 1, pp. 28–33, 2003.

[11] J. Syrjänen, M. Iivanainen, M. Kallio, H. Somer, and V. V. Valtonen, "Three different pathogenic mechanisms for paraparesis in association with bacterial infections," *Annals of Clinical Research*, vol. 18, no. 4, pp. 191–194, 1986.

[12] M. E. Carey, "Infections of the spine and spinal cord," in *Neurological Surgery*, J. R. Youmans, Ed., pp. 3759–3781, WB Saunders, Philadelphia, Pa, USA, 3rd edition, 1990.

[13] D. C. Wirtz, I. Genius, J. E. Wildberger, G. Adam, K.-W. Zilkens, and F. U. Niethard, "Diagnostic and therapeutic management of lumbar and thoracic spondylodiscitis—an evaluation of 59 cases," *Archives of Orthopaedic and Trauma Surgery*, vol. 120, no. 5-6, pp. 245–251, 2000.

[14] F. Vorbeck, M. Morscher, A. Ba-Ssalamah, and H. Imhof, "Infectious spondylitis in adults," *Radiologe*, vol. 36, no. 10, pp. 795–804, 1996.

[15] H. Wessling and P. De Las Heras, "Cervicothoracolumbar spinal epidural abscess with tetraparesis. Good recovery after nonsurgical treatment with antibiotics and dexamethasone. Case report and review of the literature," *Neurocirugia*, vol. 14, no. 6, pp. 529–533, 2003.

[16] O. Eser, A. Aslan, Ö. Şahin, and H. Fidan, "Progressif paraparezi ile gelen lumbosakral spinal epidural abse," *Turkiye Klinikleri Journal of Medical Sciences*, vol. 26, pp. 471–473, 2006.

35

On-Treatment Elevation in Hepatic Transaminases during HCV Treatment with Ombitasvir, Paritaprevir, Dasabuvir, Ritonavir, and Ribavirin

Madelyne Bean,[1,2] Lydia Tang,[3] Shyam Kottilil,[3] Kimberly L. Beavers,[4] and Eric G. Meissner[1]

[1]Division of Infectious Diseases, Department of Medicine, Medical University of South Carolina,
135 Rutledge Avenue Suite 1209, MSC 752, Charleston, SC 29425, USA

[2]Department of Pharmacy Services, Medical University of South Carolina, 150 Ashley Avenue, Charleston, SC 29425, USA

[3]Institute of Human Virology, University of Maryland School of Medicine, 725 West Lombard Street, Baltimore, MD 21201, USA

[4]Division of Gastroenterology and Hepatology, Department of Medicine, Medical University of South Carolina,
114 Doughty Street Suite 249, MSC 702, Charleston, SC 29425, USA

Correspondence should be addressed to Eric G. Meissner; meissner@musc.edu

Academic Editor: Tomoyuki Shibata

Eradication of chronic hepatitis C virus (HCV) infection is now possible with all oral antiviral medications, including the combination of ombitasvir, paritaprevir, dasabuvir, and ritonavir (PrOD) with or without ribavirin. While high rates of sustained virologic response (SVR) can be achieved, a small subset of patients experience on-treatment liver enzyme elevations, in particular women using concurrent estradiol-containing oral contraceptive medications (OCPs). Herein, we describe four cases of liver enzyme elevations within 2-3 weeks of PrOD initiation in African-American men infected with HCV genotype 1a or 1b. Three patients with varying degrees of hepatic fibrosis received a full treatment course without medication modification, achieved SVR, and experienced resolution of liver enzyme abnormalities. One patient with cirrhosis was switched mid-treatment to an alternate HCV regimen, experienced subsequent resolution of liver enzyme abnormalities, and achieved SVR. In summary, these cases suggest that all HCV patients treated with PrOD, independent of gender or concurrent medications, should have laboratory monitoring for liver enzyme elevations, with a particular emphasis on early monitoring in cirrhotic patients.

1. Introduction

Eradication of chronic hepatitis C virus (HCV) infection is now possible with all oral regimens composed of directly acting antiviral (DAA) agents. The combination of ombitasvir (an HCV NS5A inhibitor), paritaprevir (an NS3/4A protease inhibitor), dasabuvir (a nonnucleoside NS5B polymerase inhibitor), and ritonavir (collectively referred to as PrOD) with or without ribavirin is FDA approved for treatment of genotype 1a/1b in patients with HCV monoinfection and HIV/HCV coinfection [1]. High rates of sustained virologic response (SVR) are routinely achieved, with treatment duration and concomitant ribavirin use dependent upon genotype-1 subtype and presence of cirrhosis [2–5].

An increase in serum levels of aspartate transaminase (AST) and alanine transaminase (ALT) greater than 5 times the upper limit of normal (ULN) has been observed in a minority (~1%) of patients treated with PrOD in clinical trials [1]. Women taking concomitant estradiol-containing oral contraceptive pills (OCPs) during PrOD treatment have thus far been the primary identified risk group for liver enzyme elevation [1]. In HCV monoinfected subjects, on-treatment AST/ALT elevations were noted to be typically asymptomatic, with onset in the first 4 weeks of treatment and decline within

8 weeks during continued treatment [1]. In a small study of 63 HIV/HCV patients, only 1 patient treated with PrOD and ribavirin for 24 weeks had an AST value greater than 5 times the ULN, while 15 of 17 patients with bilirubin increases 3–10x ULN were taking concomitant atazanavir for HIV [5].

Although hepatic transaminase elevation during PrOD treatment is well reported, there are as yet no published reports describing in detail the temporal changes in AST/ALT that can occur to help guide expectations for clinicians and aid in patient management. With the recent report of hepatic decompensation in a subset of cirrhotic patients treated with PrOD, particularly those with more advanced cirrhosis [6], understanding the clinical characteristics of this uncommon side effect is imperative. Here, we describe the detailed clinical course for 4 African-American male patients treated with PrOD with or without ribavirin who developed on-treatment elevation in AST/ALT, all of whom demonstrate a clinical scenario similar to that described for women on OCPs, and all of whom achieved SVR with treatment.

2. Case Presentation

2.1. Case 1. A 62-year-old presented with treatment-naïve, HCV genotype 1b infection, and well-controlled HIV coinfection on a regimen of emtricitabine, tenofovir, atazanavir, and ritonavir with a CD4 count of 580 cells/mm^3 and an HIV viral load < 40 copies/mL. Liver biopsy in 2004 revealed stage 0 disease, liver staging by Fibrosure in 2012 suggested F3-F4 disease (measured while taking atazanavir), and a 1.9 cm liver biopsy in 2013 again revealed stage 0 disease. Additional noninvasive staging revealed a FIB4 score of 2.3 and an APRI score of 0.89. Ultrasonography revealed normal liver size and echogenicity, with no evidence of portal hypertension or splenomegaly. Baseline labs included HCV viral load 61,251 IU/mL, platelets 158,000/mm^3, ALT 83 IU/mL, AST 56 IU/mL, albumin 4.0 g/dL, and total bilirubin 2.0 IU/mL (bilirubin elevation likely due to atazanavir). He had no other significant past medical history or medication use, other than receiving azithromycin for chlamydia urethritis 3 days prior to initiating PrOD therapy for 12 weeks without ribavirin. Safety labs obtained at week 1 of treatment revealed an elevation in AST/ALT over pretreatment values (Figure 1(a)). During continued treatment, he remained asymptomatic and had frequent laboratory checks, including direct bilirubin to monitor for drug-induced liver injury, as baseline indirect bilirubin was elevated due to atazanavir. By week 7 hepatic transaminases had declined markedly from their peak (Figure 1(a)). No medication modifications were made during PrOD treatment, and he achieved SVR 12 weeks after treatment with liver enzymes in the normal range.

2.2. Case 2. A 61-year-old presented with treatment-naïve, HCV genotype 1a monoinfection with liver biopsy 3 years prior to treatment revealing stage 1-2 fibrosis and FibroScan 2 months prior to treatment showing a stiffness score of 9.5 kPa, suggesting F2-F3 disease. Additional noninvasive staging revealed a FIB4 score of 2.3 and an APRI score of 0.68. Baseline labs included HCV viral load 11.6 million IU/mL, platelets 162,000/mm^3, ALT 52 U/L, AST 44 U/L, albumin

4.4 g/dL, and total bilirubin 0.9 mg/dL. Past medical history included spinal fusion surgery, hypertension (not on medications), and hyperlipidemia (on pravastatin 40 mg daily, a dose that did not require modification) [1]. PrOD was initiated for 12 weeks with weight-based ribavirin. At week 4 of treatment, an elevation in AST/ALT over baseline values was observed (Figure 1(b)). He reported mild side effects from therapy including fatigue, headache, insomnia, and itching that all resolved by week 4 of treatment. PrOD and ribavirin therapy were continued, he remained asymptomatic, and 12 weeks after treatment AST/ALT were in the normal range and HCV RNA was undetectable, indicating SVR.

2.3. Case 3. A 63-year-old presented with treatment-naïve, genotype 1a HCV monoinfection, with liver biopsy 4 years prior to treatment revealing stage 2-3 disease. Prior to treatment, noninvasive staging revealed a FIB4 score of 1.6 and an APRI score of 0.35. Baseline labs included HCV viral load 1.1 million IU/mL, platelets 194,000/mm^3, ALT 28 U/L, AST 27 U/L, albumin 4.1 g/dL, and total bilirubin 1.5. Past medical history included hypertension, for which he took amlodipine and hydrochlorothiazide. PrOD was initiated for 12 weeks with weight-based ribavirin. At week 2 of treatment, labs revealed an elevation in AST/ALT over baseline values (Figure 1(c)). He was asymptomatic and treatment was continued without dose modification. By week 3, hepatic transaminases were declining and normalized by week 8. Hemoglobin and hematocrit remained stable throughout the treatment course and the patient achieved SVR.

2.4. Case 4. An 82-year-old presented with treatment-naïve, genotype 1a HCV monoinfection with FibroScan 4 months prior to treatment revealing a stiffness score of 14 kPa, suggesting cirrhosis. Noninvasive staging scores were FIB4 4.6 and APRI 1.3. Liver ultrasound revealed changes consistent with cirrhosis and no concerning masses. Pretreatment labs included HCV viral load 46,382 IU/mL, platelets 160,000/mm^3, ALT 86 U/L, AST 84 U/L, albumin 3.6 g/dL, and total bilirubin 1.5 U/L. Past medical history included hypertension (on hydrochlorothiazide), chronic idiopathic peripheral neuropathy (on gabapentin), and cecal adenocarcinoma treated surgically. Patient evaluation at treatment initiation did not reveal any signs of decompensated cirrhosis. Treatment with PrOD with weight-based ribavirin was initiated. At week 2, safety labs revealed unchanged AST/ALT values and a slight increase in total bilirubin (Figure 1(d)), as well as a decline in hemoglobin and hematocrit from 15.3/45.2 g/L to 13.5/38.3 g/L, respectively. He was asymptomatic and treatment was continued without dose modification. By week 4 of treatment, AST/ALT had increased while total bilirubin remained stable (Figure 1(d)) and he reported mild foot swelling, not present prior to treatment initiation. Physical exam confirmed bilateral 1+ pitting edema on the dorsum of his feet. At week 5 of treatment, hemoglobin and hematocrit had declined to 11.7/35.4, respectively, and bilateral pedal edema had increased to 2+. Ribavirin dose was reduced from 1200 mg/day to 600 mg/day. By week 7 of treatment, AST/ALT had increased further (Figure 1(d)), hemoglobin and hematocrit remained stable, and creatinine had increased

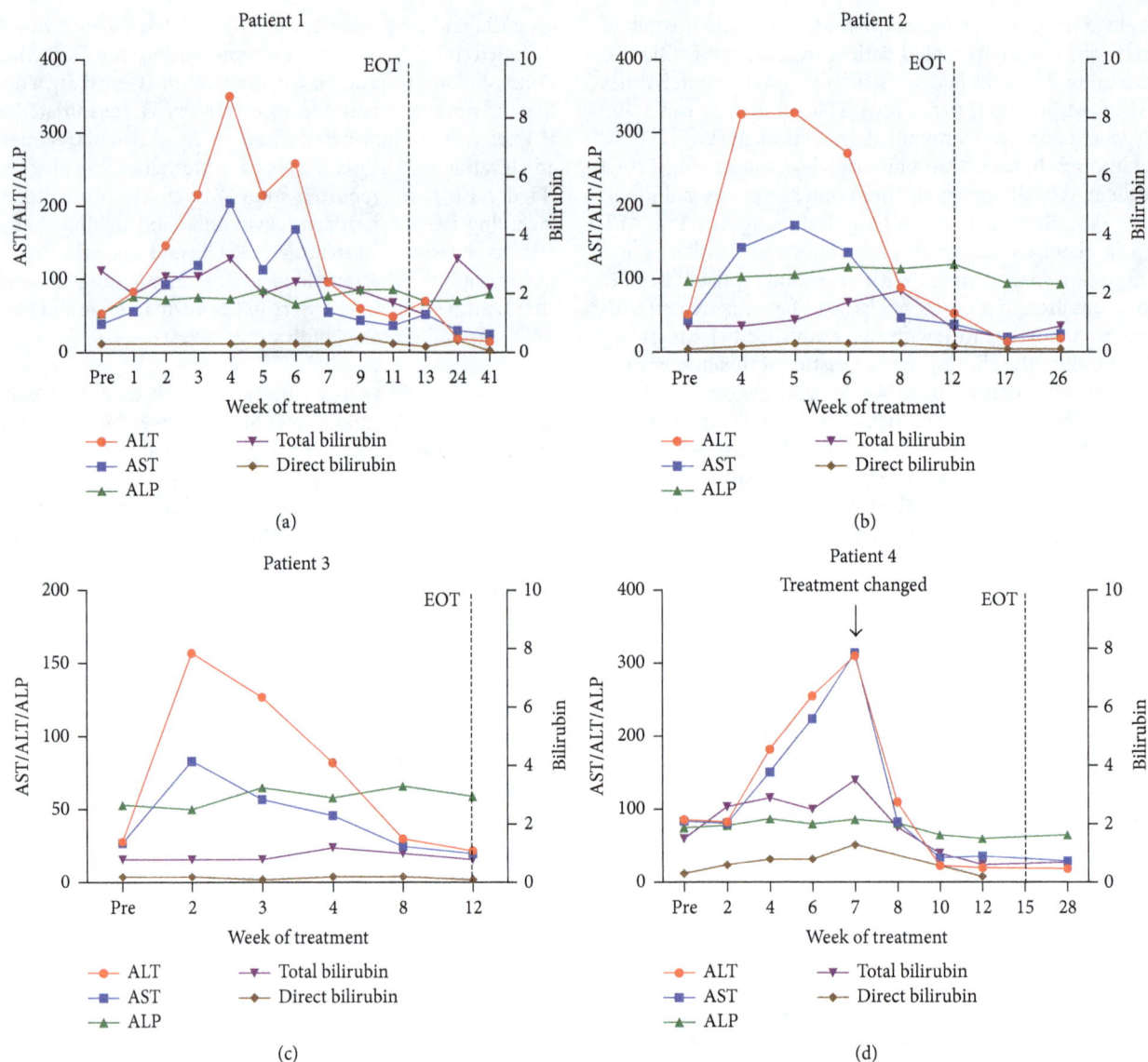

FIGURE 1: Liver enzyme progression for individual patients. EOT: end of treatment; ALP: alkaline phosphatase.

from 1.34 at baseline to 2.15 mg/dL. He remained asymptomatic and had stable foot swelling that was relieved by use of compression stockings. PrOD and ribavirin therapy were stopped and the patient continued HCV therapy with ledipasvir-sofosbuvir. At week 10 of total HCV therapy (week 3 of ledipasvir-sofosbuvir) serum creatinine and AST/ALT had returned to baseline and remained normal thereafter (Figure 1(d)). He completed a total of 8 weeks of ledipasvir-sofosbuvir following the 7 weeks of PrOD and ribavirin. Foot swelling persisted throughout treatment but had resolved by 28 weeks after initiation of treatment when SVR was achieved.

3. Discussion

Herein, we present a detailed clinical description of AST/ALT elevations that can occur during PrOD therapy, with or without ribavirin, for chronic HCV genotype-1 infection. Although caution is recommended with concomitant use

of estradiol-containing oral contraceptive medications [1], all 4 subjects in our series were African-American males with advancing age and differing degrees of hepatic fibrosis, including 1 patient with cirrhosis. All completed HCV treatment, with therapy modification in 1 case, and all achieved SVR. No medications or comorbidities were shared amongst these patients in terms of an alternate etiology for the observed pattern of hepatic transaminases.

Aside from a higher risk of AST/ALT elevations reported in women taking concomitant estrogen therapy during PrOD therapy, there are no reports of other specific patient factors related to an increased incidence of enzyme alterations that may help clinicians target patients for close monitoring or anticipate liver enzyme elevations. This report indicates and suggests that these abnormalities can occur in African-American men with advanced age and highlights the importance of close lab monitoring during treatment in cirrhotic patients in light of new FDA warnings for risk of liver toxicity with PrOD use. To determine whether age, race, and gender are significant risk factors for ALT elevation during PrOD therapy would require observation in a larger cohort of treated patients. Of note, none of our patients had a liver enzyme pattern suggestive of drug-induced liver injury. For case 4, therapy was switched during the peak of AST/ALT elevation and within the reported typical window of lab abnormality resolution, and thus it is challenging to know whether hepatic transaminases would have resolved without a switch in therapy.

In summary, these cases suggest that all PrOD patients should have monitoring as early as week 2 of treatment to monitor for abnormalities, with a particular emphasis on early monitoring in cirrhotic patients. While the patients with advanced liver disease who experienced liver injury associated with PrOD suggested that elevated transaminases were not as prominent a feature of their presentation as that reported in the package insert [6], close monitoring in the setting of cirrhosis remains a recommendation. For HIV/HCV coinfected patients on antiretroviral therapy containing atazanavir, direct bilirubin should be utilized to monitor for drug-induced liver injury given elevations in indirect bilirubin as a result of atazanavir use. Importantly, these cases also highlight that AST/ALT elevations for those without cirrhosis did not have an apparent clinical consequence and all patients progressed to achieve SVR.

Competing Interests

Dr. Meissner receives institutional research support from Gilead Sciences.

References

[1] Viekira Pak, AbbVie, Inc, Chicago, Ill, USA, December 2014.

[2] J. J. Feld, K. V. Kowdley, E. Coakley et al., "Treatment of HCV with ABT-450/r-ombitasvir and dasabuvir with ribavirin," *The New England Journal of Medicine*, vol. 370, no. 17, pp. 1594–1603, 2014.

[3] F. Poordad, C. Hezode, R. Trinh et al., "ABT-450/r-ombitasvir and dasabuvir with ribavirin for hepatitis C with cirrhosis," *New England Journal of Medicine*, vol. 370, no. 21, pp. 1973–1982, 2014.

[4] P. Ferenci, D. Bernstein, J. Lalezari et al., "ABT-450/r-ombitasvir and dasabuvir with or without ribavirin for HCV," *The New England Journal of Medicine*, vol. 370, no. 21, pp. 1983–1992, 2014.

[5] M. S. Sulkowski, O. J. Eron, D. Wyles et al., "Ombitasvir, paritaprevir co-dosed with ritonavir, dasabuvir, and ribavirin for hepatitis C in patients co-infected with HIV-1 a randomized trial," *JAMA-Journal of the American Medical Association*, vol. 313, no. 12, pp. 1223–1231, 2015.

[6] U.S. Food and Drug Administration (FDA), FDA Drug Safety Communication: FDA warns of serious liver injury risk with hepatitis C treatments Viekira Pak and Technivie, October 2015, http://www.fda.gov/Drugs/DrugSafety/ucm468634.htm.

36

Granulomatous Lobular Mastitis Associated with *Mycobacterium abscessus* in South China: A Case Report and Review of the Literature

Ye-sheng Wang,[1] **Qi-wei Li,**[1] **Lin Zhou,**[1] **Run-feng Guan,**[1] **Xiang-ming Zhou,**[1] **Ji-hong Wu,**[1] **Nan-yan Rao,**[2] **and Shuang Zhu**[1]

[1]*Guangdong Province Key Laboratory for Biotechnology Drug Candidates, School of Biosciences and Biopharmaceutics, Guangdong Pharmaceutical University, Guangzhou, Guangdong 510006, China*
[2]*Sun Yat-sen Memorial Hospital of Zhongshan University, Guangzhou, Guangdong 510120, China*

Correspondence should be addressed to Nan-yan Rao; raonany@126.com and Shuang Zhu; 15683727@qq.com

Academic Editor: Tomoyuki Shibata

Mycobacteria, which are known as rapidly growing bacteria, are pathogens that are responsible for cutaneous or subcutaneous infections that especially occur after injection, trauma, or surgery. In this report, we describe a species of *Mycobacterium abscessus* that was isolated from a breast abscess in a patient who was previously diagnosed with granulomatous lobular mastitis (GLM). This current case is the first ever presented case of GLM associated with *M. abscessus* documented in South China. The case presentation highlights the role of *M. abscessus* in GLM. The association of *M. abscessus* and GLM is discussed and a summary of breast infection due to *Mycobacteria* is given.

1. Introduction

Granulomatous lobular mastitis (GLM), also known as idiopathic granulomatous mastitis, was first described by Kessler and Wolloch in 1972 [1]. GLM is a rare inflammatory condition of the breast with unknown etiology and variable treatment options [2–5]. Clinically, GLM may be present as a firm, red, tender lesion that suggests the presence of an abscess [6], or as a hard mass closely resembling a malignancy [7]. Although the majority GLM cases appear aseptic [8–10], case reports of documented coinfections with *Mycobacterium abscessus* have been reported in Turkey [11] and the United States [12]. To our knowledge, the present case is the first ever presented case of GLM associated with *M. abscessus* that is documented in South China.

2. Case Report

A 29-year-old female from South China with a history of swelling, discharge, and chronic abscesses of the right breast for more than 10 days presented to the Department of Breast Surgery in the Second Affiliated Hospital, Sun Yat-sen University, Guangzhou, China. About one month prior, the patient had noted a painful mass in the right breast and a mini-invasive operation was performed. The patient did not have a history of fever, night sweats, weight loss, and respiratory symptoms. In addition, there was no family history of breast cancer and no personal history of tuberculosis. The patient was referred to an outpatient surgery clinic, where a breast ultrasound demonstrated a duct ectasia hypoechoic lobulated mass measuring 16.7 mm × 9.8 mm in the lower quadrant of the right breast and palpable lymph nodes in the ipsilateral axilla. Blood tests showed that full blood count, renal function, liver function, thyroid function, and blood glucose were all within normal limits. The patient was treated with a variety of antibiotics, including doxycycline, clindamycin, and amoxicillin-clavulanic acid for 10 days, without success. The patient underwent drainage of the right breast and 1 ml of purulent fluid was aspirated.

Specimens were sent for routine bacteriology, acid-fast bacteria stain, Gram stain, fungal stains, and culture. Acid-fast bacilli were not found, and Gram staining of the pus

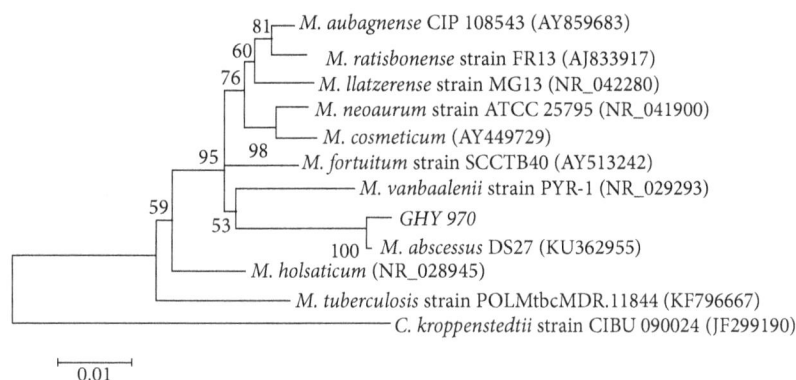

FIGURE 1: Phylogenetic tree based on 16S rDNA gene sequences of GHY 970.

showed that numerous polymorphonuclear leukocytes were present, however, without any organisms. The pus was plated on Columbia agar containing 5% sheep blood and incubated at 37°C in air supplemented with 5% CO_2. Three days after incubation, the presence of strain GHY 970 was confirmed. The colonies that were present on the blood agar plates were identified with 16S rDNA PCR and phylogenetic analysis. Genomic DNA was extracted with the TIANamp Genomic DNA Kit (cat. No. #DP304-02), according to the manufacturer's guidelines. Bacterial 16S rDNAs were amplified by PCR using the combination of a universal primer 1492r (5′ GGT TAC CTT GTT ACG ACT T 3′) and bacterial primer 27f (5′ AGA GTT TGA TCC TGG CTC AG 3′). PCR was performed using a thermal cycler with the following cycling parameters: 95°C for 5 min as initial denaturation followed by 30 cycles of 94°C for 30 s, 55°C for 30 s, 72°C for 1 min, and 72°C for 7 min as final extension. After purification, the amplified products were sent to BGI Company for sequencing analysis. Homology search was performed using BLAST (https://www.ncbi.nlm.nih.gov) and the differences in nucleotide sequences between various bacteria were determined using the sequence alignment editor "BioEdit". Products were further analyzed by MEGA 6.0. The Neighbor-Joining (NJ) tree was constructed using the Kimura-two-parameter (K2P) distance model. Phylogenetic analysis of the 16S rDNA gene sequence of strain GHY 970 revealed the species of *M. abscessus* (Figure 1). NCBI data search indicated >99% sequence identity to the *M. abscessus* DS27 (KU362955). Because the patient's treatment with antibiotics was discontinued, a new breast nodule appeared in the right breast, and the patient was treated with a combination of rifampicin, isoniazid, and pyrazinamide. After 3 months of treatment, the mass in the right breast and axillary lymph nodes had totally disappeared. The entire treatment therapy was completed by 6 months and, at follow-up after 1 year, there were no signs of recurrence or any other issues.

3. Discussion

M. abscessus, a rapidly growing type of *Mycobacterium*, is abundant in natural and processed water sources as well as in sewage and soil. *M. abscessus* primarily affects pulmonary,

soft tissue and causes disseminated infections [13]. *M. abscessus* may be present in cases following trauma or surgery after contamination of the wound, medical device implantation, and injection site abscesses. *Mycobacteria* encompass a broad range of Gram-positive bacilli that are often part of the skin microbiome. Therefore, trying to distinguish between colonization, infection, and contamination is challenging. GLM caused by *M. abscessus* is extremely rare and only occurs in few cases. We have summarized several cases of breast infection that are due to other *Mycobacteria* after nipple piercing: four cases of *M. fortuitum* [14–17] and one case of either *M. holsaticum, M. agricund,* or *M. brurnae* (Table 1) [18]. Taken together, breast abscesses can be caused by these organisms either before or after surgery.

In the case presented here, *M. abscessus* was isolated from breast abscess from a patient with GLM. Only few published reports that focus on *M. abscessus* associated with breast infections are available and, to our knowledge, this is the first case of GLM caused by *M. abscessus* in South China. Literature studies confirmed that *Mycobacterium* was not the only bacterial strain that associates with GLM. Previous studies in the USA and Canada showed that *Corynebacteria* are commonly detected in GLM [19, 20]. In addition, a recent study performed in China demonstrated that the predominance of *Corynebacteria*, especially *C. kroppenstedtii*, was observed in GLM [21]. In another study it was shown that breast tissue is not sterile but instead contains a diverse population of bacteria. The sources of these bacteria are unknown [22]. Thus, the *M. abscessus* found in this case may be one of the organisms associated with GLM. Therefore, to elucidate the pathological role of this organism in GLM, further research is warranted.

This case presentation was retrospective and, therefore, lacks a complete data set. However, we found that, in this patient, *M. abscessus* was associated with GLM. In the initial treatment approach of this patient, treatment with a variety of antibiotics was not successful. This could be due because the patient may be resistant to antibiotics. Therefore, antibiotic treatment was stopped and the patient underwent further clinical examination. It was suggested by clinicians and clinical microbiologists that the source of the *Mycobacteria* found in this case could be the nonpathogenic components of

TABLE 1: Cases of breast infection caused by *Mycobacteria* reported in the literature.

Case	Author, year	Age/ sex	Area (race)	Presentation	Surgery	Organism	Length of therapy	Outcome
1	Trupiano, 2001	17/f	American	Mass	Resection	*M. abscessus*	None	Complete response
2	Jacobs, 2002	35/f	German	Mass	Open biopsy	*M. holsaticum, M. agricund, M. brurnae*	10 days	Complete response
3	Lewis, 2004	29/f	American	Mass	Core needle and open biopsy	*M. fortuitum*	6 months	Complete response
4	Bengualid, 2008	17/f	American	Abscess	Incision and drainage	*M. fortuitum*	6 to 12 months	Relapse after 3 months
5	Yasar, 2011	38/f	Turks	Mass	Fine needle aspirations	*M. abscessus*	4 months	Complete response
6	Betal, 2011	51/f	Caucasian	Abscess	Incision and drainage	*M. fortuitum*	6 months	Complete response
7	Abbass, 2014	21/f	Canadian	Mass	Aspiration	*M. fortuitum*	6 months	Complete response
8	Present study, 2016	29/f	Chinese	Mass	Core needle and open biopsy	*M. abscessus*	1 year	Complete response

the normal microbiota of the skin flora. After the appearance of a new breast nodule, the patient was cured successfully with rifampicin, isoniazid, and pyrazinamide. Thus, this case presentation highlights the role of *M. abscessus* in GLM and should be targeted for optimal treatment therapy of GLM.

In addition to our study, eight cases of *Mycobacteria* were reviewed. *M. abscessus* and other *Mycobacteria* should be kept in mind when patients with chronic breast or soft tissue infections including recurrent breast abscess do not respond to standard antibiotic therapy. In conclusion, we report a patient with a breast abscess that is caused by *M. abscessus*. Drainage and a prolonged course of rifampicin, isoniazid, and pyrazinamide therapy were essential for successful treatment.

Competing Interests

The authors declare that they have no conflict of interests.

References

[1] E. Kessler and Y. Wolloch, "Granulomatous mastitis: a lesion clinically simulating carcinoma," *American Journal of Clinical Pathology*, vol. 58, no. 6, pp. 642–646, 1972.

[2] A. F. Azlina, Z. Ariza, T. Arni, and A. N. Hisham, "Chronic granulomatous mastitis: diagnostic and therapeutic considerations," *World Journal of Surgery*, vol. 27, no. 5, pp. 515–518, 2003.

[3] A. Akcan, H. Akyildiz, M. A. Deneme, H. Akgun, and Y. Aritas, "Granulomatous lobular mastitis: a complex diagnostic and therapeutic problem," *World Journal of Surgery*, vol. 30, no. 8, pp. 1403–1409, 2006.

[4] M. M. Baslaim, H. A. Khayat, and S. A. Al-Amoudi, "Idiopathic granulomatous mastitis: a heterogeneous disease with variable clinical presentation," *World Journal of Surgery*, vol. 31, no. 8, pp. 1677–1681, 2007.

[5] B. Al-Khaffaf, F. Knox, and N. J. Bundred, "Idiopathic granulomatous mastitis: a 25-year experience," *Journal of the American College of Surgeons*, vol. 206, no. 2, pp. 269–273, 2008.

[6] J. Pouchot, E. Foucher, M. Lino, J. Barge, and P. Vinceneux, "Granulomatous mastitis: an uncommon cause of breast abscess," *Archives of Internal Medicine*, vol. 161, no. 4, pp. 611–612, 2001.

[7] C. H. Yip, G. Jayaram, and M. Swain, "The value of cytology in granulomatous mastitis: a report of 16 cases from Malaysia," *Australian and New Zealand Journal of Surgery*, vol. 70, no. 2, pp. 103–105, 2000.

[8] A. Fletcher, I. M. Magrath, R. H. Riddell, and I. C. Talbot, "Granulomatous mastitis: a report of seven cases," *Journal of Clinical Pathology*, vol. 35, no. 9, pp. 941–945, 1982.

[9] A. Sellitto, A. Santoriello, U. De Fanis et al., "Granulomatous lobular mastitis: another manifestation of systemic lupus erythematosus?" *The Breast Journal*, vol. 19, no. 3, pp. 331–332, 2013.

[10] B. Bercot, C. Kannengiesser, C. Oudin et al., "First description of NOD2 variant associated with defective neutrophil responses in a woman with granulomatous mastitis related to corynebacteria," *Journal of Clinical Microbiology*, vol. 47, no. 9, pp. 3034–3037, 2009.

[11] K. K. Yasar, F. Pehlivanoglu, G. Sengoz, and N. Cabioglu, "Successfully treated *Mycobacterium abscessus* mastitis: a rare cause of breast masses," *Indian Journal of Medical Microbiology*, vol. 29, no. 4, pp. 425–427, 2011.

[12] J. K. Trupiano, B. A. Sebek, J. Goldfarb, L. R. Levy, G. S. Hall, and G. W. Procop, "Mastitis due to *Mycobacterium abscessus* after body piercing," *Clinical Infectious Diseases*, vol. 33, no. 1, pp. 131–134, 2001.

[13] B. Petrini, "Mycobacterium abscessus: an emerging rapid-growing potential pathogen," *APMIS*, vol. 114, no. 5, pp. 319–328, 2006.

[14] C. G. Lewis, M. K. Wells, and W. C. Jennings, "*Mycobacterium fortuitum* breast infection following nipple-piercing, mimicking carcinoma," *Breast Journal*, vol. 10, no. 4, pp. 363–365, 2004.

[15] V. Bengualid, V. Singh, H. Singh, and J. Berger, "*Mycobacterium fortuitum* and anaerobic breast abscess following nipple piercing: case presentation and review of the literature," *Journal of Adolescent Health*, vol. 42, no. 5, pp. 530–532, 2008.

[16] D. Betal and F. A. MacNeill, "Chronic breast abscess due to *Mycobacterium fortuitum*: a case report," *Journal of Medical Case Reports*, vol. 5, article 188, 2011.

[17] K. Abbass, M. K. Adnan, R. J. Markert, M. Emig, and N. A. Khan, "Mycobacterium fortuitum breast abscess after nipple piercing," *Canadian Family Physician*, vol. 60, no. 1, pp. 51–52, 2014.

[18] V. R. Jacobs, K. Golombeck, W. Jonat, and M. Kiechle, "Three case reports of breast abscess after nipple piercing: underestimated health problems of a fashion phenomenon," *Zentralblatt fur Gynakologie*, vol. 124, no. 7, pp. 378–385, 2002.

[19] G. B. Taylor, S. D. Paviour, S. Musaad, W. O. Jones, and D. J. Holland, "A clinicopathological review of 34 cases of inflammatory breast disease showing an association between corynebacteria infection and granulomatous mastitis," *Pathology*, vol. 35, no. 2, pp. 109–119, 2003.

[20] T. J. Hieken, J. Chen, T. L. Hoskin et al., "The microbiome of aseptically collected human breast tissue in benign and malignant disease," *Scientific Reports*, vol. 6, Article ID 30751, 2016.

[21] H. Yu, H. Deng, J. Ma et al., "Clinical metagenomic analysis of bacterial communities in breast abscesses of granulomatous mastitis," *International Journal of Infectious Diseases*, vol. 53, pp. 30–33, 2016.

[22] C. Urbaniak, J. Cummins, M. Brackstone et al., "Microbiota of human breast tissue," *Applied and Environmental Microbiology*, vol. 80, no. 10, pp. 3007–3014, 2014.

37

Nigerian Female with Skin Lesions in the Leg and Face: Herpetic Sycosis Folliculitis

Dominique Dilorenzo, Naganna Channaveeraiah, Patricia Gilford, and Bruce Deschere

Orange Park Medical Center Family Medicine GME, 2021 Professional Center Drive, Suite 100, Orange Park, FL 32073, USA

Correspondence should be addressed to Naganna Channaveeraiah; ncgs@hotmail.com

Academic Editor: Larry M. Bush

Nongenital HSV 1 presents outside the mucus membrane. Our patient had unusual presentation that caused diagnostic dilemma. 30-year-old native Nigerian female coming with fiancée to the United States presented to our service one day after arrival through ER with a lesion on her right ankle. She was diagnosed with cellulitis, started on antibiotics, and admitted to hospital. She had fever of 39.1°C. Head and neck exam showed multiple sized lesions over tongue and palate and inner aspect of lower lip. Abdomen and genital exam was normal. Skin exam showed lesions over the face and lesions over the lateral aspect of the right leg. There was ulcerated lesion over the right lateral malleolus with surrounding erythema and edema. Her tests showed elevated ESR of 98; HIV test was negative; CT scan of the ankle showed no abscess or osteomyelitis. TB quantiferon was indeterminate; AFB stain and culture were negative; HSV IgM was elevated at 1 : 16; RPR was negative; ANA was negative; malaria screen was negative, and blood cultures were negative for bacteria, fungus, and virus. Debrided wound had no growth of bacteria or fungus or virus. This case illustrates the unusual presentation of the HSV1 outside the mucus membrane and how it can be confused with other conditions that required extensive tests. Therapeutic trail with antiviral medications resolved lesions over the leg and face.

1. Presenting History

A 30-year-old female native of Sokoto, Western Nigeria, coming to the United States with fiancée for the first time presented to us one day after arrival at the hospital emergency room with a painful ulcerated lesion on her right ankle [1–7].

2. History Review

According to the patient, she noticed this lesion over the right ankle 10 days ago; she visited her pharmacist and there was a questionable history of trauma. The pharmacist in Nigeria performed incision and drainage of the pus and removal of unhealthy tissue at the lesion and started her on Trypsin, Amoxicillin/Clavulanate, and unknown pain medication. The pain from right ankle persisted and she went to community hospital and was treated with wound cleaning and other antibiotics. Patient then noticed bullous lesions over face and enlarging mouth ulceration.

3. Review of Systems

The patient was positive for fever, mouth ulcers, and stress and negative for weakness in any limbs, cough, eye pain, blurry vision, and history of keloid.

4. Past Medical History

The past medical history was significant for sickle cell trait.

5. Family History

The family history was noncontributory.

6. Personal History

Patient lives with her fiancé and has never been pregnant. She is a nonsmoker and denies alcohol or illicit substance use. Vaccinations status is not clear. Patient had no known history of BCG vaccination.

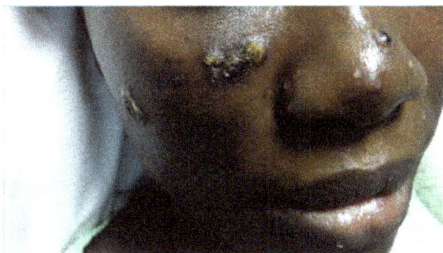

FIGURE 1

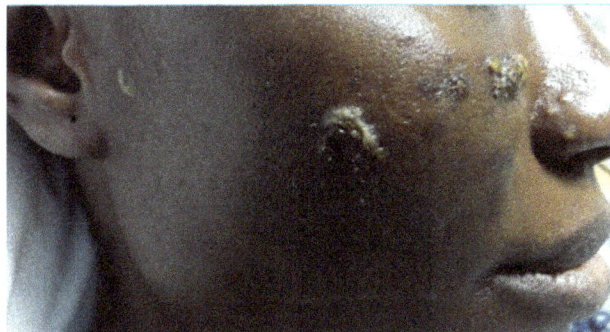

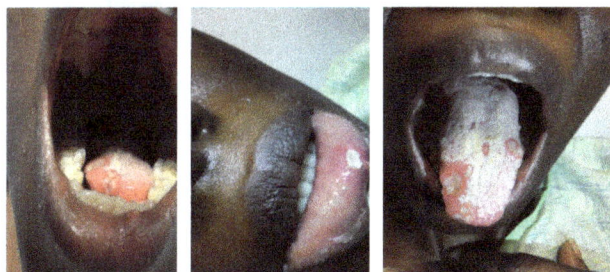

FIGURE 2

7. Physical Examination

She is an African female. She was pleasant and in no distress. She had fever of 39.1°C, regular pulse of 73, BP of 121/74, and saturating 100% on room air. HEENT showed dry oral mucosa, multiple sized ulcerated lesions over tongue and palate and inner aspect of lower lip (Figure 2); no lymphadenopathy was found in neck, and the eye exam was normal. Lung and cardiovascular examinations were normal. Abdomen and genital exam was normal. Neuroexam was normal. Skin exam on the face showed multiple pustules, some with crusts and ulceration on elevated base measuring from 2 mm to 10 mm (Figure 1). One pustule measured 6 mm over the lateral aspect of the right leg. Ulcerated lesion was found over the right lateral malleolus measuring 3 cm × 4 cm with surrounding erythema and edema (Figure 3), and pulses were intact.

8. Investigations

CBC and BMP were within normal limits; ESR was elevated at 98 (normal rage 0–29 in females). HIV test was negative. X-ray of the ankle showed no bony abnormalities but a large soft tissue defect overlying the lateral malleolus with soft tissue swelling extending extensively along the dorsum of the foot. CT scan of the lower extremity and ankle showed no abscess or osteomyelitis. TB quantiferon was read as indeterminate high. Debrided tissue from the wound was tested with AFB stain. The acid-fast Bacilli (AFB) test was negative on the stain and culture. PCR was negative for *M. Ulcerans*. HSV IgM was elevated at 1 : 16 (normal; nonreactive); RPR was negative; ANA was negative; malaria screen was negative; and blood cultures were negative for bacteria, fungus, and virus.

9. Initial Admission Diagnosis and Hospital Course

The initial admission diagnosis of the patient was cellulitis. Infectious disease consultant was called in to help in the management as the history was not clear on the day of presentation to the hospital.

She was started on broad spectrum antibiotics in the ER (Vancomycin and Zosyn). She had the surgical debridement of the wound in the leg. After surgery, topical enzymatic debridement was done with Santyl to her foot wound and wound vac was applied. Colchicine was started for the possibility of Behcet's syndrome but was stopped after one day when the patient's symptoms did not improve and pathology tests were negative. Dermatology recommended Valtrex for oral lesions. Patient's face and oral lesions began to resolve after the first dose. Vancomycin was discontinued due to high levels which started affecting the renal function. All cultures were negative and antibiotics were discontinued. Wound vacuum was removed from right ankle before discharge from the hospital. Patient followed up in the ambulatory clinic and wounds have healed very well.

10. Discussion

10.1. Herpes Ulcers. HSV 1 IgM blood titers were elevated in this patient. In addition to cellulitis at the site of the right ankle, the patient had history of small mouth ulcers but had never presented with skin lesions outside the mouth. Once patient was treated with acyclovir, mouth and facial lesions healed and ankle ulcer began to heal more quickly. Nongenital herpes simplex virus type 1 is a common infection usually transmitted during childhood via nonsexual contact or during adulthood through sexual contact. Oral mucosa or lips are usually involved in these infections. The primary lesion may range from being asymptomatic to being very painful, which can lead to poor nutritional intake. The recurrence of symptoms may be due to stress, fever, sun exposure, extreme temperatures, UV radiation, immunosuppression, or trauma. Other forms of herpes include herpetic keratitis infection of the eye, herpetic whitlow lesion found on hand or digits, and herpetic sycosis follicular infection. Treatment with oral acyclovir, valacyclovir, or famciclovir is effective for treatment and recurrence; see Table 1 (1).

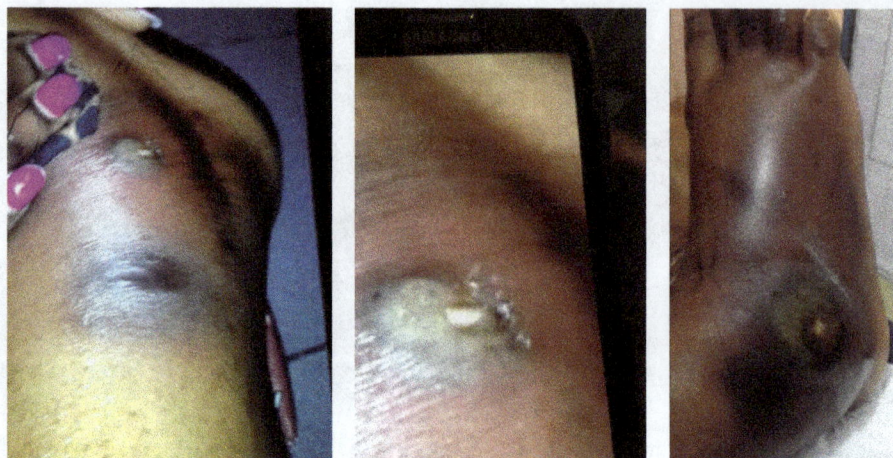

FIGURE 3

TABLE 1: Multiple ulcer causing conditions with etiology and characteristics.

Condition	Etiology	Characteristics
(1) HSV ulcer	Herpes simplex virus type 1	Small, painful blister, vesicles, crusting, ulcer
(2) Buruli ulcer	*Mycobacterium ulcerans*	Painless nodule breaks down days to weeks forming ulcer
(3) Behcets ulcer	Autoimmune vasculitis	Oral apthous ulcers, cutaneous lesions with varying types
(4) Erythema multiforme (drug induced)	NSAIDS, sulfonamides, antiepileptics, antibiotics	Target lesion with central bullae, erythematous base
(5) Syphilitic ulcer	*Treponema pallidum*	Painless, circumferential ulcer

10.2. Buruli Ulcer. Buruli ulcer is a common ulceration found in tropical Africa, New Guinea, Malaysia, and Australia caused by *mycobacterium ulcerans*; see Table 1 (2). Mycobacterium ulcerans represents the third most common mycobacterial disease in intertropical areas. Clinical features consist of small mobile skin nodules that generally enlarge over days to weeks; lesions may resolve spontaneously but most will progress. Lesions generally are not painful and have no systemic inflammatory response. Eventually the papule breaks down at the center and forms an ulcer. Diagnosis consists of positive acid-fast bacilli culture from necrotic ulcer; PCR testing and punch biopsies can also be performed. Treatment of ulcer involves surgery to debride necrotic tissue. *Mycobacterium ulcerans* is generally sensitive to clarithromycin, rifampicin, and ethambutol.

10.3. Behcet's Syndrome. Behcet's syndrome is a group of symptoms that occur together with unknown clear cause; see Table 1 (3). Clinical manifestations of Behcet's syndrome include oral ulceration, genital ulceration, uveitis, skin lesions including erythema nodosum, folliculitis, ulceration, hyperirritability or lethargy, arthritis, vasculitis, GI lesions, CV lesions, neurologic lesions, epididymitis, and family history. Diagnosis is based on clinical symptoms. Treatment includes use of colchicine and azathioprine and symptomatic treatment.

10.4. Erythema Multiforme. Erythema multiforme is an acute and immune-mediated condition with the most common cause being drugs; see Table 1 (4). Drugs that cause reaction are NSAIDS, sulfonamides, antiepileptics, and antibiotics, but drug reaction is less than 10% of etiology. Clinical course is generally acute and self-limiting. Clinical symptoms include history of malaise, fever, myalgia, and cutaneous lesions involving round, erythematous, edematous papules surrounded by areas of blanching, which may appear as targetoid lesion with symmetrical distribution on extremities. There is not any available diagnostic test. Treatment in EM involves discontinuation of all inciting factors.

10.5. Syphilis. Syphilis is a bacterial infection caused by the *Treponema pallidum*; see Table 1 (5). Syphilis is primarily transmitted through sexual contact and can also be transmitted through vertical transmission from mother to fetus. Primary syphilis is the first stage and typically presents clinically with a painless ulcer or chancre 14–28 days after initial exposure. Secondary syphilis presents with development of a flat maculopapular rash and can present with patches in mucosal membranes, headache, fatigue, lymphadenopathy, sore throat, and fever 6–8 weeks after development of chancre. Diagnosis is based on history and clinical symptoms, which can be diagnosed using VDRL and RPR. Treatment involves use of penicillin or doxycycline.

11. Conclusions

This was an unusual presentation of herpes simplex virus infection. Patient was examined extensively but was only found to have HSV IgM and significant improvement of symptoms after starting antiviral therapy. After patient completed first course of antiviral therapy right ankle ulceration had delayed healing and once therapy was restarted the wound healing improved. Since she recently travelled to the United States, other diagnoses like Buruli ulcer and syphilitic ulcer took the center stage of diagnostic workup.

Competing Interests

The authors declare that there is no conflict of interests regarding the publication of this paper.

References

[1] R. P. Ustaine and R. Tinitigan, "Nongenital herpes simplex virus," *American Family Physician*, vol. 82, no. 9, pp. 1075–1082, 2010.

[2] B. S. Thomas, T. C. Bailey, J. Bhatnagar et al., "*Mycobacterium ulcerans* infection imported from Australia to Missouri, USA, 2012," *Emerging Infectious Diseases*, vol. 20, no. 11, pp. 1876–1879, 2014.

[3] P. D. Johnson, T. P. Stinear, and J. A. Hayman, "Mycobacterium ulcerans-a mini-review," *Journal of Medical Microbiology. Monash Medical Centre*, vol. 48, no. 6, pp. 511–513, 1999.

[4] A. C. Chi, B. W. Neville, J. W. Krayer, and W. C. Gonsalves, "Oral manifestations of systemic disease," *American Family Physician*, vol. 82, no. 11, pp. 1381–1388, 2010.

[5] C. Mulryan, "Syphilis: recognizing the 'great Pretender," *Practice Nursing*, vol. 24, no. 5, 2013.

[6] P. Maccallum, J. C. Tolhurst, G. Buckle, and H. A. Sissons, "A new mycobacterial infection in man," *The Journal of Pathology and Bacteriology*, vol. 60, no. 1, pp. 93–122, 1948.

[7] E. Marion, K. Carolan, A. Adeye, M. Kempf, A. Chauty, and L. Marsollier, "Buruli ulcer in South Western Nigeria: a retrospective cohort study of patients treated in Benin," *PLoS Neglected Tropical Diseases*, vol. 9, no. 1, Article ID e3443, 2015.

38

An Uncommon Feature of Chronic Granulomatous Disease in a Neonate

Razieh Afrough,[1] Sayyed Shahabeddin Mohseni,[2] and Setareh Sagheb[1]

[1]*Department of Pediatrics, Tehran University of Medical Sciences, Tehran, Iran*
[2]*Department of Dermatology, Tehran Medical Sciences Branch, Islamic Azad University, Tehran, Iran*

Correspondence should be addressed to Setareh Sagheb; dr.ssagheb@yahoo.com

Academic Editor: Larry M. Bush

Chronic Granulomatous Disease (CGD) represents recurrent life-threatening bacterial and fungal infections and granuloma formation with a high mortality rate. CGD's sign and symptoms usually appear in infancy and children before the age of five; therefore, its presentation in neonatal period with some uncommon features may be easily overlooked. Here we describe a case of CGD in a 24-day-old boy, presenting with a diffuse purulent vesiculopustular rash and multiple osteomyelitis.

1. Introduction

Chronic Granulomatous Disease (CGD) is a rare inherited disease of phagocytic system that leads to recurrent and severe bacterial and fungal infections with a high mortality rate [1, 2]. CGD is characterized by granuloma and abscess formation in the skin, liver, lungs, spleen, and lymph nodes. These granuloma and abscess are caused by the inability of macrophages to kill ingested organisms [2, 3]. Infants with CGD encounter life-threatening infections, so prompt diagnosis and treatment with broad spectrum antibiotics are crucial [4, 5]. CGD's sign and symptoms usually appear in infancy and children before the age of five [3]; therefore, its presentation in neonatal period with some uncommon features may be easily overlooked. We report a 24-day-old boy with an uncommon presentation of CGD.

2. Case Presentation

A 24-day-old boy was referred to our hospital with vesiculopustular rash in the periorbita, genitalia, foot, and sacroiliac regions. The patient was born to a 26-year-old primigravida woman after a full term gestation without any complications during pregnancy. His father and mother were cousins. His birth weight was 2700 gr. He was admitted to NICU due to respiratory distress and was discharged after 4 days with a healthy condition. Ten days after his birth, he developed a vesiculopustular rash progressively in periorbita, genitalia, foot, and sacroiliac regions.

Fourteen days later, he was referred to our hospital and was admitted for further evaluation and treatment. There was no complaint of poor feeding or fever. In physical examination, his weight was 2950 gr. He was not ill or toxic. Neonatal reflexes were normal.

Asymmetric vesiculopustular lesions partially ruptured with erosions and crusted ulcers were seen. They were found in the left periorbital region, scrotum, penis, and sacroiliac region and on the medial malleolus of the left ankle, with some necrosis having extension into the dorsal surface of the foot (Figure 1).

We also found conjunctivitis with purulent discharge and dactylitis in the left foot. Examinations of other organs were normal (Figure 2).

Routine laboratory tests, smear, and culture from lesions and lumbar puncture were performed (Tables 1 and 2). Chest X-ray was normal at the time of admission, so lung CT scan was not performed.

Gram positive cocci were seen in direct smear from skin lesions, and culture was also positive for *Staphylococcus aureus*. Tzanck smear was negative for the Herpes Simplex

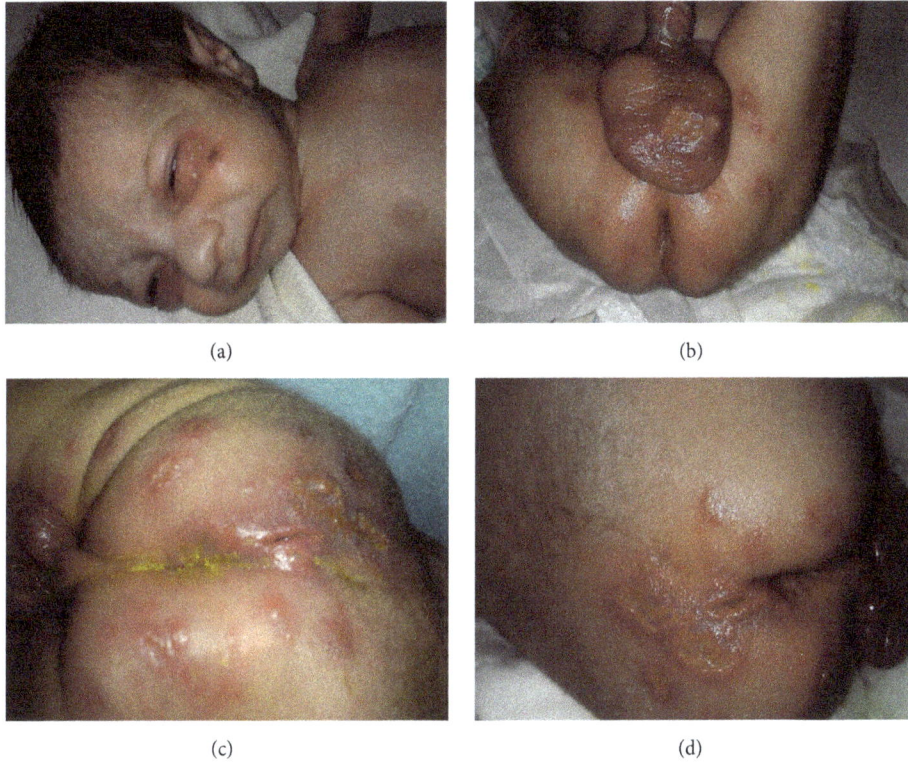

(a)

(b)

(c)

(d)

FIGURE 1: Vesiculopustular lesions ((a)–(d)).

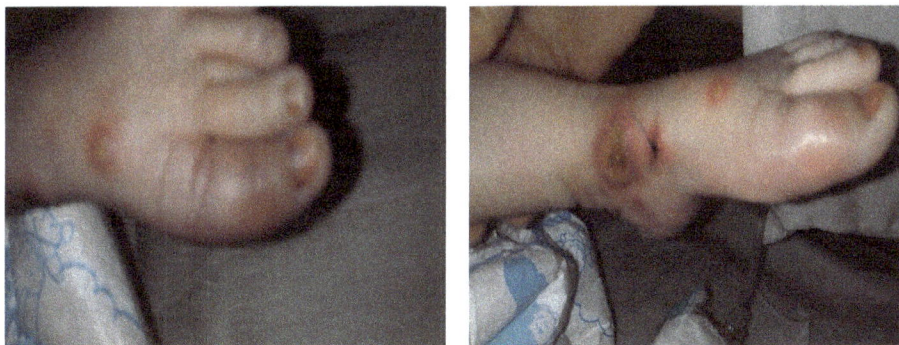

FIGURE 2: Dactylitis in the left foot.

TABLE 1: Results of the routine laboratory tests.

Parameter	Before treatment	After treatment	Units
WBC	15.2	11.3	K/μL
Neut	55	41	%
Lymph	31.6	32.8	%
Mono	11.9	21.9	%
Eos	1.6	4	%
RBC	4.23	3.75	M/μL
Hgb	13.3	11.5	g/dL
Platelet	112	582	K/μL
CRP	56.2	22	mg/L

TABLE 2: Results of the lumbar puncture.

Parameter	Value
Protein	45 mg/dL
Glucose	57 mg/dL
WBC	1/μL
RBC	700/μL
Smear	Negative
Culture	Negative
PCR for HSV	Negative

Virus (HSV). Samples were sent to determine the specific mutation, but the results are not available yet.

We started our treatment with a combination of broad spectrum antibiotics (meropenem and vancomycin) and local treatment with saline irrigation and sterile dressing and

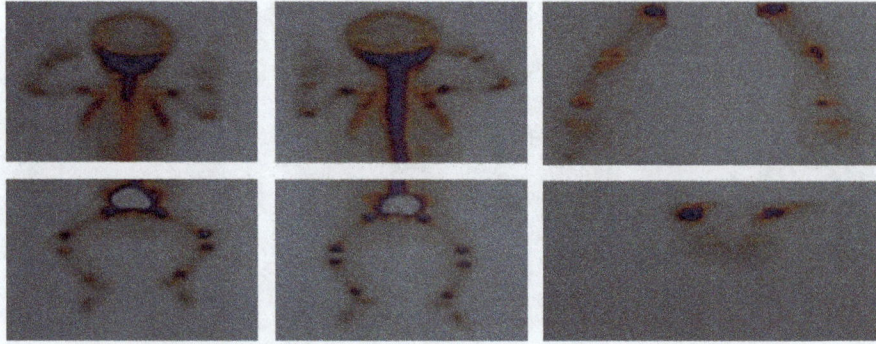

FIGURE 3: Osteomyelitis of the left ankle, right elbow, and right wrist.

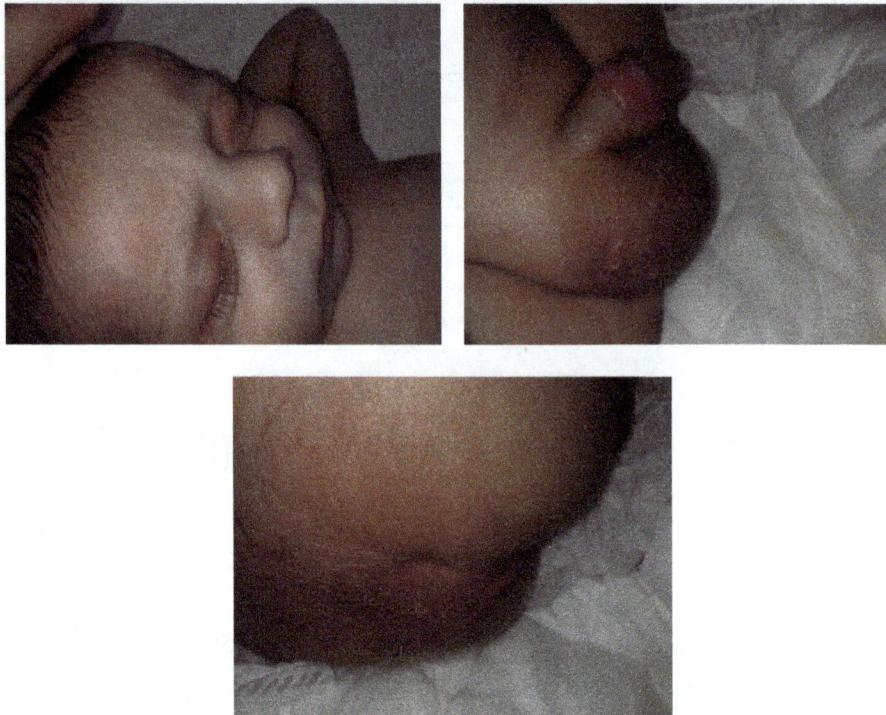

FIGURE 4: lesions after treatment.

then modified it to vancomycin and amikacin when culture results were available.

According to the severity and extension of the lesions, a consult with a dermatologist and an immunologist was requested. Skin biopsy showed necrotizing granulomatous tissue reaction, with infectious etiology. Nitroblue tetrazolium (NBT) and Dihydrorhodamine (DHR) tests were performed for confirming diagnosis. Osteomyelitis of the left ankle, right elbow, and right wrist was seen in Tc99m whole body scan (Figure 3).

BCGiosis or tuberculosis was ruled out by biopsy of phalanx.

After a few days of treatment, lesions were significantly improved. Treatment with intravenous antibiotics continued for six weeks, and then he was discharged with antibiotic (trimethoprim-sulfamethoxazole) and antifungal prophylaxis (Figure 4).

3. Discussion

Chronic Granulomatous Disease (CGD) is an inherited rare disorder of the immune system and represents with recurrent infections and granuloma formation at different sites [5, 6]. Pneumonia, liver abscess, lymphadenitis, osteomyelitis, and skin (cellulitis or abscesses) are the most important clinical manifestations [4–7].

We have encountered an infant with multiple diffuse vesiculopustular lesions with multiple osteomyelitis but there was no evidence of pneumonia and lymphadenitis. *Staphylococcus aureus*, gram negative *Enterobacteriaceae*, and *Aspergillus* species are the most common pathogens [5, 6]. In our patient, Gram positive cocci were seen in direct smear, and culture was positive for *Staphylococcus aureus*. We started our treatment with broad spectrum antibiotics and then modified them to vancomycin and amikacin based on culture results. Diagnosis of CGD is based on the DHR test. This test evaluates neutrophil superoxide production via NADPH oxidase complex [4]. Due to diffused and delayed heeling lesions, the NBT and DHR tests were used as diagnostic tests for CGD. As infants with CGD encounter life-threatening infections, early diagnosis and prompt treatment with antibiotics are crucial during acute infections. Antibacterial and antifungal prophylaxes are considered for reducing infections in CGD [5, 6]. Immunotherapy with interferon-γ is sometimes taken and hematopoietic stem cell transplant is also considered in severe forms [8, 9]. In our patient, treatment with intravenous antibiotics continued for 6 weeks and then he was discharged with antibiotic and antifungal prophylaxis.

Previous studies presented multifocal abscess [10] and invasive pulmonary aspergillosis [11] as clinical manifestation of CGD during neonatal periods.

In our case, multiple diffuse vesiculopustular lesions with multiple osteomyelitis were considered as a clinical presentation of CGD.

Despite the rare incidence of CGD during neonatal period, it should be considered in the differential diagnosis of a newborn with clinical features of skin cellulitis or abscesses and multiple osteomyelitis in the absence of appropriate response to treatment with antibiotics.

Competing Interests

The authors have no conflict of interests to disclose.

Acknowledgments

The authors would like to thank Mr. Sayyed Ourmazd Mohseni for his help in editing this manuscript.

References

[1] S. F. Tafti, P. Tabarsi, N. Mansouri et al., "Chronic granulomatous disease with unusual clinical manifestation, outcome, and pattern of inheritance in an Iranian family," *Journal of Clinical Immunology*, vol. 26, no. 3, pp. 291–296, 2006.

[2] B. Martire, R. Rondelli, A. Soresina et al., "Clinical features, long-term follow-up and outcome of a large cohort of patients with Chronic Granulomatous Disease: An Italian Multicenter Study," *Clinical Immunology*, vol. 126, no. 2, pp. 155–164, 2008.

[3] S. Kliegman and S. St. Geme, *Nelson Textbook of Pediatrics, 2-Volume Set*, chapter 128, Elsevier, 20th edition, 2015.

[4] J. Ben-Ari, O. Wolach, R. Gavrieli, and B. Wolach, "Infections associated with chronic granulomatous disease: linking genetics to phenotypic expression," *Expert Review of Anti-Infective Therapy*, vol. 10, no. 8, pp. 881–894, 2012.

[5] J. W. Leiding and S. M. Holland, "Chronic granulomatous disease," GeneReviews, Bookshelf, February 2016.

[6] M. Chiriaco, I. Salfa, G. Di Matteo, P. Rossi, and A. Finocchi, "Chronic granulomatous disease: clinical, molecular, and therapeutic aspects," *Pediatric Allergy and Immunology*, vol. 27, no. 3, pp. 242–253, 2016.

[7] S. Kliegman and S. St Geme, *Nelson Textbook of Pediatrics*, vol. 2, chapter 130, 20th edition, 2016.

[8] A. Rawat, S. Bhattad, and S. Singh, "Chronic granulomatous disease," *The Indian Journal of Pediatrics*, vol. 83, no. 4, pp. 345–353, 2016.

[9] T. Cole, M. S. Pearce, A. J. Cant, C. M. Cale, D. Goldblatt, and A. R. Gennery, "Clinical outcome in children with chronic granulomatous disease managed conservatively or with hematopoietic stem cell transplantation," *Journal of Allergy and Clinical Immunology*, vol. 132, no. 5, pp. 1150–1155, 2013.

[10] A.-M. Armanian, P. Iravani, M. Mohammadizadeh, and H. Rahimi, "Multifocal abscess in a neonate: neonatal chronic Granulomatous disease—case report," *The Southeast Asian Journal of Case Report and Review*, vol. 3, no. 4, pp. 856–867, 2014.

[11] S. Saito, A. Oda, M. Kasai et al., "A neonatal case of chronic granulomatous disease, initially presented with invasive pulmonary aspergillosis," *Journal of Infection and Chemotherapy*, vol. 20, no. 3, pp. 220–223, 2014.

39

A Rare Case of Disseminated Pyogenic Gonococcal Infection in an Immunocompetent Woman

Iordanis Romiopoulos,[1] Athina Pyrpasopoulou,[1,2] Anna Varouktsi,[2]
Elisavet Simoulidou,[2] Konstantina Kontopoulou,[3] Ekaterini Karantani,[4]
Vivian Georgopoulou,[5] Konstantinos Kitsios,[6] Apostolos Mamopoulos,[7]
Charalampos Antachopoulos,[1] Asterios Karagiannis,[2] and Emmanuel Roilides[1]

[1]Infectious Diseases Unit, 3rd Department of Pediatrics, Faculty of Medicine, Aristotle University School of Health Sciences,
  Hippokration General Hospital, Thessaloniki, Greece
[2]2nd Propaedeutic Department of Internal Medicine, Faculty of Medicine, Aristotle University School of Health Sciences,
  Hippokration General Hospital, Thessaloniki, Greece
[3]Laboratory of Microbiology, Gennimatas General Hospital, Thessaloniki, Greece
[4]Laboratory of Microbiology, Hippokration General Hospital, Thessaloniki, Greece
[5]Laboratory of Radiology, Hippokration General Hospital, Thessaloniki, Greece
[6]Department of Medicine, Gennimatas Hospital, Thessaloniki, Greece
[7]3rd Department of Obstetrics and Gynecology, Faculty of Medicine, Aristotle University School of Health Sciences,
  Hippokration General Hospital, Thessaloniki, Greece

Correspondence should be addressed to Emmanuel Roilides; roilides@med.auth.gr

Academic Editor: Fariborz Mansour-ghanaei

We present a case of previously healthy, immunocompetent, 41-year-old woman who developed systemic inflammatory response syndrome secondary to *Neisseria gonorrhoeae* bacteremia. Clinical course was complicated by the simultaneous formation of multiple muscular abscesses, epidural abscess, and septic spondylodiscitis. The patient responded well to prolonged ceftriaxone treatment and was released 10 weeks after initial admission. Spinal lesions and/or pyomyositis individually constitute rare complications of disseminated gonococcal infection. This case, combining both manifestations, is to our knowledge unique. Apropos, diversity of the clinical presentation, and therapeutic challenges for this historical disease are discussed for the practicing physician.

1. Introduction

Gonococcal disease is generally asymptomatic or mildly symptomatic [1]. Disseminated disease and distal septic complications such as spinal abscesses and pyomyositis have been very rarely reported [2]. We describe the case of a female, who developed disseminated disease accompanied by severe systemic inflammatory response syndrome (SIRS), pyomyositis, and spinal lesions including septic spondylodiscitis and epidural abscess with neurological symptoms. To our knowledge, this is the first case reported of such extensive complications including spinal lesions and pyomyositis.

2. Case Presentation

A 41-year-old woman was referred to the 3rd Department of Obstetrics and Gynecology of Hippokration General Hospital for further investigation and treatment of pyogenic pelvic inflammatory disease. The patient's past history included bowel obstruction at the age of 8 months with no more data available and 3 caesarian sections; she was taking no chronic medication.

Symptoms started 9 days before referral with intense low back pain of abrupt onset for which she had consulted an orthopedic surgeon and had been prescribed nonsteroidal

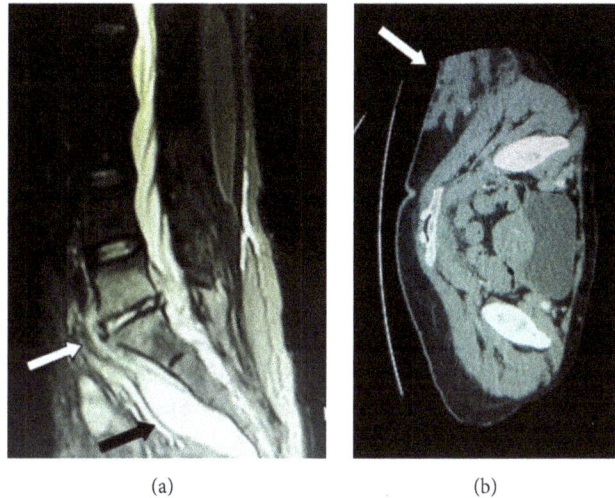

FIGURE 1: (a) Presacral epidural inflammatory fluid collection (abscess) (black arrow) and adjacent spondylodiscitis that developed at the level of L5-S1 vertebrae (white arrow). Due to its small size the epidural abscess was successfully managed with antibiotics alone. (b) Large abscess of the right buttock (white arrow) that was drained under CT scan guidance.

anti-inflammatory drugs (NSAIDS) without response. Two days later (day 1) the patient was admitted to the Department of Medicine, Gennimatas Hospital, with fever (38.2°C) and abdominal pain, localized in the right upper quadrant and the epigastrium. Laboratory tests revealed leukocytosis (WBC 14,900/μL, 96% neutrophils), thrombocytopenia (60,000/μL), markedly elevated C-reactive protein (330 mg/L), and mildly affected liver chemistry (SGOT 60 U/L, SGPT 84 U/L, γGT 104 U/L, ALP 160 U/L, total bilirubin 2.79 mg/dL, and direct bilirubin 2.62 mg/dL). Initial blood and urine cultures did not grow any pathogen. Despite the normal abdominal ultrasound findings, the patient was treated empirically for potential cholecystitis with intravenous cefoxitin, 1 g tid.

The following day (day 2) the clinical course was further complicated by arthritis of the right shoulder, the right elbow, and the right ankle, which improved with administration of NSAIDS. Abdominal pain, however, worsened involving the lower abdomen, and tenderness of the right thigh developed, which was aggravated by movement. Computed tomography scan of the abdomen revealed no liver and biliary lesions but increased size and calcifications of the uterus, thickening of the perirectal fasciae, formation of perirectal abscesses, collection of fluid in the epidural and presacral space with presence of air, and presence of air within the subcutaneous tissue of the anterior abdominal wall. Given the formation of perirectal abscesses in the setting of a fever with abdominal pain and arthritis, the patient underwent colonoscopy on day 5 and a potential diagnosis of inflammatory bowel disease was excluded. On day 6 the patient had an episode of self-limited vaginal bleeding (her last menstrual cycle being 2 weeks previously). The cervical swab was positive for Gram-negative, coffee bean-shaped diplococci and culture grew Neisseria gonorrhoeae. No other pathogens were isolated. Serological tests for HIV and syphilis were negative. The patient denied previously extramarital sexual activity or prior sexually transmitted diseases. She was living with

her husband who refused examination for gonorrhoea. Her last sexual intercourse was reported to be 1 month before admission.

On day 7, new blood cultures incubated into the BacT/ALERT automated system (Biomérieux, Marcy-l'Étoile, France) revealed high bacterial load, evidenced by the fact that positive signal was elicited as early as two hours after incubation. A Gram-negative diplococcus was seen on microscopy. The isolate was identified as N. gonorrhoeae on the automated system Vitek II (Biomérieux). Due to absence of N. gonorrhoeae susceptibility card the antimicrobial susceptibility testing was performed by Kirby Bauer disc diffusion method and revealed susceptibility to ceftriaxone, clindamycin, and ciprofloxacin but resistance to azithromycin.

On the same day the patient was referred to Hippokration Hospital for further evaluation and management of pyogenic pelvic inflammatory disease. At referral she was septic with a temperature of 39.5°C, hypoalbuminemic (2.0 g/dL), and markedly oedematous. A quadruple intravenous antibiotic regimen was initiated (ceftriaxone 2 g q12 h, clindamycin 600 mg q6 h, gentamicin 6 mg/kg q24 h, and azithromycin 600 mg q24 h); the patient gradually responded and became afebrile within a week. On day 8, she developed a hemorrhagic maculopapular rash in her lower extremities, painful palpable lumps in the right thigh, and shin and splinter hemorrhages. Endocarditis was excluded by transesophageal echocardiography. Magnetic resonance imaging confirmed the presence of a presacral epidural inflammatory collection with associated septic spondylodiscitis of the 5th lumbar and 1st sacral vertebrae and abscesses of multiple muscles (pyomyositis) including psoas, gluteus maximus, and quadratus femoris, the largest among them measuring 12.1 cm × 6.7 cm (Figures 1(a) and 1(b)).

On day 20, this large abscess was drained and 160 mL of purulent fluid was removed under CT scan guidance. Gram stain and cultures of the fluid were negative. In the setting of a disseminated gonococcal disease with multiple complications, the possibility of an underlying immunodeficiency was investigated by quantitative analysis of immunoglobulins and components of complement, with normal findings. The antibiotic regimen was gradually deescalated to only intravenous ceftriaxone, which was continued for 6 weeks. CRP levels normalized very slowly and finally the patient was discharged with oral ciprofloxacin 500 mg bid for a month.

3. Discussion

The case described in this report has several unusual and interesting features. The clinical course of the infection in an otherwise immunocompetent woman escalated from asymptomatic gonorrhoea to disseminated gonococcal disease. At this point, Fitz-Hugh-Curtis syndrome, also known as acute perihepatitis, characterized by inflammation of the peritoneum and the perihepatic tissues [3] was considered in relation to gonococcal disease. The syndrome can be underdiagnosed because of subtle CT liver and peritoneal findings. Of note, cefoxitin used to treat probable cholecystitis did not prove efficient against gonococcal syndrome although it is considered in vitro active. This underlies the fact that the efficacy of an antibiotic is not determined only by antibiotic pharmacodynamics but is based on pharmacokinetics/pharmacodynamics index, which was possibly not fulfilled in this case [4]. On the other hand, although azithromycin was resistant in vitro, it was included in the therapeutic regimen at least for a potential broader and enhanced activity given the rapid evolution of the clinical condition. Septic arthritis is a well-characterized late complication of the bacteremic stage of the disease; the spinal vertebrae however become affected very rarely [5]. Our patient may have developed this complication due to preexisting degenerative lesions of the spine and the adjacent inflammatory fluid collection that developed in the course of the disease.

Disseminated gonococcal disease is generally rare (1–3%) and has been reported mostly in immunocompromised patients with complement or other immunological deficiencies [6–9]. There are only few published cases of disseminated pyogenic gonococcal infection either as spondylitis [5] or as pyomyositis [10].

The prevalence of gonococcal pyomyositis is extremely low. In 1992, a review included 100 cases of pyomyositis in North America over a period of 20 years, of which no case was gonococcal [11]. Gonococcal pyomyositis has been reported in 6 patients [10, 12–16]. The involved muscular sites were thigh and calf [10], biceps brachii [12, 14], and obturator internus [13, 15]. On the other hand, an axial skeleton involvement in the setting of a disseminated gonococcal infection is maybe an even more rare complication. In 1976, Seruzier et al. published probably the first case of gonococcal spinal infection in a 47-year-old male with spondylodiscitis at the level of 9th and 10th thoracic vertebra [17]. In 2004, Van Hal and Post reported a thoracic epidural mass at 6th to 7th vertebra [18] and more recently Low et al. reported a case of gonococcal spinal epidural abscess extended from the 6th cervical to the 2nd thoracic vertebra without cord compression [5].

Our case is unique because, to our knowledge, disseminated gonococcal disease of an excessively suppurative form affecting both spine and multiple muscles has not been previously reported. The intensity of the symptomatology in this otherwise healthy individual, the complications that she developed, and the delayed response to appropriate treatment necessitated increased medical care and prolonged hospitalization.

N. gonorrhoeae has always been and probably will remain a major health problem, which rarely may involve difficult-to-manage spine and muscular septic complications. Awareness of the diversity of the clinical presentation and therapeutic challenges for this historical disease remains therefore important for the practicing physician.

Competing Interests

The authors have no conflict of interest.

Acknowledgments

The authors thank the patient who gave them written informed consent for the publication of this case report.

References

[1] P. A. Cook, J. Evans-Jones, H. Mallinson et al., "Comparison of patients diagnosed with gonorrhoea through community screening with those self-presenting to the genitourinary medicine clinic," *BMJ Open*, vol. 4, no. 3, Article ID e004862, 2014.

[2] A. Belkacem, E. Caumes, J. Ouanich et al., "Changing patterns of disseminated gonococcal infection in france: cross-sectional data 2009–2011," *Sexually Transmitted Infections*, vol. 89, no. 8, pp. 613–615, 2013.

[3] X. Muschart, "A case report with Fitz-Hugh-Curtis syndrome, what does it mean?" *Acta Clinica Belgica*, vol. 70, no. 5, pp. 357–358, 2015.

[4] W. Belda Jr., P. E. N. F. Velho, L. J. Fagundes, and M. Arnone, "Evaluation of the in vitro activity of six antimicrobial agents against Neisseria gonorrhoeae," *Revista do Instituto de Medicina Tropical de Sao Paulo*, vol. 49, no. 1, pp. 55–58, 2007.

[5] S. Y. Y. Low, C. W. M. Ong, P.-R. Hsueh, P. A. Tambyah, and T. T. Yeo, "Neisseria gonorrhoeae paravertebral abscess: case report," *Journal of Neurosurgery: Spine*, vol. 17, no. 1, pp. 93–97, 2012.

[6] K. E. Miller, "Diagnosis and treatment of Neisseria gonorrhoeae infections," *American Family Physician*, vol. 73, no. 10, pp. 1779–1784, 2006.

[7] O. Amir, V. D. Nguyen, and B. J. Barnett, "Acute human immunodeficiency virus infection presenting as disseminated gonococcal infection," *Southern Medical Journal*, vol. 96, no. 3, pp. 284–286, 2003.

[8] H. D. Keiser, "Recurrent disseminated gonococcal infection in a patient with hypocomplementemia and membranoproliferative glomerulonephritis," *Journal of Clinical Rheumatology*, vol. 3, no. 5, pp. 286–289, 1997.

[9] R. T. Ellison, J. G. Curd, P. F. Kohler, L. B. Reller, and F. N. Judson, "Underlying complement deficiency in patients with disseminated gonococcal infection," *Sexually Transmitted Diseases*, vol. 14, no. 4, pp. 201–204, 1987.

[10] A. Jitmuang, A. Boonyasiri, N. Keurueangkul, A. Leelaporn, and A. Leelarasamee, "Gonococcal subcutaneous abscess and pyomyositis: a case report," *Case Reports in Infectious Diseases*, vol. 2012, Article ID 790478, 4 pages, 2012.

[11] L. Christin and G. A. Sarosi, "Pyomyositis in North America: case reports and review," *Clinical Infectious Diseases*, vol. 15, no. 4, pp. 668–677, 1992.

[12] R. L. Swarts, L. A. Martinez, and H. G. Robson, "Gonococcal pyomyositis," *Journal of the American Medical Association*, vol. 246, no. 3, article 246, 1981.

[13] S. G. Gurbani, C. T. Cho, K. R. Lee, and L. Powell, "Gonococcal abscess of the obturator internal muscle: use of new diagnostic tools may eliminate the need for surgical intervention," *Clinical Infectious Diseases*, vol. 20, no. 5, pp. 1384–1386, 1995.

[14] P. J. Haugh, C. S. Levy, E. Hoff-Sullivan, M. Malawer, Y. Kollender, and V. Hoff, "Pyomyositis as the sole manifestation of disseminated gonococcal infection: case report and review," *Clinical Infectious Diseases*, vol. 22, no. 5, pp. 861–863, 1996.

[15] D. Birkbeck and J. T. Watson, "Obturator internus pyomyositis. A case report," *Clinical Orthopaedics and Related Research*, no. 316, pp. 221–226, 1995.

[16] N. O. Owino, D. Goldmeier, and R. A. Wall, "Gonococcal septicaemia presenting as a subcutaneous abscess," *British Journal of Venereal Diseases*, vol. 57, no. 2, pp. 143–144, 1981.

[17] E. Seruzier, F. Blanquart, J. F. Lemeulant, and P. Deshayes, "Gonococcal spondylodiscitis," *La Nouvelle Presse Medicale*, vol. 5, no. 9, p. 2166, 1976.

[18] S. J. Van Hal and J. J. Post, "An unusual cause of an epidural abscess," *Medical Journal of Australia*, vol. 180, no. 1, pp. 40–41, 2004.

40

Forgotten but Not Gone! Syphilis Induced Tenosynovitis

**Felicia Ratnaraj, David Brooks, Mollie Walton,
Arun Nagabandi, and Mahmoud Abu Hazeem**

CHI Health Creighton University Medical Center, Omaha, NE, USA

Correspondence should be addressed to Felicia Ratnaraj; feliciaratnaraj@creighton.edu

Academic Editor: Antonella Marangoni

Objective. Tenosynovitis, inflammation of a tendon and its synovial sheath, is a rare manifestation of secondary syphilis and if diagnosed early is reversible. *Background.* A 52-year-old male with past medical history of untreated syphilis presented with gradual onset of swelling and pain of the right fourth metacarpophalangeal joint (MCP). He reported a history of painless penile lesions after having sexual intercourse with a new partner approximately five months ago which was treated with sulfamethoxazole/trimethoprim. An RPR done at that time came back positive with a high titer; however, patient was lost to follow-up. On examination, patient had an edematous, nonerythematous right fourth proximal interphalangeal (PIP) joint. Urgent irrigation, debridement, and exploration of the right hand into the tendon sheath were performed. With his history of syphillis, an RPR was done, which was reactive with a titer of 1 : 64. A confirmatory FTA-ABS test was completed, rendering a positive result. Based on his history of untreated syphilis, dormancy followed by clinical scenario of swelling of the right fourth finger, and a high RPR titer, he was diagnosed with secondary syphilis manifesting as tenosynovitis.

1. Introduction

Tenosynovitis, inflammation of a tendon and its synovial sheath, is a rare manifestation of secondary syphilis that if diagnosed early is entirely reversible. The causes of tenosynovitis can be divided into those of noninfectious or infectious etiology. Examples of noninfectious tenosynovitis include de Quervain's and stenosing tenosynovitis (trigger-finger). Infectious tenosynovitis is often caused by bacterial inoculation of the tendon via direct trauma, contiguous spread, or hematogenous spread.

2. Case Presentation

A 52-year-old male with a past medical history of untreated syphilis presented with gradual onset of swelling and pain of the right fourth finger, as well as palmar tenderness proximal to the right fourth metacarpophalangeal joint (MCP). He denied any allergies, surgeries, recent trauma, or fevers. He did report a history of a painless penile lesion after having sexual intercourse with a new partner approximately five months ago. The lesion had resolved spontaneously after

being treated with sulfamethoxazole/trimethoprim by his primary care physician. Rapid plasma reagin (RPR) was ordered. A few days later, the result came back positive with a high titer. However, since the patient was asymptomatic, he was lost to follow-up for additional treatment.

At the time of this case presentation, patient had an edematous, nonerythematous right fourth PIP joint. There was tenderness to palpation of the right fourth PIP, extending proximally to the MCP joint. A tender, nonerythematous nodule was appreciated upon palpation of the hand proximal to the right fourth MCP joint. The patient was started on broad spectrum antibiotics to be treated empirically for possible infectious tenosynovitis. X-ray of right hand (Figure 1) showed severe degenerative changes at the fourth proximal interphalangeal joint with medial subluxation of the middle phalanx, subchondral cyst formation, and periosteal reaction. Urgent irrigation, debridement, and exploration of the right hand into the tendon sheath and exploration of all digits of the tendon were performed by plastic surgery.

After surgery, magnetic resonance imaging (MRI) (Figures 2 and 3) of the right hand showed severe degenerative changes of the right fourth PIP with soft tissue edema

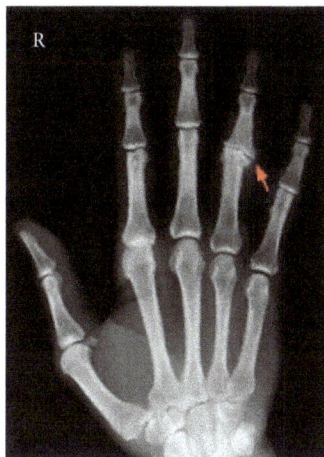

FIGURE 1: X-ray of right hand, severe degenerative changes at the fourth PIP joint with medial subluxation of the middle phalanx, and periosteal reaction.

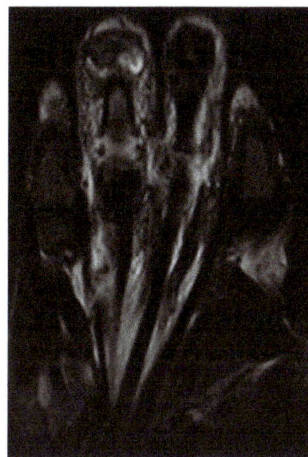

FIGURE 3: MRI coronal view, edema along tendons.

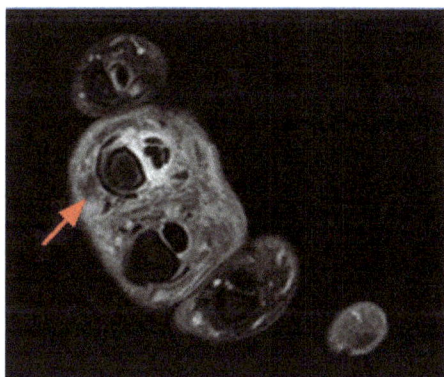

FIGURE 2: MRI axial view, postcontrast tenosynovitis.

extending along the palmar aspect of the digit into the wrist and tenosynovitis of the concerned flexor pollicis longus tendon. Blood cultures were negative for bacterial growth, white blood count was 7.8×10^9/L, and patient was afebrile. Due to his history of syphilis infection, Hepatitis, HIV, and RPR were ordered. HIV and hepatitis panels were negative, but RPR was reactive with a titer of 1 : 64. Fluorescent treponemal antibody absorption (FTA-ABS) test was completed, rendering a positive result, and confirming the diagnosis of syphilis.

Based on his history of untreated syphilis followed by a dormancy period, his clinical presentation, and laboratory findings, the patient was diagnosed with secondary syphilis manifesting as tenosynovitis. He was given a dose of benzathine penicillin 2.4 million units IM, and his partner was encouraged to undergo further testing for syphilis.

As an outpatient, he followed up with occupational therapy for whirlpool treatments with good improvement in his range of motion. Complete resolution of symptoms was achieved four weeks after being discharged from the hospital.

3. Discussion

While any tendon can be targeted in tenosynovitis, the wrist and hand are most commonly affected. The causes of tenosynovitis can be divided into noninfectious or infectious etiology. Examples of noninfectious tenosynovitis include de Quervain's syndrome and stenosis tenosynovitis (trigger-finger). Infectious tenosynovitis is caused by bacterial inoculation of the tendon via direct trauma, contiguous spread, or hematogenous spread [1].

Infectious tenosynovitis can present in a variety of ways. Pang et al. conducted a retrospective study on 75 patients with tenosynovitis and found that the most common presenting symptom was digit swelling. Other presenting symptoms included pain with passive finger extension, a flexed finger posture, and tenderness to digit palpation [1]. Late signs of tenosynovitis that may present are crepitus and swelling localized to the sheath of the infected tendon.

The diagnosis of tenosynovitis is made based on history and clinical presentation. However, MRI can aid in making the diagnosis and assessing damage of associated joint. With tenosynovitis, an MRI will show thickening of the tenosynovium [2]. Compared to conventional radiography, MRI is more sensitive in the detection of tenosynovium inflammation and bony erosion [3]. Alternatively, ultrasound is a modality that is highly sensitive at detecting tenosynovitis. However, it is not as sensitive as MRI in detecting bony erosions [4].

The literature on syphilis induced tenosynovitis, a form of infectious tenosynovitis, is scarce. A literature review performed using the keywords "tenosynovitis" and "syphilis" returned two studies from 1979 and 1984 [5, 6]. Musculoskeletal complaints, such as tenosynovitis, were observed in up to one-third of patients with secondary syphilis [5]. It involved a variety of joints including the wrists, fingers, knees, and ankles. Patients also presented with arthritis with effusions of the tendon sheaths without erythema or tenderness [5]. On physical exam, most of the patients in these studies had generalized lymphadenopathy and a generalized nonpruritic papulosquamous rash [6]. In both studies, treatment of patients with penicillin G led to rapid resolution of musculoskeletal symptoms [5, 6].

This case is an example of infectious tenosynovitis caused by secondary syphilis. Syphilis is a chronic venereal disease with varied and often subtle clinical manifestations. In 2013, the number of primary and secondary syphilis cases reported to the CDC was 17,375, a 10.9% increase from 2012 [7]. However, the rates of syphilis are likely much higher. Primarily due to variations of completeness and accuracy of reporting, reported rates are generally varied and imprecise. Even in the United States, where the importance of reporting is emphasized and rates have been followed for years, it is estimated that as few as half of the actual cases are reported [8].

The causative agent of syphilis is the bacterium *Treponema pallidum*, hereafter referred to as *T. pallidum*. These spirochetes are typically transmitted via direct contact with an infected lesion, entering the host through disrupted epithelium at sites of minor trauma during sexual intercourse [8]. Untreated, acquired syphilis progresses through three stages, with each stage displaying distinct clinical and pathologic manifestations. Primary syphilis, the earliest stage, manifests approximately three weeks after exposure. It is defined by the presence of a firm, nontender, raised, red lesion, known as a chancre, at the site of invasion on the penis, cervix, vaginal wall, or anus. This characteristic chancre heals within three to six weeks with or without therapy [4].

Hematogenous dissemination of *T. pallidum* causes the widespread findings in secondary syphilis, characterized by mucocutaneous and multisystem involvement. The skin lesions of this stage are maculopapular, scaly, or pustular in nature, typically appearing on the palms or soles of the feet. Depending on the type of surface, lesions may assume various appearances. Moist areas of the skin, such as the anogenital region, inner thighs, and axillae may show condylomata lata, broad-based, elevated plaques. Silvery-gray superficial erosions form on mucous membranes, particularly those in the mouth, pharynx, and external genitalia. As in primary syphilis, the lesions of secondary syphilis are superficial and painless and contain the inciting spirochetes. They too are infectious. Lymphadenopathy, mild fever, malaise, and weight loss are also common to this stage. Symptoms of secondary syphilis may last several weeks. Even without treatment, the signs of primary and secondary syphilis resolve spontaneously, and patients then enter the latent stage of infection [4].

After a variable period of latency, usually five years or more, the manifestations of the tertiary stage develop in approximately one-third of untreated patients [4]. There are three main manifestations, which may occur alone or in combination: cardiovascular syphilis, neurosyphilis, and benign tertiary (gummatous) syphilis. Syphilitic aortitis, a form of cardiovascular syphilis, accounts for the majority of cases of tertiary syphilis. Symptomatic neurosyphilis manifests in a variety of ways, including chronic meningovascular disease, tabes dorsalis, and a general paresis. Benign tertiary syphilis is characterized by the formation of gummas, white-gray rubbery lesions, in various sites throughout the body. Although any organ can be affected, gummas occur primarily in skin, mucous membranes, subcutaneous tissue, bone, and joints. Since the use of effective antibiotics, gummas are now very rare and are seen mainly in individuals with acquired immune deficiency syndrome (AIDS) [4].

While clinical staging is useful in guiding therapeutic decisions, it is imprecise. Patients with late stages of disease may have no recollection of signs of earlier stages, possibly because most syphilitic lesions are painless or because some patients may not have clinically apparent primary or secondary lesions. Of note, there is considerable overlap between stages [8].

T. pallidum is too slender to be detected using Gram stain, although it can be visualized by silver stain, dark-field examination, and immunofluorescence. Therefore, serologic testing is the most widely used laboratory technique for the diagnosis of syphilis [8, 9]. Serologic testing should include the use of both nontreponemal and treponemal tests. Either test can be used as the initial screening test. Confirmatory testing is necessary due to the potential for a false positive screening test result. For example, false positive VDRL tests results are not uncommon and are often seen in association with acute infections, collagen vascular diseases, drug addiction, pregnancy, hypergammaglobulinemia, and lepromatous leprosy [4]. Nontreponemal tests, which test for reagin antibodies, are based upon the reactivity of serum from infected patients to a cardiolipin-cholesterol-lecithin antigen. Although the nontreponemal tests are nonspecific, they have traditionally been used for initial syphilis screening due to their relatively low cost, ease of use, and ability to be quantified for the purpose of following response to therapy. Such tests include Rapid Plasmin Reagin (RRR), Venereal Disease Research Laboratory (VDRL), and Toluidine Red Unheated Serum Test (TRUST). Treponemal tests have historically been more complex and expensive to perform than nontreponemal tests. Therefore, they have traditionally been used as confirmatory tests for syphilis when the nontreponemal tests are reactive. However, newer automated versions of these tests enhance simplicity and facilitate ease of use. As a result, these tests are increasingly used to screen for syphilis, rather than as confirmatory tests. Such tests include the Fluorescent treponemal antibody absorption (FTA-ABS), Microhemagglutination test for antibodies to *T. pallidum* (MHA-TP), and *T. pallidum* enzyme immunoassay (TP-EIA). As a group, these tests are based upon the detection of antibodies directed against specific treponemal antigens; therefore, they tend to be more specific than nontreponemal tests. The TP-EIA test has become the favored treponemal test in many laboratories, particularly those with large volumes of testing. Although both nontreponemal and treponemal tests are subject to occasional false positive results in patients without syphilis, sequential use of the two tests greatly improves the accuracy of serologic diagnosis [8].

The treatment of choice for *T. pallidum* is penicillin G with a goal of achieving and maintaining serum penicillin concentration of more than 0.03 ug per mL for 7–14 days. Typically, this can be achieved by a single IM injection of 2.4 million units of benzathine penicillin G in patients with primary, secondary, and early latent syphilis. For patients with penicillin allergies or lacking access to IM penicillin, a single, 2-gram oral dose of azithromycin has been shown to be equally effective in treating primary and secondary syphilis [10].

Competing Interests

The authors declare that they have no competing interests.

References

[1] H.-N. Pang, L.-C. Teoh, A. K. T. Yam, J. Y.-L. Lee, M. E. Puhaindran, and A. B.-H. Tan, "Factors affecting the prognosis of pyogenic flexor tenosynovitis," *The Journal of Bone & Joint Surgery—American Volume*, vol. 89, no. 8, pp. 1742–1748, 2007.

[2] F. M. McQueen, "The MRI view of synovitis and tenosynovitis in inflammatory arthritis: implications for diagnosis and management," *Annals of the New York Academy of Sciences*, vol. 1154, pp. 21–34, 2009.

[3] M. Backhaus, T. Kamradt, D. Sandrock et al., "Arthritis of the finger joints: a comprehensive approach comparing conventional radiography, scintigraphy, ultrasound, and contrast-enhanced magnetic resonance imaging," *Arthritis & Rheumatism*, vol. 42, no. 6, pp. 1232–1245, 1999.

[4] A. J. McAdam and A. H. Sharpe, "Infectious diseases," in *Robbins and Cotran Pathologic Basis of Disease*, V. Kumar, A. K. Abbas, N. Fausto, S. L. Robbins, and R. S. Cotran, Eds., pp. 374–376, Elsevier Saunders, Philadelphia, Pa, USA, 2010.

[5] S. J. McPhee, "Secondary syphilis: uncommon manifestations of a common disease," *The Western Journal of Medicine*, vol. 140, no. 1, pp. 35–42, 1984.

[6] A. J. Reginato, H. R. Schumacher, S. Jimenez, and K. Maurer, "Synovitis in secondary syphilis," *Arthritis and Rheumatism*, vol. 22, no. 2, pp. 170–176, 1979.

[7] CDC 2014 Syphilis, "Atlanta (GA): Centers for Disease Control and Prevention," 2014, http://www.cdc.gov/std/stats13/syphilis.htm.

[8] E. W. Hook III and C. M. Marra, "Acquired syphilis in adults," *The New England Journal of Medicine*, vol. 326, no. 16, pp. 1060–1069, 1992.

[9] A. E. Singh and B. Romanowski, "Syphilis: review with emphasis on clinical, epidemiologic, and some biologic features," *Clinical Microbiology Reviews*, vol. 12, no. 2, pp. 187–209, 1999.

[10] G. Riedner, M. Rusizoka, J. Todd et al., "Single-dose azithromycin versus penicillin G benzathine for the treatment of early syphilis," *The New England Journal of Medicine*, vol. 353, no. 12, pp. 1236–1244, 2005.

41

Identification of *Dietzia* spp. from Cardiac Tissue by 16S rRNA PCR in a Patient with Culture-Negative Device-Associated Endocarditis: A Case Report and Review of the Literature

Praveen Sudhindra,[1] Guiqing Wang,[2] and Robert B. Nadelman[1]

[1] *Division of Infectious Diseases, New York Medical College, Valhalla, NY 10595, USA*
[2] *Department of Pathology, New York Medical College, Valhalla, NY 10595, USA*

Correspondence should be addressed to Praveen Sudhindra; praveen.raghavendra@gmail.com

Academic Editor: Oguz R. Sipahi

The genus *Dietzia* was recently distinguished from other actinomycetes such as *Rhodococcus*. While these organisms are known to be distributed widely in the environment, over the past decade several novel species have been described and isolated from human clinical specimens. Here we describe the identification of *Dietzia natronolimnaea/D. cercidiphylli* by PCR amplification and sequencing of the 16S rRNA encoding gene from cardiac tissue in a patient with culture-negative device-associated endocarditis.

1. Introduction

Blood culture-negative endocarditis is a term used to describe definite or probable endocarditis where three or more aerobic and anaerobic blood cultures collected over 48 hours do not yield growth despite prolonged incubation. 2.5% to 31% of all cases of endocarditis end up being culture negative [1]. The wide variation can be accounted for by the use of varying diagnostic and sampling criteria as well as the distribution of fastidious zoonotic agents that are known to cause endocarditis. The use of implantable cardiac devices such as pacemakers and defibrillators have added another dimension to the problem. The rate of device-associated infection has been estimated to be 1.5–2.4% [2]. We describe a case of device-associated culture-negative endocarditis in which a *Rhodococcus*-like organism, recently classified in a separate genus, was identified by a broad range PCR and DNA sequencing of the 16S rRNA gene performed on cardiac tissue.

2. Case Report

A 58-year-old man was admitted with a three-month history of daily fevers and night sweats. The fevers were preceded by oral canker sores, all but one of which had resolved at the time of presentation. He also had weight loss that he could not quantify and a poor appetite. He denied any other associated symptoms. An automated implantable cardioverter defibrillator (AICD) had been placed several years earlier for primary prevention of ventricular tachycardia. Two weeks prior to admission, the patient had seen his primary care physician and underwent imaging and blood tests, including two sets of blood cultures that were negative. He was not prescribed any antibiotics. Two days prior to presentation he was seen by his cardiologist, who performed a transesophageal echocardiogram at another hospital. The study revealed global left ventricular dysfunction and mobile echo densities on the atrial aspect of the AICD lead. Additional blood cultures were drawn following which the patient was transferred for further management. Three more sets of blood cultures were drawn after which intravenous vancomycin and gentamicin were administered.

Past medical history was significant for chronic atrial fibrillation that was managed by AV nodal ablation and a pacemaker that had been upgraded to an AICD three years prior to presentation. In addition, he had psoriasis, gout, and obstructive sleep apnea. Home medications included rivaroxaban, allopurinol, amlodipine, atorvastatin,

TABLE 1: A PubMed search performed in June 2016 using the terms "Dietzia", "Dietzia and infection" revealed the following published case reports identifying *Dietzia* spp. from human clinical specimens. This excludes the 24 isolates which retrospectively reclassified organisms initially identified as *Rhodococcus equi*.

Organism (date of publication)	Source
Dietzia maris (1999) [3]	Blood culture drawn from in-dwelling catheter and from catheter tip culture
Dietzia maris (2001) [4]	Biopsy from site of prosthetic hip joint infection, by 16S rRNA sequencing
Dietzia maris (2006) [5]	Culture of specimen from aortic wall and pericardial liquid in a patient with aortitis
Dietzia maris (2007) [6]	Skin of 8 healthy human control subjects, by 16S rRNA sequencing
Dietzia cinnamea (2006) [7]	Perianal swab culture of bone marrow transplant recipient
Dietzia papillomatosis (2008) [8]	Skin culture from a patient with confluent and reticulated papillomatosis
Dietzia spp. (2012) [9]	Pacemaker pocket infection, by 16S rRNA sequencing
Dietzia cinnamea (2012) [10]	Culture of wound from dog bite
Dietzia aurantiaca (2012) [11]	CSF culture
Dietzia papillomatosis (2013) [12]	Blood culture in a 2-year-old with fever, rash, and recent VP shunt placement for syringomyelia

furosemide, carvedilol, lisinopril, alprazolam, meloxicam, and omeprazole. The patient lived with his wife, owned a cable company, and had never smoked or used illicit drugs. He drank alcohol occasionally. He did not have any pets or animal contact. He had travelled extensively throughout the United States, but not in the past year.

On examination the temperature was 100.9°F, blood pressure 125/56 mmHg, pulse 59 beats per minute, and an oxygen saturation 94% while breathing ambient air. There was a solitary 2-3 mm ulcer in the right buccal mucosa with a clean base and mild surrounding erythema. The lungs were clear to auscultation and heart sounds were normal without an audible murmur or rub. The pacemaker pocket on the left upper chest had a healed incision and was not tender or erythematous. There were healing psoriatic lesions on the lower abdomen, back, thighs, and forearms. Examination of the fingertips revealed pitting, but no splinter hemorrhages.

Laboratory data were significant for a leukocyte count of $5,900 \, \text{cells/mm}^3$, hemoglobin of 13.9 g/dL, platelet count of $161,000/\text{mm}^3$, and a creatinine of 0.94 mg/dL. Urine dipstick revealed 2+ protein (100 mg/dL). ELISA for antibody to human immunodeficiency virus was negative. Liver function assays were within normal limits. Chest roentgenogram showed an AICD, with clear lungs.

Five days after admission, the patient underwent pacemaker lead extraction, excision of the left atrial appendage, closure of a patent foramen ovale, and epicardial pacemaker lead placement. All blood cultures were negative. Serologies for *Bartonella* spp., *Legionella* spp., *Brucella* spp., and *Coxiella burnetii* were negative as were fungal blood cultures, as well as bacterial, fungal, and mycobacterial cultures of the vegetation and atrial tissue. Nasopharyngeal swab for respiratory pathogen multiplex PCR (including *Mycoplasma pneumoniae*, *Chlamydophila pneumoniae,* and *Bordetella pertussis*) was negative.

Intravenous ceftriaxone was added to the patient's regimen as he remained intermittently febrile a week after admission. Serum IgA antibody to *C. pneumoniae* was positive at a titer of 1 : 128 as was IgM at a titer of 1 : 64; IgG was negative.

A broad range PCR and DNA sequencing targeting 16S rRNA gene was performed on the excised atrial tissue by using the MicroSEQ 500 16S rDNA Sequencing Kit (Life Technologies, Grand Island, NY). The yielded DNA sequence revealed a 100% identity for *Dietzia natronolimnaea*. A subsequent Basic Local Alignment Search Tool (BLAST) search revealed that *D. cercidiphylli* has an identical 16S rRNA sequence and cannot be distinguished from *D. natronolimnaea* using the MicroSEQ 500 Sequencing Kit. PCR was not performed on the vegetation itself, since there was insufficient sample remaining after cultures were performed. Pathological examination of the atrial tissue revealed mild chronic endocarditis and reactive changes in the myocardium, thus satisfying the Modified Duke's criteria for diagnosing infective endocarditis.

Intravenous vancomycin, gentamicin, and ceftriaxone were continued for an additional 10 days at which time the patient developed acute kidney injury; this was attributed to cephalosporin- related allergic interstitial nephritis. All three antibiotics were discontinued and intravenous daptomycin and ciprofloxacin were administered. The creatinine improved, following which the patient was discharged with instructions to complete a four-week course of intravenous daptomycin and oral ciprofloxacin. Attempts made to contact the patient subsequently in order to follow up on his response to therapy were unsuccessful.

3. Discussion

The genus *Dietzia* was first assigned in 1995 to organisms previously classified as rhodococci [13]. They are aerobic, Gram-positive, nonsporing, catalase positive nonacid fast actinomycetes. Since their identification and classification, a number of new species have been isolated from the environment and from human specimens. *Dietzia natronolimnaea* is one of 13 *Dietzia* species currently described. It was first isolated from an East African Soda Lake located in the Kenyan Tanzanian Rift Valley. It is alkaliphilic, growing best at a pH of 9.0 (range 6–10) and at salt concentrations up to 10% [13, 14].

The first report implicating *Dietzia* spp. in human disease was published in 1999 (Table 1). It described the isolation of *Dietzia maris* from the blood of an immunocompromised patient with catheter associated septic shock [3]. Subsequently there have been three other case reports implicating *Dietzia maris* in human infection, one associated with a prosthetic hip joint infection, another from the blood of a patient with respiratory failure, and the third from the pericardial fluid of a patient with aortitis [4, 5]. *D. maris* has also been isolated from the skin of asymptomatic subjects [8]. Two other species—*Dietzia papillomatosis* and *Dietzia cinnamea*—were recovered from a blood culture and a dog bite wound, respectively [10, 12]. Finally, a case of late pacemaker pocket infection was reported, in which 16S rRNA PCR performed on specimens collected from the pocket revealed *Dietzia* spp.; further identification was not attempted [9].

Two studies retrospectively identified *Dietzia* spp. from human clinical specimens by sequencing the 16S rRNA genes and performing biochemical analysis (CAMP test) on isolates initially classified as *Rhodococcus equi* [15, 16]. The first study identified 8 out of 15 isolates as belonging to the genus *Dietzia*. The sources of the clinical specimens were not mentioned. Two of these were identified as *Dietzia natronolimnaea*. The second study followed a similar methodology to identify 16 human clinical isolates previously classified as *Rhodococcus equi*. Nine of these isolates were identified as *D. natronolimnaea/D. cercidiphylli*, and the investigators were unable to distinguish between the two species since the 16S rRNA gene sequences were identical. The isolates were obtained from a wide range of sites including wounds, vaginal, peritoneal, and lung biopsies, blood cultures, and a heart valve.

Both studies also found that the isolates were susceptible to a wide range of antibiotics, including vancomycin, amikacin, amoxicillin-clavulanic acid, ampicillin, ceftriaxone, clarithromycin, ciprofloxacin, imipenem, and linezolid. Some of the *D. maris* and *D. natronolimnaea* isolates were found to be resistant to trimethoprim/sulfamethoxazole. Susceptibilities were tested using the Etest Diffusion gradient method (AB Biodisk, Solna, Sweden).

The increasing identification of this genus from human clinical specimens probably reflects a combination of rising awareness about these organisms as well as more sensitive microbiological diagnostic tools, such as 16S rRNA sequencing. This technique relies on amplifying and sequencing conserved bacterial 16S rRNA genes, which are then compared to known bacterial nucleotide sequences made available either by the manufacturer (MicroSeq ID 16S rDNA Full Gene Library V1.0, http://www3.appliedbiosystems.com/cms/groups/web/documents/softwaredownloads/cms_234268.pdf) or by other approved sources. In principle, several thousand bacterial species could be identified based on this technique. It is an attractive tool to identify fastidious organisms that are difficult to culture in the lab as well as to clarify the identity of organisms that are seen on special stains of biopsy specimens, but fail to grow when cultured. The method does have limitations, especially in identifying organisms at the species level, since percentage differences in sequences that constitute separate species are not always agreed upon [17, 18].

The most common reason for blood culture-negative endocarditis is the administration of antibiotics prior to obtaining blood cultures [14, 19]. Our patient had at least 4 sets of blood cultures obtained prior to the administration of antibiotics. The blood cultures were drawn on two different occasions about 10 days apart. Since infective endocarditis is known to be associated with continuous, low grade bacteremia, one would have expected to diagnose endocarditis due to most agents known to cause subacute bacterial endocarditis (e.g., *Streptococci* or *Enterococcus* spp.). The HACEK group of organisms were previously difficult to isolate by routine blood culture methods, but with modern culture techniques these organisms are usually isolated within three to five days [20, 21].

We do not believe that the positive *C. pneumoniae* serology in our patient indicates infection with this organism. Guidelines for diagnosis of acute respiratory tract infections due to *C. pneumoniae* suggest a cutoff of 1:16 for IgM titers and 1:512 for IgG. IgM antibodies are expected to appear within 2-3 weeks of primary infection, while IgG antibodies may take 6–8 weeks to become detectable [22]. Our patient had been symptomatic for about 12 weeks prior to testing; therefore one would have expected IgG antibodies to be detectable. In addition, PCR performed on a nasopharyngeal swab specimen and the 16S rRNA PCR assay performed on excised atrial tissue were negative for *C. pneumoniae*. The specificity and reproducibility of these serological tests have been questioned, with a high rate of asymptomatic infection and cross-reactivity with serologies for *Mycoplasma*, *Bartonella*, and *Yersinia* [23, 24]. The applicability of these criteria to the diagnosis of endocarditis is also questionable. *C. pneumoniae* was identified on cardiac tissue by PCR in most cases where the diagnosis of endocarditis due to this organism was made [25]. The lack of follow-up serologic testing was a potential limitation in this case. In the unlikely event that *C. pneumoniae* played an etiologic role, the patient was treated with oral ciprofloxacin, which has activity against this organism.

Contamination during specimen collection, transport, and storage are always concerns when atypical organisms are identified from clinical specimens, even more so when nontraditional and highly sensitive microbiological methods are used. Some species of *Dietzia* may be part of human skin flora and in one case may have caused infection of a pacemaker pocket [6, 9]. We cannot rule out the possibility of PCR contamination in view of negative culture results in our patient. No serological test is currently available for detection of antibodies specific to infection with this organism. However, the DNA sequence of a single PCR amplicon from the excised atrial tissue of this patient shared 100% identity with that of a *D. natronolimnaea/D. cercidiphylli* strain.

Pathologic findings satisfied the Modified Duke's criteria for the diagnosis of infective endocarditis, classifying it as "Definite Infective Endocarditis"; however, not all clinical criteria were met since this was a case of culture-negative, device-associated endocarditis. The antimicrobial regimen was selected after considering the then current guideline recommendations by Baddour et al. [26] as well as available clinical and epidemiological data. We also considered the rarity of *Dietzia* infections, relative paucity of information regarding the course of disease caused by these organisms and long term response to antibiotics, as well as the high likelihood that the patient would require a new implantable cardiac device after completing antibiotic therapy. Therefore, we selected a regimen which was likely to be convenient for outpatient therapy, well tolerated, and treat most *Enterococci, Staphylococci, Streptococci,* and HACEK organisms.

The etiologic role of *Dietzia natronolimnaea/D. cercidiphylli* in this case of culture-negative device-associated endocarditis is supported by the multiple reported instances where *Dietzia* spp. were isolated from blood cultures as well as one instance each where organisms were identified from heart valve, aortic wall, and pericardial fluid (Table 1). Potential portals of entry may have been the psoriatic lesions on our patient's skin (cultures of the patient's skin were not performed) or from the pacemaker pocket site following implantation of the AICD.

This case serves to illustrate the potential value of PCR and DNA sequencing in diagnosing culture-negative endocarditis and the potential role of *Dietzia* spp. in causing this infection. Developing serological tests could help in clarifying the role played by these organisms in human disease.

Competing Interests

The authors declare that there is no conflict of interests regarding the publication of this article.

References

[1] A. Katsouli and M. G. Massad, "Current issues in the diagnosis and management of blood culture-negative infective and noninfective endocarditis," *Annals of Thoracic Surgery*, vol. 95, no. 4, pp. 1467–1474, 2013.

[2] A. J. Greenspon, J. D. Patel, E. Lau et al., "16-year trends in the infection burden for pacemakers and implantable cardioverter-defibrillators in the United States : 1993 to 2008," *Journal of the American College of Cardiology*, vol. 58, no. 10, pp. 1001–1006, 2011.

[3] P. Bemer-Melchior, A. Haloun, P. Riegel, and H. B. Drugeon, "Bacteremia due to *Dietzia maris* in an immunocompromised patient," *Clinical Infectious Diseases*, vol. 29, no. 5, pp. 1338–1340, 1999.

[4] O. Pidoux, J.-N. Argenson, V. Jacomo, and M. Drancourt, "Molecular identification of a *Dietzia maris* hip prosthesis infection isolate," *Journal of Clinical Microbiology*, vol. 39, no. 7, pp. 2634–2636, 2001.

[5] G. Reyes, J.-L. Navarro, C. Gamallo, and M.-C. De Las Cuevas, "Type A aortic dissection associated with *Dietzia maris*," *Interactive Cardiovascular and Thoracic Surgery*, vol. 5, no. 5, pp. 666–668, 2006.

[6] I. Dekio, H. Sakamoto, H. Hayashi, M. Amagai, M. Suematsu, and Y. Benno, "Characterization of skin microbiota in patients with atopic dermatitis and in normal subjects using 16S rRNA gene-based comprehensive analysis," *Journal of Medical Microbiology*, vol. 56, no. 12, pp. 1675–1683, 2007.

[7] A. F. Yassin, H. Hupfer, and K. P. Schaal, "*Dietzia cinnamea* sp. nov., a novel species isolated from a perianal swab of a patient with a bone marrow transplant," *International Journal of Systematic and Evolutionary Microbiology*, vol. 56, no. 3, pp. 641–645, 2006.

[8] A. L. Jones, R. J. Koerner, S. Natarajan, J. D. Perry, and M. Goodfellow, "*Dietzia papillomatosis* sp. nov., a novel actinomycete isolated from the skin of an immunocompetent patient with confluent and reticulated papillomatosis," *International Journal of Systematic and Evolutionary Microbiology*, vol. 58, no. 1, pp. 68–72, 2008.

[9] S. Perkin, A. Wilson, D. Walker, and E. McWilliams, "Dietzia species pacemaker pocket infection: an unusual organism in human infections," *BMJ Case Reports*, vol. 2012, 2012.

[10] J. J. Hirvonen, I. Lepistö, S. Mero, and S.-S. Kaukoranta, "First isolation of *Dietzia cinnamea* from a dog bite wound in an adult patient," *Journal of Clinical Microbiology*, vol. 50, no. 12, pp. 4163–4165, 2012.

[11] P. Kämpfer, E. Falsen, A. Frischmann, and H.-J. Busse, "*Dietzia aurantiaca* sp. nov., isolated from a human clinical specimen," *International Journal of Systematic and Evolutionary Microbiology*, vol. 62, no. 3, pp. 484–488, 2012.

[12] P. Rammer, H. Calum, C. Moser et al., "*Dietzia papillomatosis* bacteremia," *Journal of Clinical Microbiology*, vol. 51, no. 6, pp. 1977–1978, 2013.

[13] F. A. Rainey, S. Klatte, R. M. Kroppenstedt, and E. Stackebrandt, "*Dietzia*, a new genus including *Dietzia maris* comb. nov., formerly *Rhodococcus maris*," *International Journal of Systematic Bacteriology*, vol. 45, no. 1, pp. 32–36, 1995.

[14] R. J. Koerner, M. Goodfellow, and A. L. Jones, "The genus *Dietzia*: a new home for some known and emerging opportunist pathogens," *FEMS Immunology and Medical Microbiology*, vol. 55, no. 3, pp. 296–305, 2009.

[15] H. Niwa, B. A. Lasker, H. P. Hinrikson et al., "Characterization of human clinical isolates of *Dietzia* species previously misidentified as *Rhodococcus equi*," *European Journal of Clinical Microbiology and Infectious Diseases*, vol. 31, no. 5, pp. 811–820, 2012.

[16] L. Pilares, J. Agüero, J. A. Vázquez-Boland, L. Martínez-Martínez, and J. Navas, "Identification of atypical Rhodococcus-like clinical isolates as *Dietzia spp.* by 16S rRNA gene sequencing," *Journal of Clinical Microbiology*, vol. 48, no. 5, pp. 1904–1907, 2010.

[17] P. C. Y. Woo, S. K. P. Lau, J. L. L. Teng, H. Tse, and K.-Y. Yuen, "Then and now: use of 16S rDNA gene sequencing for bacterial identification and discovery of novel bacteria in clinical microbiology laboratories," *Clinical Microbiology and Infection*, vol. 14, no. 10, pp. 908–934, 2008.

[18] J. M. Janda and S. L. Abbott, "16S rRNA gene sequencing for bacterial identification in the diagnostic laboratory: pluses, perils, and pitfalls," *Journal of Clinical Microbiology*, vol. 45, no. 9, pp. 2761–2764, 2007.

[19] L. Slipczuk, J. N. Codolosa, C. D. Davila et al., "Infective endocarditis epidemiology over five decades: a systematic review," *PLoS ONE*, vol. 8, no. 12, Article ID e82665, 2013.

[20] A. Apisarnthanarak, R. M. Johnson, A. C. Braverman, W. M. Dunne, and J. R. Little, "*Cardiobacterium hominis* bioprosthetic mitral valve endocarditis presenting as septic arthritis," *Diagnostic Microbiology and Infectious Disease*, vol. 42, no. 1, pp. 79–81, 2002.

[21] D. M. Arnold, F. Smaill, T. E. Warkentin, L. Christjanson, and I. Walker, "*Cardiobacterium hominis* endocarditis associated with very severe thrombocytopenia and platelet autoantibodies," *American Journal of Hematology*, vol. 76, no. 4, pp. 373–377, 2004.

[22] S. Kumar and M. R. Hammerschlag, "Acute respiratory infection due to *Chlamydia pneumoniae*: current status of diagnostic

methods," *Clinical Infectious Diseases*, vol. 44, no. 4, pp. 568–576, 2007.

[23] M. Maurin, F. Eb, J. Etienne, and D. Raoult, "Serological cross-reactions between *Bartonella* and *Chlamydia* species: implications for diagnosis," *Journal of Clinical Microbiology*, vol. 35, no. 9, pp. 2283–2287, 1997.

[24] C. L. Hyman, P. M. Roblin, C. A. Gaydos, T. C. Quinn, J. Schachter, and M. R. Hammerschlag, "Prevalence of asymptomatic nasopharyngeal carriage of *Chlamydia pneumoniae* in subjectively healthy adults: assessment by polymerase chain reaction-enzyme immunoassay and culture," *Clinical Infectious Diseases*, vol. 20, no. 5, pp. 1174–1178, 1995.

[25] R. Gdoura, S. Pereyre, I. Frikha et al., "Culture-negative endocarditis due to *Chlamydia pneumoniae*," *Journal of Clinical Microbiology*, vol. 40, no. 2, pp. 718–720, 2002.

[26] L. M. Baddour, W. R. Wilson, A. S. Bayer et al., "Infective endocarditis: diagnosis, antimicrobial therapy and management of complications," *Circulation*, vol. 111, pp. e394–e434, 2005.

42

Bacteremia Caused by *Kocuria kristinae* from Egypt: Are There More? A Case Report and Review of the Literature

Reem M. Hassan,[1] **Dina M. Bassiouny,**[1] **and Yomna Matar**[2]

[1]*Department of Clinical and Chemical Pathology, Faculty of Medicine, Cairo University, Cairo, Egypt*
[2]*Department of Psychiatry, Faculty of Medicine, Cairo University, Cairo, Egypt*

Correspondence should be addressed to Reem M. Hassan; reem.mostafa@kasralainy.edu.eg

Academic Editor: Pau Montesinos Fernández

Kocuria kristinae is opportunistic Gram-positive cocci from the family Micrococcaceae. It is usually considered part of the normal flora that rarely is isolated from clinical specimens. Here, we report a case of *Kocuria kristinae* bacteremia; to the best of our knowledge, this is the first report from Egypt.

1. Introduction

Kocuria are Gram-positive, coccoid actinobacteria that occur in tetrads belonging to the family Micrococcaceae, suborder Micrococcineae, order Actinomycetales [1]. They are widely distributed in nature and can also be found frequently as normal skin and oral cavity flora in humans and other mammals. The genus contains 18 species, only five of which are known to be opportunistic pathogens [2].

Few reports on *Kocuria* spp. clinical infections exist in the literature. They were reported to cause catheter-related bacteremia in immunocompromised patients and those with chronic illness, peritonitis, cholecystitis, and urinary tract infection in patients with indwelling urinary catheters [3–6].

The underestimated prevalence of this organism is due to its misidentification as coagulase-negative staph and absence of guidelines for its clinical evaluation as a pathogen as it can be a common source of contamination in clinical specimens [7, 8].

2. Case Report

A 70-year-old female patient diagnosed with bipolar disease was admitted to the psychiatry department in Cairo University Hospital (Kasr Al-Ainy). The patient develops manic/depressive episodes every now and then and was in an episode of mania for which she received treatment for 2 weeks, regular antipsychotic regimen (risperidone, depakine, and quetiapine). A peripheral cannula was introduced for intravascular fluids. The patient was not controlled with regular treatment and received aqueous intramuscular injection of clopixol 200 mg, after which she developed bilateral lower limb weakness, disturbed conscious level a day later, and fever. Weakness progressed to hypotonia and external rotation, with no rigidity and equivocal plantar reflex. Manifestations in the right limb were severer than in the left one, as there were redness, warmness, and edema of calf muscles but no pain or tenderness. The patient received clexane 40 mg prophylaxis. Examination of the patient revealed temperature 38.3°C, blood pressure 130/80 mmHg, pulse 110/min, and respiratory rate 20/min.

Radiological investigations were done in the form of CT brain, MRI brain, and echocardiogram, which were normal, and venous Duplex on lower limbs that showed recent adherent deep venous thrombosis (DVT) in right peroneal and soleal areas for which she received a higher dose of clexane (60 mg every 12 hours).

Laboratory investigations were done and results were as follows: CPK was 3200 U/L which gradually decreased later on, AST was 94 U/L, platelets were 87000 cells/cmm, Na was 134 mg/dL, K was 3.5 mg/dL, Ca++ was 0.61 mg/dL, Hb was 10 mg/dL, WBCs were 3600 cells/cmm, CRP was positive, PT and PTT were normal, and urine culture grew *E. coli* (ESBL).

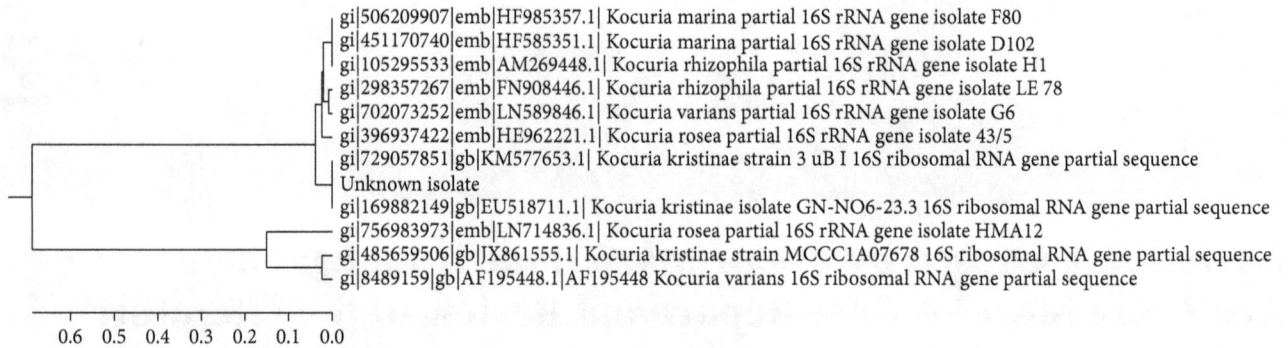

FIGURE 1: Evolutionary relationships of taxa. The evolutionary history was inferred using the UPGMA method [10].

Microbiological Methods. Blood culture was withdrawn in the BACTEC Plus aerobic/F and BACTEC Plus anaerobic/F blood culture bottles (Becton, Dickinson and Company, Spain, MD). All bottles were incubated in BACTEC 120 instrument. Blood culture grew Gram-positive cocci on blood and chocolate agar with catalase-positive, coagulase-negative, and typical pigmentation of *Kocuria* colonies (pale rose) that became more distinct after further 24 hr incubation in 4°C. Vitek2 automated identification system (bioMerieux, France) was used to identify the isolate using the Gram positive identification cards (GP cards) and the isolate was identified as *Kocuria kristinae* (99%). Susceptibility testing was done using the modified Kirby-Bauer disc diffusion method; the organism was found to be sensitive to cefoxitin, gentamicin, amikacin, ciprofloxacin, levofloxacin, and linezolid but resistant to vancomycin, teicoplanin, rifampicin, amoxicillin/clavulanate, and clindamycin. Phenotypic identification was confirmed by performing a molecular assay, namely, 16S rRNA gene sequencing, as previously described using the primer sets 536f 5′CAGCAGCCGCGGTAATAC and RP2 5′eACGGCACCTTGTTACGACTT (AccuOligo, Bioneer, Daejeon, Korea), BigDye® Terminator v3.1 cycle sequencing kit (Applied Biosystems, Foster City, CA, USA), and the BigDye Xterminator™ purification kit (Applied Biosystems, Foster City, CA, USA), and then run on Applied Biosystems 3500 Genetic Analyzer (Applied Biosystems, Foster City, CA, USA). Sequences were analyzed with AutoAssembler software (KB_3500_POP7_BDTv3.mob) and compared using the basic local alignment search tool. Also, a neighbor-joining phylogenetic tree with the 16S rRNA gene sequences of all *Kocuria* species using MEGA6 program (Figure 1) was constructed [9–12].

3. Discussion

By reviewing the literature, 20 reports on *Kocuria* infections in humans were found, most of which were in immunocompromised hosts with few reports in otherwise healthy people. The five opportunistic *Kocuria* spp. are *K. kristinae*, *K. rhizophila*, *K. rosea*, *K. varians*, and *K. marina* [3, 13–16].

K. kristinae was first described in 1974 (previously known as *Micrococcus kristinae*). The bacterium is facultative anaerobic, nonmotile, catalase-positive, and coagulase-negative and

is known to cause catheter-related bacteremia and infective endocarditis [2, 17].

In the present case report, we describe a case of catheter-related blood stream infection caused by *K. kristinae*, complicated by DVT, which was the case in other reported infections caused by *Kocuria* spp. As the patient had a concomitant urinary tract infection (caused by *E. coli*), the presented fever could be caused either by one of the organisms or even by the DVT. The patient was not known to be immunocompromised except for antipsychotic drugs which with prolonged use can cause impaired liver functions with mild state of immune system disturbance.

Infection with this organism takes place mostly in immunocompromised patients like *K. kristinae* bacteremia that occurred in a patient suffering from ovarian cancer. This patient had multiple febrile episodes through a period of six months, all of which grew the organism from several blood cultures and central venous lines (CVLs) [18].

K. kristinae was also described as the cause of acute peritonitis in a patient with end-stage renal failure that had CAPD for two years. The source of contamination was suspected to be touch of the catheter that led to access of bacteria into the peritoneal cavity [4, 19].

An immunocompetent pregnant female developed severe *K. kristinae* intravascular infections with suppurative thrombosis that led to septic pulmonary emboli. These complications followed catheter-related blood stream infection [3].

A recent report of *K. kristinae* bacteremia discussed an infant with a history of prolonged diarrhea complicated with black hairy tongue symptoms [20].

A different access route of *K. kristinae* infection was recently documented in an elderly diabetic patient who developed endocarditis after amputation of a forefoot ulcer and the central venous catheter was not involved [21].

Many recent studies, including ours, correctly identified *Kocuria* spp. using the Vitek-2 ID-GPC Gram-positive identification card, perhaps due to the recently introduced larger database that allows the identification of additional taxa [22].

Misidentification among members of the *Kocuria* genus cannot be ruled out as other studies have reported such situations [5, 13, 14].

As a consequence to the absence of evidence-based guidelines for managing *Kocuria* infections, cases are managed depending on previous experience or similar cases in the literature. These reports suggested the removal of offending catheter and the use of an antibiotic either alone or in combination. Only one report by Szczerba proposed amoxicillin/clavulanate along with drugs like ceftriaxone, cefuroxime, doxycycline, and amikacin as a first-line therapy against micrococcal infections [23].

Also, there are no specific criteria for interpreting sensitivity assays with Kocuria isolates and only a few investigated the resistance mechanisms expressed in this genus as the one report that postulated decreased cell wall permeability and multidrug efflux pump expressed in these organisms [2]. Another study identified proteins that may be involved in efflux mechanisms [24].

To summarize, Kocuria kristinae bacteremia should be considered especially in liable patients and on repeated isolation. Introduction of newer diagnostic techniques to the microbiology lab leads to better identification of rare pathogens and underestimated ones. Proper diagnosis is the key to better treatment strategies.

Consent

Informed consent was obtained from the participant included in the study.

Competing Interests

The authors declare no competing interests.

References

[1] E. Stackebrandt, C. Koch, O. Gvozdiak, and P. Schumann, "Taxonomic dissection of the genus Micrococcus: Kocuria gen. nov., Nesterenkonia gen. nov., Kytococcus gen. nov., Dermacoccus gen. nov., and Micrococcus cohn 1872 gen. emend," International Journal of Systematic Bacteriology, vol. 45, no. 4, pp. 682–692, 1995.

[2] V. Savini, C. Catavitello, G. Masciarelli et al., "Drug sensitivity and clinical impact of members of the genus Kocuria," Journal of Medical Microbiology, vol. 59, no. 12, pp. 1395–1402, 2010.

[3] R. Dunn, S. Bares, and M. Z. David, "Central venous catheter-related bacteremia caused by Kocuria kristinae: case report and review of the literature," Annals of Clinical Microbiology and Antimicrobials, vol. 10, article 31, 2011.

[4] A. Carlini, R. Mattei, I. Lucarotti, A. Bartelloni, and A. Rosati, "Kocuria kristinae: an unusual cause of acute peritoneal dialysis-related infection," Peritoneal Dialysis International, vol. 31, no. 1, pp. 105–107, 2011.

[5] E. S. K. Ma, C. L. P. Wong, K. T. W. Lai, E. C. H. Chan, W. C. Yam, and A. C. W. Chan, "Kocuria kristinae infection associated with acute cholecystitis," BMC Infectious Diseases, vol. 5, article 60, 2005.

[6] R. Tewari, M. Dudeja, A. K. Das, and S. Nandy, "Kocuria kristinae in catheter associated urinary tract infection: a case report," Journal of Clinical and Diagnostic Research, vol. 7, no. 8, pp. 1692–1693, 2013.

[7] R. Ben-Ami, S. Navon-Venezia, D. Schwartz, Y. Schlezinger, Y. Mekuzas, and Y. Carmeli, "Erroneous reporting of coagulase-negative staphylococci as Kocuria spp. by the Vitek 2 system,"

Journal of Clinical Microbiology, vol. 43, no. 3, pp. 1448–1450, 2005.

[8] W. E. Kloos, T. G. Tornabene, and K. H. Schleifer, "Isolation and characterization of micrococci from human skin, including two new species: Micrococcus lylae and Micrococcus kristinae," International Journal of Systematic Bacteriology, vol. 24, no. 1, pp. 79–101, 1974.

[9] R. M. Hassan, M. G. El Enany, and H. H. Rizk, "Evaluation of broad-range 16S rRNA PCR for the diagnosis of bloodstream infections: two years of experience," Journal of Infection in Developing Countries, vol. 8, no. 10, pp. 1252–1258, 2014.

[10] P. H. A. Sneath and R. R. Sokal, Numerical Taxonomy, Freeman, San Francisco, Calif, USA, 1973.

[11] K. Tamura, M. Nei, and S. Kumar, "Prospects for inferring very large phylogenies by using the neighbor-joining method," Proceedings of the National Academy of Sciences of the United States of America, vol. 101, no. 30, pp. 11030–11035, 2004.

[12] K. Tamura, G. Stecher, D. Peterson, A. Filipski, and S. Kumar, "MEGA6: molecular evolutionary genetics analysis version 6.0," Molecular Biology and Evolution, vol. 30, no. 12, pp. 2725–2729, 2013.

[13] K. Becker, F. Rutsch, A. Uekötter et al., "Kocuria rhizophila adds to the emerging spectrum of micrococcal species involved in human infections," Journal of Clinical Microbiology, vol. 46, no. 10, pp. 3537–3539, 2008.

[14] F. Altuntas, O. Yildiz, B. Eser, K. Gündogan, B. Sumerkan, and M. Çetin, "Catheter-related bacteremia due to Kocuria rosea in a patient undergoing peripheral blood stem cell transplantation," BMC Infectious Diseases, vol. 4, article 62, 2004.

[15] C.-Y. Tsai, S.-H. Su, Y.-H. Cheng, Y.-L. Chou, T.-H. Tsai, and A.-S. Lieu, "Kocuria varians infection associated with brain abscess: a case report," BMC Infectious Diseases, vol. 10, article 102, 2010.

[16] Y. L. Ja, H. K. Si, S. J. Haeng et al., "Two cases of peritonitis caused by Kocuria marina in patients undergoing continuous ambulatory peritoneal dialysis," Journal of Clinical Microbiology, vol. 47, no. 10, pp. 3376–3378, 2009.

[17] C. C. Lai, J. Y. Wang, S. H. Lin et al., "Catheter-related bacteraemia and infective endocarditis caused by Kocuria species," Clinical Microbiology and Infection, vol. 17, no. 2, pp. 190–192, 2011.

[18] G. Basaglia, E. Carretto, D. Barbarini et al., "Catheter-related bacteremia due to Kocuria kristinae in a patient with ovarian cancer," Journal of Clinical Microbiology, vol. 40, no. 1, pp. 311–313, 2002.

[19] C. Y. Cheung, N. H. Y. Cheng, K. F. Chau, and C. S. Li, "An unusual organism for CAPD-related peritonitis: Kocuria kristinae," Peritoneal Dialysis International, vol. 31, no. 1, pp. 107–108, 2011.

[20] E. K. Oncel, M. S. Boyraz, and A. Kara, "Black tongue associated with Kocuria (Micrococcus) kristinae bacteremia in a 4-month-old infant," European Journal of Pediatrics, vol. 171, no. 3, p. 593, 2012.

[21] R. Citro, C. Prota, L. Greco et al., "Kocuria kristinae endocarditis related to diabetic foot infection," Journal of Medical Microbiology, vol. 62, no. 6, pp. 932–934, 2013.

[22] M. Boudevrijns, J. Vandeven, J. Verhaegen, R. Ben-Ami, and Y. Carmeli, "Vitek 2 automated identification system and Kocuria kristinae," Journal of Clinical Microbiology, vol. 43, no. 11, p. 5832, 2005.

[23] I. Szczerba, "Susceptibility to antibiotics of bacteria from genera Micrococcus, Kocuria, Nesterenkonia, Kytococcus and Derma-coccus," *Medycyna Doswiadczalna i Mikrobiologia*, vol. 55, no. 1, pp. 75–80, 2003 (Polish).

[24] H. Takarada, M. Sekine, H. Kosugi et al., "Complete genome sequence of the soil actinomycete *Kocuria rhizophila*," *Journal of Bacteriology*, vol. 190, no. 12, pp. 4139–4146, 2008.

43

A Case of Tuberculous Meningitis with Paradoxical Response in a 14-Year-Old Boy

Murat Özer,[1] Yasemin Özsürekci,[2] Ali Bülent Cengiz,[2] Nagehan Emiralioğlu,[3] Deniz Doğru,[3] Kader Karlı Oğuz,[4] Onur Akça,[4] and Özgür Özkayar[5]

[1]Department of Pediatrics, Hacettepe University Faculty of Medicine, Ankara, Turkey
[2]Pediatric Infectious Diseases, Hacettepe University Faculty of Medicine, Ankara, Turkey
[3]Pediatric Chest Diseases, Hacettepe University Faculty of Medicine, Ankara, Turkey
[4]Department of Radiology, Hacettepe University Faculty of Medicine, Ankara, Turkey
[5]Department of Pathology, Hacettepe University Faculty of Medicine, Ankara, Turkey

Correspondence should be addressed to Murat Özer; muratozer@hacettepe.edu.tr

Academic Editor: Sandeep Dogra

A clinical or radiological worsening of already existing lesions or an emergence of new lesions after beginning treatment in patients with tuberculosis (TB) is referred to as the paradoxical response. This has aroused suspicion regarding the accuracy of diagnosis, the possibilities of treatment failure, or the presence of another underlying disease, and thus it is an important topic for clinicians to understand. In this article, the development of a paradox reaction in a 14-year-old male patient diagnosed with and treated for tuberculosis meningitis is reported. This pediatric patient with a healthy immune system is treated with steroids successfully and reported to elucidate the importance of managing the paradox of TB progression in spite of the appropriate anti-TB medications.

1. Introduction

In tuberculosis (TB) patients, the clinical or radiological worsening of already existing lesions or new lesions appearing after treatment is called a paradoxical response [1]. Paradoxical responses are especially seen in lungs, lymph nodes, and the central nervous system affected by TB [2]. There is scarce data about the incidence of paradoxical reactions in HIV-negative children in literature. In 115 HIV-negative children with pulmonary and extrapulmonary TB, 12 patients (10%) developed a paradoxical reaction [3]. Therefore, awareness of clinicians about the clinical nature of this situation is important, particularly in patients with treatment failure or underlying diseases [2]. It poses serious problems in the management of central nervous system (CNS) TB. There is always a question of development of drug resistant TB when there is worsening of the patient and often paradoxical reaction leads to inappropriate increment or addition of more toxic newer antitubercular drugs with several adverse consequences [4]. Herein, the case of a child

with TB meningitis with a normal immune system, who was observed to have paradoxical responses, was reported to emphasize this situation and increase clinicians' awareness.

2. Case Report

Two months before being admitted to our hospital, a 14-year-old male patient was admitted to another hospital because of headache, vomiting, and fever. An emerging hemiparesis persisted on the left side of the patient. When his family history was questioned, the patient's father was treated 1.5 years ago for lung TB (caused by resistant *Mycobacterium tuberculosis* bacilli); however, it was learned that prophylaxis was not given to the patient. Tuberculosis meningitis was diagnosed according to physical examination and laboratory findings and radiological findings in magnetic resonance imaging (MRI) of brain. Anti-TB treatments (isoniazid, rifampicin, ethambutol, and pyrazinamide) and 0.5 mg/kg of prednisolone were started for CNS TB. Complaints improved with the treatment, and the prednisolone was decreased

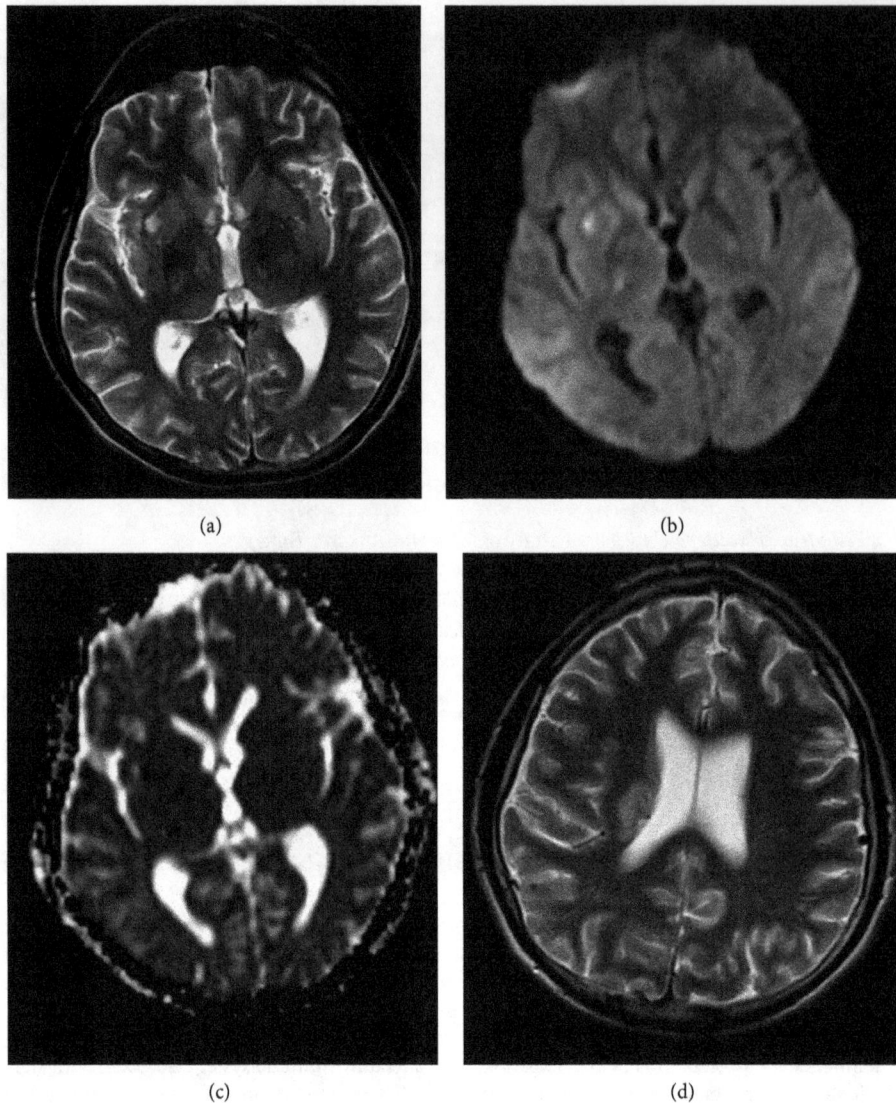

FIGURE 1: Instant diagnosis T2A (a), diffusion image (b = 1000 s/mm^2) (b), ADC (c) map, and T2A image 15 days after diagnosis (d). Acute ischemic lesions in the right thalamus, globus pallidus, and lateral putamen (b, c), increases of bilateral hypothalamic T2 intensity (a), and corona radiata intensity increment after 15 days (d). After IVKM there was no inclusion of a parenchymal contrast.

gradually. He was discharged at 38th day of the treatment with a plan of follow-up outpatient clinic visits.

One week later, after 45 days of the anti-TB treatment, the patient was admitted into our hospital because of a severe headache. In the initial evaluation, the patient was conscious, cooperative, and oriented, and his vitals parameters were normal. A Bacillus Calmette-Guerin (BCG) scar was present. He had right-central facial paralysis and strength loss, specifically on the left half of the body. Dysmetria, tremor, and prominent loss of fine motor coordination were all present in the upper left extremity. Other physical examination findings were normal. In laboratory examinations, complete blood count (CBC) test, C-reactive protein (CRP), and erythrocyte sedimentation rate were in normal limits. Additionally, the test for antibodies against the human immunodeficiency virus (HIV) was negative and biochemical analysis of serum

was normal. Cerebrospinal fluid (CSF) samples were microscopically normal and CSF opening pressure was 16 cm of water, the CSF protein level was 198 mg/dL (15–40), and the CSF glucose level was 46 mg/dL (60–80) (with a simultaneous blood glucose level of 72 mg/dL). No organisms were recovered in aerobic CSF culture. There was not any evidence for TB in the anteroposterior chest X-ray. MRI findings of the cerebral and cerebellar regions were a wide edema area in the frontotemporal white matter and a chronic infarct sequel area shown in the leptomeningeal region. In comparison with previous MRI, it was shown that the same lesion had clearly enlarged (Figures 1, 2, and 3). Moxifloxacin and clarithromycin were added to the isoniazid, rifampicin, ethambutol, and pyrazinamide treatment on account of the possible existence of resistant *M. tuberculosis* such as father's pattern. On the other hand, oral prednisolone (1 mg/kg/day)

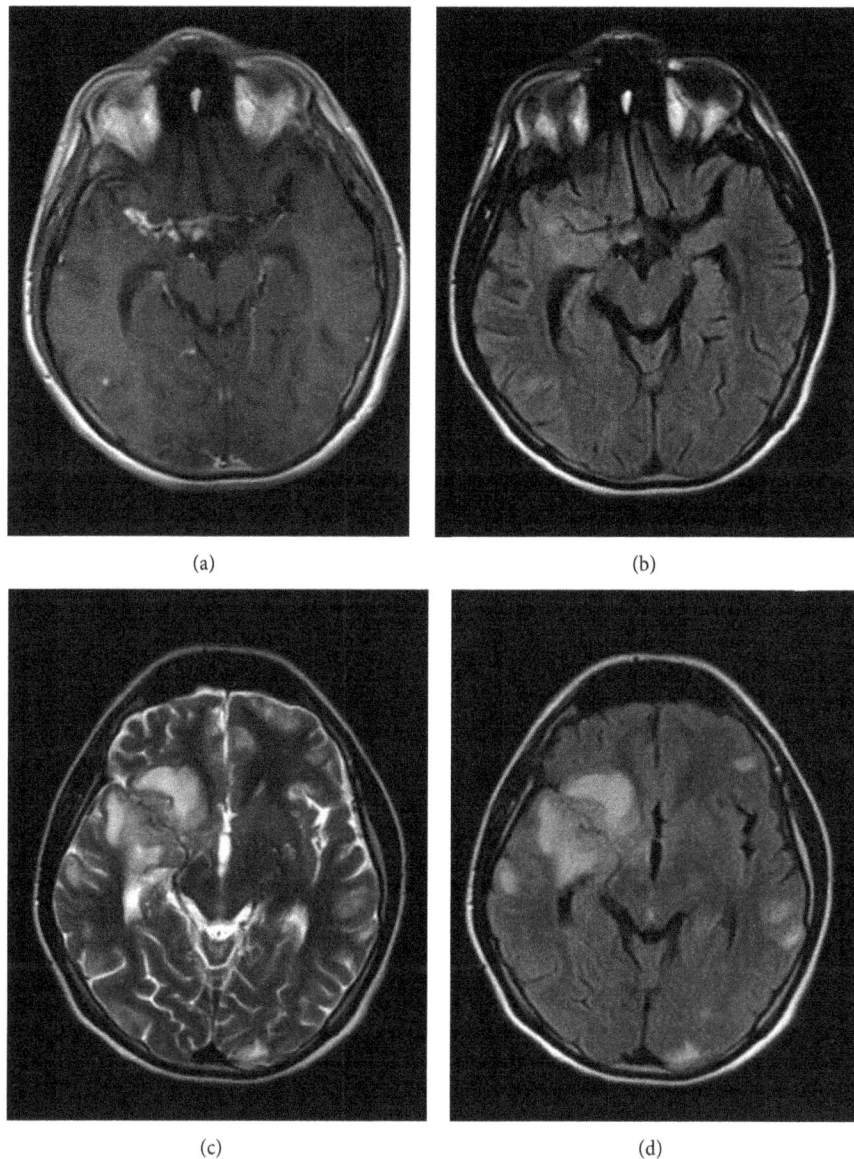

FIGURE 2: A contrast of an initial diagnosis against its progression after one month T1A (a), FLAIR (b), a diagnosis 45 days later with T2A (c), and FLAIR (d) images. A meningeal contrast is involved and a thickening compatible with a diagnosis of basal meningitis is visible in the neighborhood of the right sylvian fissure and basal cisterns (a) and increments of parenchymal T2 intensity in that region (b). Instead of antituberculosis treatments working, on the forty-fifth day mark, parenchymal lesions have been proven to grow and new lesions have appeared (c, d).

was added to the management protocol because of the prospect of the paradoxical response. A brain biopsy was performed to confirm the diagnosis and a lymphohistiocytic reaction, giant cell formation, and a granulomatous response, which is characterized by abortive granulomas, but does not include caseous necrosis, are all seen in the microscopic examination of the tissue (Figure 4). Polymerase chain reaction (PCR) of the brain tissue was positive for *M. tuberculosis*. Tissue cultures were negative in terms of aerobic microorganism, fungus, and *M. tuberculosis*. The primary immunologic workup including lymphocyte subgroups, immunoglobulins, and slide nitroblue tetrazolium (NBT) test was normal as well as interleukin- (IL-) 12 receptor B1 expression and interferon (IFN) gamma functions. A decreasing size of tuberculoma

was detected in the control MRI. The patient's complaints were minimized under the medication of isoniazid, ethambutol, rifampicin, moxifloxacin, and clarithromycin. The patient participated in physiotherapy and rehabilitation program in addition to symptomatic treatments for spasticity and was discharged after 45 days of hospitalization. Tuberculoma was not revealed in the cranial MRI of the patient one month later. Steroid treatment was decreased at 8 weeks and interrupted at 12 weeks after discharge.

3. Discussion

In 1955, a paradoxical response under TB treatment was first identified by Choremis and his friends on lung graph

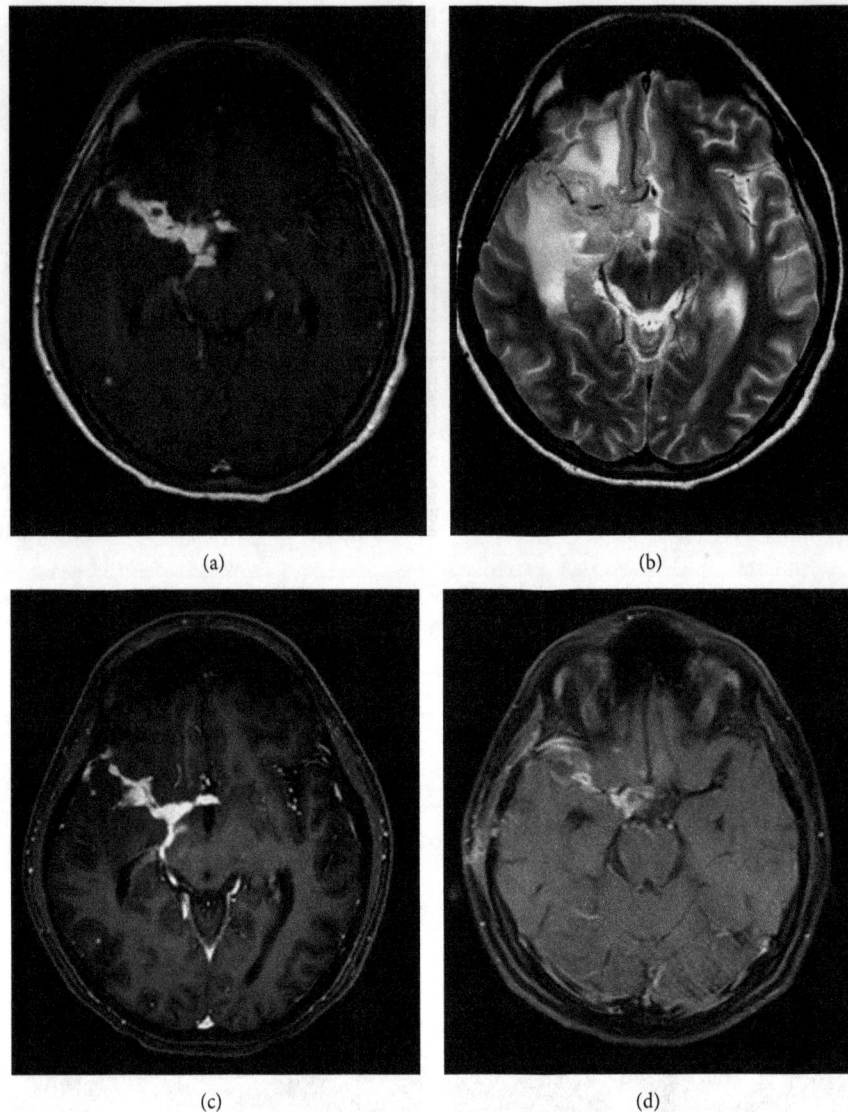

FIGURE 3: Contrasted T1A (a) and T2A (b) images 60 days after the diagnosis, contrasted T1A (c) image of 75 days later, and contrasted T1A (d) image of 90 days after the diagnosis. Considerable progression of the basal meningitis and parenchymal tuberculomas was seen after the 60th day instead of tuberculosis regression (a, b). A contrast is seen in the scattered parenchymal tuberculoma (a). After this examination, the patient began taking a steroid. There is a reduction of the basal meningitis and tuberculoma at the contrasted T1A image after 15 days on the steroid treatment. (c) A disappearance of tuberculomas, regression of contrast involvement, and exudate on the right sylvian fissure are seen on the contrasted T1A image 30 days after the steroid treatment.

imaging results of a child who was being treated for TB [5]. In 1974, Thrush and Barwick, for the first time, documented paradoxical reaction in a patient with CNS TB, who had multiple tuberculomas and developed a new tuberculoma during treatment with anti-TB drugs [6]. In 1980, Lees and coworkers described the first report of paradoxical reaction of TB meningitis in 2 female patients, who paradoxically developed multiple cerebral tuberculoma and basal arachnoiditis [7]. There is limited pediatric data about the paradoxical response, which confuses physicians on the accuracy of the diagnosis leading to invasive diagnostic modalities such as brain biopsy and being forced to add unnecessary antimicrobial new drugs as in our patient. Understanding of the clinical

nature of this response will let us avoid adverse outcomes of diagnostic and therapeutic modalities. Therefore, we share the hope that the increase in reports of the concept of paradoxic response which has been made possible by the awareness of pediatricians will throw light on appropriate management of children with TB.

Paradoxical deterioration mostly occurs in patients with extrapulmonary and disseminated TB, like miliary TB and TB meningitis. The CNS and the respiratory system remain the most common sites of involvement during paradoxical deterioration reported in literature. For the CNS manifestations, patients may have headache, mental confusion, focal seizures, cranial nerve palsies, and cortical signs such as

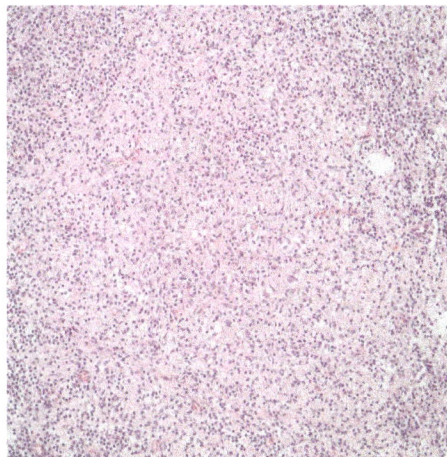

FIGURE 4: H&E, 200x. The lymphohistiocytic reaction and abortive granuloma structures.

hemiparesis, paraparesis, and hemianaesthesia as a result of the enlargement or development of intracranial tuberculomas and hydrocephalus [8]. Our patient presented with severe headache and hemiparesis caused by enlargement of the CNS lesion too. The reason why a paradoxical response occurs is not known exactly. Various hypotheses have been suggested to explain this unusual phenomenon. One of them is that this response occurs as a result of decreased penetration of antitubercular drugs into the brain. Restoration of blood brain barrier with appropriate treatment is proposed to result in reactivation of latent foci. However, this hypothesis cannot explain the development or enlargement of intracranial tuberculoma which is treated with isoniazid and pyrazinamide, both of which freely cross the blood brain barrier in the absence of inflamed meninges. Enlargement of lymph nodes (which do not have the barrier like blood brain barrier) in patients on anti-TB therapy further goes against the hypothesis. The most likely explanation for paradoxical response is interplay between host's immune response and the direct effect of mycobacterial products [4]. A paradoxical response can occur 3–12 weeks after the initiation of a TB treatment; however, it can take as long as 18 months [9]. It was seen in our patient 8 weeks after the treatment with several CNS symptoms.

A paradoxical response is commonly seen in 6–30% of patients being treated for TB [8], particularly in adult and immunocompromised patients. This situation is seen very rarely in children and the earliest age at which it has occurred was 21-day-old child who was treated for congenital lung TB [10]. Although few adult paradoxical responses are reported in Turkey, a paradoxical reaction has never been reported in children who were diagnosed with TB meningitis. The aforementioned case is one of the rarely seen and reported cases of a child having a paradoxical reaction. Furthermore, although the reported rate of the paradoxical response in patients with HIV infection is 35%, this rate is lower than 5% in TB patients with normal immune systems [10]. HIV was negative in our case and primary immunologic workup as well as IL-12 receptor B1 expression test and IFN-gamma

functions were normal as well. Our patient did not have a mendelian susceptibility to the mycobacterial diseases. Additionally, some stated risk factors for the paradoxical reaction are anemia, hypoalbuminemia, and lymphopenia [1]. There was no mentioned risk factors in our patient. It is not necessary to change or stop anti-TB treatments, when a paradoxical response develops. Also, 95% of mycobacteria are sensitive to the treatments [10], but resistance to anti-TB drugs is still important, especially in our country where proliferation of resistant TB strains is an ongoing process [1].

Paradoxical reactions are treated with a systemic corticosteroid and/or surgery.

Corticosteroids decrease intracranial pressure, which is helpful in diminishing any of the disease's neurological symptoms [3]. Systemic corticosteroid treatment was added to the treatment of our patient with a good clinical response. A ventriculoperitoneal shunt implementation is a surgical alternative if a medical treatment fails; however, surgical treatment is not needed for our case.

Despite appropriate treatment, the cause of the paradoxical response in TB patients is not clear. Even though his father was diagnosed with lung TB caused by a resistant form, a prophylaxis for TB was not given to our case. Firstly, it was thought that the patient would not respond to the medication because of the suspicion of the possible resistant infection as in his father's case. As a result, new antimicrobials were added to the treatment. Subsequently, a very invasive procedure such as brain biopsy was performed to confirm diagnosis due to the fact that there was no enough improvement with those new drugs. Consequently, paradoxic response may lead to a confusion in the management of the TB disease. Thus, it is clear that understanding the nature and recognizing the paradoxic response will help the clinical practice of the pediatrician to avoid unnecessary management strategies.

Competing Interests

The authors have no financial disclosures nor competing interests to declare.

References

[1] U. Gonlugur, S. Kosar, and A. Mirici, "Paradoxical radiologic progression despite appropriate anti-tuberculous therapy," *Mikrobiyoloji Bülteni*, vol. 46, no. 3, pp. 299–303, 2012.

[2] J. B. Silman, J. I. Peters, S. M. Levine, and S. G. Jenkinson, "Development of intracranial tuberculomas while receiving therapy for pulmonary fibrosis," *American Journal of Respiratory and Critical Care Medicine*, vol. 150, no. 5, pp. 1439–1440, 1994.

[3] R. K. Garg, H. S. Malhotra, and N. Kumar, "Paradoxical reaction in HIV negative tuberculous meningitis," *Journal of the Neurological Sciences*, vol. 340, no. 1-2, pp. 26–36, 2014.

[4] M. Gupta, B. K. Bajaj, and G. Khwaja, "Paradoxical response in patients with CNS tuberculosis," *The Journal of Association of Physicians of India*, vol. 51, pp. 257–260, 2003.

[5] C. B. Choremis, C. Padiatellis, D. Zoumboulakis, and D. Yannakos, "Transitory excerbation of fever and roentgenographic findingsduring treatment of tuberculosis in children," *The American Review of Tuberculosis*, vol. 72, pp. 525–536, 1955.

[6] D. C. Thrush and D. D. Barwick, "Three patients with intracranial tuberculomas with unusual features," *Journal of Neurology, Neurosurgery & Psychiatry*, vol. 37, no. 5, pp. 566–569, 1974.

[7] A. J. Lees, A. F. Macleod, and J. Marshall, "Cerebral tuberculomas developing during treatment of tuberculous meningitis," *The Lancet*, vol. 315, no. 8180, pp. 1208–1211, 1980.

[8] V. C. Cheng, P. L. Ho, R. A. Lee et al., "Clinical spectrum of paradoxical deterioration during antituberculosis therapy in non-HIV-infected patients," *European Journal of Clinical Microbiology and Infectious Diseases*, vol. 21, no. 11, pp. 803–809, 2002.

[9] T. Karagoz, H. Altinoz, T. Senol, O. Kula, T. Yarkin, and O. Yazicioglu, "Paradoxical response to antituberculous therapy," *Turkish Respiratory Journal*, vol. 4, pp. 17–20, 2007.

[10] J. A. Park, S. S. Park, and S. E. Park, "A paradoxical reaction during antituberculosis therapy for congenital tuberculosis," *International Journal of Infectious Diseases*, vol. 13, no. 5, pp. e279–e281, 2009.

44

Multiple Renal Abscesses due to ESBL Extended-Spectrum Beta-Lactamase-Producing *Escherichia coli* Causing Acute Pyelonephritis and Bacteremia: A Case Report with a Good Outcome (No Drainage Required)

Abdalla Khalil,[1] Musaad Qurash,[2] Asem Saleh,[1] Rasha Ali,[1] and Mohamed Elwakil[3]

[1]*Internal Medicine Department, International Medical Center (IMC) Hospital, Jeddah, Saudi Arabia*
[2]*Radiology Department, IMC Hospital, Jeddah, Saudi Arabia*
[3]*Emergency Medicine Department, IMC Hospital, Jeddah, Saudi Arabia*

Correspondence should be addressed to Abdalla Khalil; abdallak59@gmail.com

Academic Editor: Peter Olumese

Extended-spectrum beta-lactamase-producing Enterobacteriaceae urinary tract infections are challenging infections with increased mortality, morbidity, and failure of therapy. A 44-year-old Saudi male diabetic patient was seen at the ER of IMC Hospital with features of acute pyelonephritis: fever, burning urine, and left flank pain for three days. He was treated for cystitis at the Endocrine Clinic two weeks prior to his ER visit with nitrofurantoin and levofloxacin orally according to urine culture and sensitivity result. The patient was admitted, received IV meropenem, and continued to be febrile for three days. His urine and blood culture at ER grew the same ESBL-producing *E. coli* as in his urine culture from the Endocrine Clinic. His abdomen CT scan showed two left renal abscesses at the upper and middle poles. His temperature resolved on the fourth day of IV therapy. Intravenous meropenem was continued for 4 weeks after inserting PICC line and the patient was followed up by home healthcare. He was feeling better with occasional left flank pain and repeated abdomen CT scan showed complete resolution of both renal abscesses.

1. Introduction

Community and hospital acquired extended-spectrum beta-lactamase- (ESBL-) producing Enterobacteriaceae are prevalent worldwide [1].

ESBL-producing *Escherichia coli* (*E. coli*) and *Klebsiella pneumoniae* infections carry a higher mortality rate, higher risk of developing bacteremia, and failure of therapy compared to non-ESBL-producing isolates [2, 3].

Catheter acquired urinary tract infection is one of the most common healthcare acquired infections [4].

Prevalence surveys report that urinary catheter is the most common indwelling device, with 17.5% of the patients in European hospitals [4] and 23.6% in United States hospitals [5] having a catheter related infection.

Overall frequency of ESBLs from all isolates of Enterobacteriaceae in the United States was 16 percent in *K. pneu-*

moniae, 11.9 percent in *E. coli*, 10 percent in *K. oxytoca*, and 4.8 percent in *P. mirabilis* [6].

Prevalence is even higher in isolates from Asia, Latin America, and the Middle East [7], reaching 60 percent in *K. pneumoniae* isolates from Argentina and 48 percent in *E. coli* isolates from Mexico [8].

Renal abscess is a rare complication for complicated urinary tract infections due to Enterobacteriaceae.

We are presenting a case of multiple renal abscesses secondary to a complicated urinary tract infection (pyelonephritis and bacteremia) caused by ESBL *E. coli* in a diabetic morbidly obese middle-aged Saudi male patient. These abscesses responded to intravenous therapy with meropenem.

2. Case Report

A 45-year-old Saudi male known to have type II diabetes mellitus, mixed hyperlipidaemia, essential hypertension, and

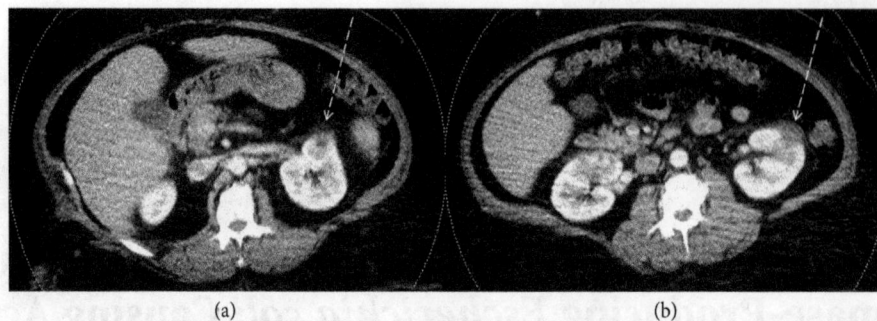

FIGURE 1: Abdomen CT scan with intravenous contrast on the third day of admission. It showed two left renal focal pyelonephritic changes in the upper and middle poles as well as the perinephric fat infiltration and thickening of Gerota's fascia. Also, scattered small para-aortic lymph nodes are noted. The first abscess in the upper pole is 2.5 × 2.3 cm in diameter (CT scan cut on (a)), and the other one in the middle pole is 2.6 × 1.8 cm in diameter (CT scan cut on (b)).

morbid obesity was seen at the Emergency Department with fever for three days associated with chills, dysuria, frequency, and incontinence of urine. He had repeated vomiting and left flank pain for one day.

He was seen at the Endocrine Clinic 2 weeks prior to his ER visit with burning urine and frequency and was treated for cystitis. His urine culture grew ESBL extended-spectrum beta-lactamase-producing *E. coli* >100.000 colonies and he received oral nitrofurantoin 100 mg 6-hourly and levofloxacin 500 mg orally once daily. His symptoms improved for 10 days and then recurred again.

He did not have a history of urethral catheterization, renal stone, or recurrent urinary tract infection. He denied history of illicit drug intake and his last admission to a hospital was two months ago for upper endoscopy.

On examination at the ER, his temperature was 38.3°C, his pulse rate was 110/minute, and his blood pressure was 110/70 mmHg. Respiratory rate was 18/minute, oxygen saturation was 96% on room air, and weight was 187 kg and height was 172 cm (BMI: 63.2 kg/m^2).

He looked toxic and sweaty. He had tenderness at the left costovertebral angle and chest and heart exam were unremarkable.

His complete blood count showed increase in white blood cells, 12.2 × 10^9/L, with neutrophils 78% and normal hemoglobin and platelets count. Serum creatinine was normal, 100 μmol/L, and his electrolytes were normal too. Urinalysis showed positive nitrates, +3 leucocytes, white blood cells >50/HPF, red blood cells 30/HPF, and +2 ketones. Random blood glucose was 16 mmol/L, serum ketone bodies were negative, and C-reactive protein was raised, 29 mg/L (reference: 0–5 mg/L).

His previous urine culture at the Endocrine Clinic visit grew >100.000 colonies of Gram negative bacilli *E. coli* (morphology was done according to CDC algorithm) which were resistant to cefuroxime, cefepime, and ceftazidime (i.e., extended-spectrum beta-lactamase) and sensitive to meropenem, imipenem, gentamycin, and nitrofurantoin (culture sensitivity was done by MIC results obtained using automated Vitek 2 AST-GN69 and AST-XN06 cards).

His abdomen and pelvis ultrasound was unremarkable.

The patient was started on intravenous meropenem 1000 mg 8-hourly (first dose at the ER) and intravenous fluids. He was admitted to the medical unit where he continued to be febrile and had less pain at the left flank. Both his urine culture and blood culture taken at ER grew the same *E. coli* with the same sensitivity pattern as in urine culture collected at his previous Endocrine Clinic visit. He had two more repeated blood cultures after admission which came negative.

The patient had CT scan of the abdomen and pelvis on his third day of admission. It showed two left renal focal pyelonephritic changes in the upper and middle poles as well as the perinephric fat infiltration and thickening of Gerota's fascia. Also, scattered small para-aortic lymph nodes are noted. There is an abscess in the upper pole, 2.5 × 2.3 cm in diameter, and another in the middle pole, 2.6 × 1.8 cm in diameter (Figure 1).

The patient's temperature normalized on the fourth day on medication, and he started to feel better and the pain at the left flank nearly resolved. His white blood cells decreased to 6.0 × 10^9/L and his C-reactive protein decreased to 10 mg/L (reference: 0–5 mg/L).

Intravenous meropenem was continued after insertion of PICC (peripherally inserted central catheter) and the patient was educated on care of line, discharged, and followed up by a home healthcare team twice weekly. He was doing fine and afebrile during the 4-week course of antibiotic. He had occasional left flank pain that responded to simple analgesia paracetamol orally. His repeated compete blood count and C-reactive protein were in normal range. His repeated abdomen CT scan showed nearly complete resolution of the previously described abscesses with no perinephric fat stranding or collection (Figure 2).

3. Discussion

In Saudi Arabia, the prevalence of ESBLs Enterobacteriaceae isolates varies greatly in different regions.

It was shown to be 10.1% in the eastern province whereas in the central region it was 26.7% to 35.3% [9].

High level of carbapenem resistance had been observed in one study which was 20% [10]. In another study in the central

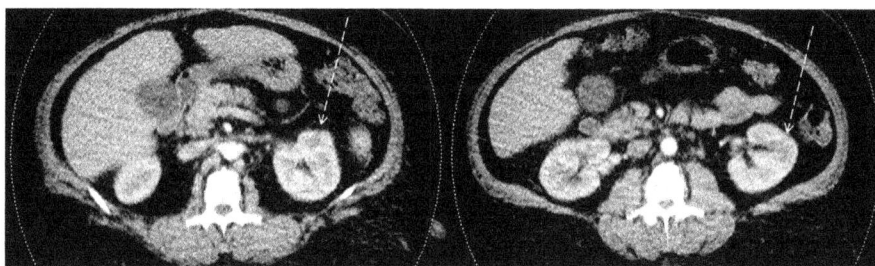

FIGURE 2: Findings. Abdomen CT scan with intravenous contrast after finishing 4 weeks of intravenous meropenem. It showed nearly complete resolution of the previously described abscesses with no perinephric fat stranding or collection.

region in Saudi Arabia, 57% of ESBL-producing *E. coli* isolates were of community origin [11].

In our electronic search (in Adult Medicine), we found only one case report of ESBL Gram negative bacilli causing renal abscesses [12].

In our present case, our patient was managed with nitrofurantoin and levofloxacin during his first visit to the Endocrine Clinic with urinary tract infection. Although the ESBL *E. coli* growing from urine culture was in vitro sensitive to nitrofurantoin, still carbapenem group of antibiotics intravenously is the drug of choice for the management of such case. His condition deteriorated after few days of partial improvement of his symptoms and he came to the ER with Gram negative ESBL (extended-spectrum beta-lactamase) *E. coli* bacteremia and failure of previous therapy.

Community acquired ESBL urinary tract infections are more challenging to manage than hospital acquired ones because treating physicians may not consider them on initiating antibiotic therapy and they will be detected later on after getting the final urine culture, that is, 48–72 hours.

We believe that we need more studies to assess the percentage of community acquired ESBL infections at other provinces of the kingdom.

Abbreviations

ER: Emergency Room
HPF: High power field
PICC: Peripherally inserted central catheter
ESBL: Extended-spectrum beta-lactamase
IV: Intravenous.

Competing Interests

The authors declare that there are no competing interests regarding the publication of this paper.

Acknowledgments

The authors are thankful to the team of microbiology at IMC Hospital.

References

[1] R. Ben-Ami, J. Rodríguez-Baño, H. Arslan et al., "A multinational survey of risk factors for infection with extended-spectrum β-lactamase-producing enterobacteriaceae in non-hospitalized patients," *Clinical Infectious Diseases*, vol. 49, no. 5, pp. 682–690, 2009.

[2] M. Melzer and I. Petersen, "Mortality following bacteraemic infection caused by extended spectrum beta-lactamase (ESBL) producing *E. coli* compared to non-ESBL producing *E. coli*," *Journal of Infection*, vol. 55, no. 3, pp. 254–259, 2007.

[3] M. Tumbarello, T. Spanu, M. Sanguinetti et al., "Bloodstream infections caused by extended-spectrum-β-lactamase- producing Klebsiella pneumoniae: risk factors, molecular epidemiology, and clinical outcome," *Antimicrobial Agents and Chemotherapy*, vol. 50, no. 2, pp. 498–504, 2006.

[4] P. Zarb, B. Coignard, J. Griskeviciene et al., "The European Centre for Disease Prevention and Control (ECDC) pilot point prevalence survey of healthcare-associated infections and antimicrobial use," *Euro Surveillance*, vol. 17, no. 46, 2012.

[5] S. S. Magill, J. R. Edwards, W. Bamberg et al., "Multistate point-prevalence survey of health care-associated infections," *New England Journal of Medicine*, vol. 370, no. 13, pp. 1198–1208, 2014.

[6] M. Castanheira, S. E. Farrell, K. M. Krause, R. N. Jones, and H. S. Sader, "Contemporary diversity of β-lactamases among enterobacteriaceae in the nine U.S. census regions and ceftazidime-avibactam activity tested against isolates producing the most prevalent β-lactamase groups," *Antimicrobial Agents and Chemotherapy*, vol. 58, no. 2, pp. 833–838, 2014.

[7] I. Morrissey, M. Hackel, R. Badal, S. Bouchillon, S. Hawser, and D. Biedenbach, "A review of ten years of the Study for Monitoring Antimicrobial Resistance Trends (SMART) from 2002 to 2011," *Pharmaceuticals*, vol. 6, no. 11, pp. 1335–1346, 2013.

[8] A. C. Gales, M. Castanheira, R. N. Jones, and H. S. Sader, "Antimicrobial resistance among Gram-negative bacilli isolated from Latin America: results from SENTRY Antimicrobial Surveillance Program (Latin America, 2008–2010)," *Diagnostic Microbiology and Infectious Disease*, vol. 73, no. 4, pp. 354–360, 2012.

[9] S. Yezli, A. M. Shibl, D. M. Livermore, and Z. A. Memish, "Prevalence and antimicrobial resistance among Gram-Negative pathogens in Saudi Arabia," *Journal of Chemotherapy*, vol. 26, no. 5, pp. 257–272, 2014.

[10] A. Kandeel, "Prevalence and risk factors of extended-spectrum β-lactamases producing *Enterobacteriaceae* in a general hospital in Saudi Arabia," *Journal of Microbiology and Infectious Diseases*, vol. 4, no. 2, pp. 50–54, 2014.

[11] F. E. Al-Otaibi and E. E. Bukhari, "Clinical and laboratory profiles of urinary tract infections caused by extended-spectrum beta-lactamase-producing Escherichia coli in a tertiary care center in central Saudi Arabia," *Saudi Medical Journal*, vol. 34, no. 2, pp. 171–176, 2013.

[12] M. K. Lim, K. W. Kim, H. K. Lee, Y. D. Woen, and Y. S. Kim, "Multiple renal abscesses caused by extended spectrum beta lactamase producing *Escherichia coli*," *Korean Journal of Nephrology*, vol. 24, no. 3, pp. 460–463, 2005 (Korean).

45

Chromobacterium violaceum Septicaemia and Urinary Tract Infection: Case Reports from a Tertiary Care Hospital in South India

Vishnu Kaniyarakkal, Shabana Orvankundil, Saradadevi Karunakaran Lalitha, Raji Thazhethekandi, and Jahana Thottathil

Government Medical College Kozhikode, Kozhikode, India

Correspondence should be addressed to Vishnu Kaniyarakkal; drkvishnu@gmail.com

Academic Editor: Gernot Walder

Chromobacterium violaceum is a gram negative oxidase positive bacillus that causes human infections infrequently. It is a normal inhabitant of soil and stagnant water of the tropical and subtropical areas. In humans, it can cause infections ranging from life threatening sepsis with metastatic abscesses to skin infections and urinary tract infections. The organism is notoriously resistant to most cephalosporins and Ampicillin. Fluoroquinolones and aminoglycosides show good in vitro susceptibility. High mortality rates associated with these infections necessitate prompt diagnosis and appropriate antimicrobial therapy. Here we present three cases of *Chromobacterium violaceum* infection from Government Medical College Kozhikode, Kerala.

1. Introduction

Chromobacterium violaceum is a gram negative, motile, oxidase positive bacillus that is temperature sensitive and widely distributed in natural aquatic environments. It grows easily on ordinary media like blood agar, MacConkey agar, and nutrient agar producing a violet antioxidant pigment known as violacein [1]. Human infections with this organism, although rare, can result in severe systemic infection by entering the bloodstream via an open wound [2]. Rapid progression to sepsis with metastatic abscesses and multidrug resistance are striking features of *Chromobacterium violaceum* infections. The microorganism, previously thought to be confined to the geographic area between latitudes 35°N and 35°S, may be expanding its habitat beyond this range due to the effects of global warming [1]. Interestingly the monobactam Aztreonam was first described as a natural metabolic product of this bacterium [3, 4].

2. Case 1 (Septicaemia)

An 11-month-old male child was referred to our hospital with complaints of high grade fever of 5-day duration, loose stools, and respiratory distress. The fever was preceded by cellulitis of the right cheek and cervical and preauricular adenitis. He was injected with Cefotaxime at the time of referral. On admission the child was febrile with pallor, cervical lymph node enlargement, and hepatosplenomegaly. Blood work-up (Table 1) showed anaemia. Peripheral smear examination reported severe microcytic hypochromic anaemia with neutropenia. Smear for malaria parasite examination was negative. X-ray examination showed multiple patchy opacities in the lungs. A provisional diagnosis of bronchopneumonia with lymphoreticular malignancy was made and the child was empirically put on Cefotaxime injection of 350 mg IV Q8H, Ampicillin injection of 350 mg IV Q6H, Vancomycin injection of 140 mg IV Q18H, and Oseltamivir of 30 mg oral BD along with other supportive measures. Second day after

TABLE 1: Results of blood tests for Case 1.

Blood test	Results	Reference range/level
Hemoglobin (gm/dl)	5.5	11–14
Platelet count (cell/mm^3)	65,000	2,00,000–5,00,000
White cell count (cell/mm^3)	2400	11,000 ± 5000
Neutrophils (%)	25.7	13–33
MCV (fl)	59	78 ± 6
MCH (pg)	18.9	27 ± 2
MCHC (gm/dl)	32.2	34 ± 2
ESR (mm/hour)	60	10

MCV, mean corpuscular volume; MCH, mean corpuscular hemoglobin; MCHC, mean corpuscular hemoglobin concentration; fl, femtoliter; pg, picogram.

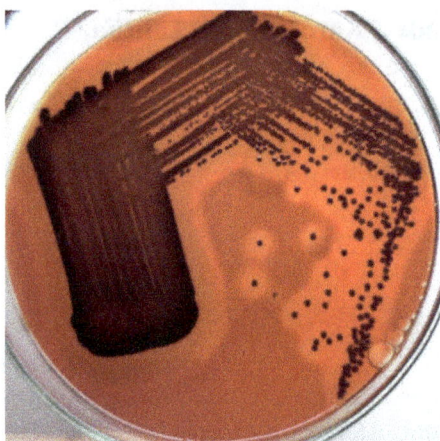

FIGURE 1: β-Hemolytic colonies on blood agar.

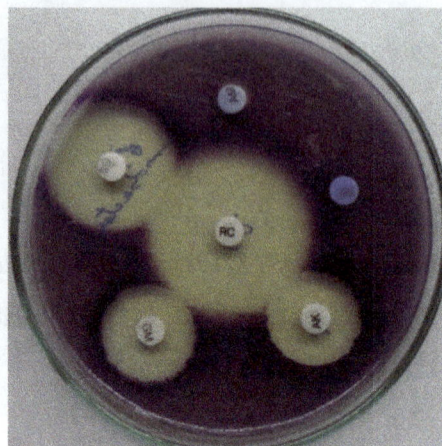

FIGURE 2: Kirby Bauer disc diffusion method.

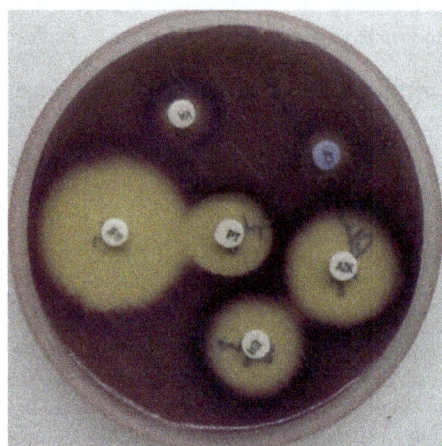

FIGURE 3: Kirby Bauer disc diffusion method.

admission, the patient's condition worsened and he was given transfusions of fresh frozen plasma and packed cells. In spite of intensive treatment, the patient succumbed to death 48 hours after admission.

A blood culture was sent at admission in brain heart infusion broth which was incubated at 37°C. Subcultures were done on blood agar, on MacConkey agar, and subsequently on nutrient agar which demonstrated numerous colonies with dark violet pigmentation (Figure 1). The organism was gram negative, motile, catalase positive, and oxidase positive. Testing of oxidase reaction by the popular method of Kovacs where the bacterial growth is smeared onto a filter paper impregnated with 1% aqueous solution of tetra methyl p-phenylene diamine dihydrochloride presented with a problem since the organism had violet pigmentation. Hence oxidase reaction was tested by the method described by Dhar and Johnson [5, 6]. The organism was identified as *Chromobacterium violaceum* based on biochemical characteristics and pigment production. It was further confirmed by Vitek-2 system Version: 07.01 (BioMerieux, France) using gram negative card. Antibiogram was done by Kirby Bauer's disk diffusion susceptibility testing technique (Figures 2 and 3) and minimal inhibitory concentration (MIC) method. The results were interpreted as per the Clinical and Laboratory Standards Institute (CLSI) guidelines for other non-Enterobacteriaceae

[7]. As the isolate was resistant to Ampicillin and intermediate sensitive to Cefotaxime (Table 2), before getting the proper antibiotic treatment, patient condition deteriorated and developed fatal septicaemia.

3. Case 2

A 2.5-year-old male child presented with painful swelling of the scalp and fever of 1-week duration. He had Kawasaki disease at the age of 7 months, measles at the age of 1.5 years, and recurrent episodes of loose stools over the past 1 month. Ultrasound examination of the scalp swelling reported it as "pyemic abscess over the scalp with underlying invasion of both parietal bones extending to extradural space through anterior fontanelle." Patient was initially treated with oral amoxicillin + Clavulanic acid and later changed to Ampicillin injection and cloxacillin injection.

Blood culture sample was sent in brain heart infusion broth to the laboratory which was incubated at 37°C. Then by subculture on blood agar, on MacConkey agar, and subsequently on nutrient agar, dark violet coloured colonies were grown on all three plates after overnight incubation at

TABLE 2: Antimicrobial susceptibility for Case 1.

Antimicrobial	MIC values	Interpretation*
Ampicillin	≥32	Resistant
Amoxicillin/Clavulanic acid	≥32	Resistant
Piperacillin/tazobactam	≥128	Resistant
Cefuroxime	≥64	Resistant
Cefotaxime	32	Intermediate
Cefoperazone/sulbactam	32	Intermediate
Ciprofloxacin	≤0.25	Sensitive
Nalidixic acid	≤2	Sensitive
Gentamicin	≤1	Sensitive
Amikacin	≤2	Sensitive
Nitrofurantoin	≤16	Sensitive
Tigecycline	≤0.5	Sensitive
Cotrimoxazole	≤20	Sensitive
Imipenem	≥16	Resistant
Meropenem	≥16	Resistant
Colistin	≥16	Resistant

*For other non-Enterobacteriaceae disc diffusion testing is not currently recommended by CLSI. Hence MIC method was used for the interpretation of antimicrobial sensitivity.

37°C. The organism was biochemically identified as *Chromobacterium violaceum*. Antimicrobial susceptibility testing showed resistance to Ampicillin and susceptibility to fluoroquinolones and aminoglycosides. Cerebrospinal fluid culture did not yield any growth.

The patient progressed to respiratory distress, hypotension, and shock and finally expired within 48 hours of admission before the results of antibiotic susceptibility testing came through.

4. Case 3

A 12-year-old school girl presented to the outpatient department with history of intermittent dysuria with fever and chills of 1-week duration. There was no history of any other concurrent illness. Patient gave a history of swimming in pond occasionally [8]. For the last three years, she had recurrent episodes of urinary tract infection. A routine urine examination showed 10–12 pus cells per high power field along with bacteria. Ultrasound examination of the abdomen revealed mild wall thickening of urinary bladder with internal echoes. Routine blood examination was within normal limits.

A mid-stream urine sample was obtained for culture in sterile bottle after following standard precautions and was inoculated on blood agar and MacConkey agar. After overnight aerobic incubation at 37°C, dark violet coloured colonies were observed on blood agar. The biochemical test characteristics were consistent with identification of *Chromobacterium violaceum*. The isolate was resistant to Ampicillin and cephalosporins and sensitive to fluoroquinolones and aminoglycosides.

The patient was empirically started on oral cefixime 200 mg BD. We received one more urine sample for culture after 5 days at the time of review, which yielded the same

organism with similar antibiotic sensitivity pattern. The result was again informed to the clinician and the importance of changing the antibiotic to fluoroquinolone was stressed. Subsequently the patient was given oral Ciprofloxacin of 500 mg BD for 7 days. A third urine culture performed at the next hospital visit a week later did not detect any bacteriuria.

5. Discussion

The scarcity of reports of human infections with *Chromobacterium violaceum* is astounding given the described ease at which the bacterium is recovered from soil and stagnant water bodies in the tropics and subtropics. The organism has a growth preference for temperatures between 20°C and 37°C. Moist soil and stagnant or slow-flowing water have been the most commonly reported sources of infection, especially in patients who have had cutaneous injury or trauma, which presumably provides a portal of entry for this pathogen. There is no age or gender predilection reported in literature and the only established predisposing disease process has been chronic granulomatous disease [3]. Identification of this organism depends primarily on the biochemical characteristics. A method of detection using multiplex polymerase chain reaction has been described by Scholz and colleagues which is yet largely confined to the realm of research and is not commercially available [1, 9].

The clinical manifestations of *C. violaceum* infections are protean. It has been associated with pneumonia, gastrointestinal tract infections, urinary tract infections, localised cutaneous lesions, localised or metastatic abscesses, osteomyelitis, meningitis, peritonitis, brain abscess, endocarditis, hemophagocytic syndrome, respiratory distress syndrome, and fulminant sepsis [3, 6, 10–12]. The genome of this bacterium has recently been completely sequenced providing a platform for detailed studies of its antiviral and bactericidal activities, cytotoxicity, and drug resistance mechanisms. The virulent strains of *C. violaceum* have elevated levels of superoxide dismutase and catalase that may protect the microorganism from phagocytic attack in humans. This might explain its pathogenicity and fatality in human infections [1, 11]. Pigment production is not a marker of pathogenicity as nonpigmented strains have also been reported to cause infections [12].

Data on antimicrobial susceptibility patterns of *Chromobacterium violaceum* is very limited owing to the rarity of isolation from clinical specimens. Most strains show resistance to penicillins and other beta-lactam antibiotics and, indeed, increased level of beta-lactamase activity has been reported in this organism [1, 11, 13]. Ciprofloxacin is the most effective antibiotic in vitro. It is also susceptible to Gentamicin and Amikacin [1, 3, 10, 11]. In all three cases described above, the patients were primarily on beta-lactam antimicrobials which explains the case fatalities in the first two. In the case of the urinary tract infection, the antibiotic was changed from 3rd generation cephalosporin to Ciprofloxacin only after the second positive culture report. The patient became asymptomatic following the change of antibiotic.

Hence in the tropics and subtropics, infection with *Chromobacterium violaceum* should be one of the differential diagnoses in sepsis, especially if it is preceded by a skin infection or cellulitis. Also, it can present as milder infections like UTI as described in the third case. The inherent resistance pattern of this organism should be borne in mind while instituting empirical antibiotic therapy.

6. Conclusion

Chromobacterium violaceum is easily isolated from natural aquatic environments of the tropics and subtropics. The traditional geographic distribution pattern of this organism is bound to change in view of the changing global climatic conditions. Human infections with this pathogen, though rare, often result in high mortality rate. Rapid diagnosis and the use of optimal antimicrobials for treatment could be life-saving. Commercial introduction of a cost effective, rapid diagnostic method is the need of the hour. The lack of awareness among clinicians regarding the pathogenesis and antimicrobial resistance pattern of this bacterium is a challenge to be tackled.

Competing Interests

The authors declare that there is no conflict of interests regarding the publication of this paper.

References

[1] C.-H. Yang and Y.-H. Li, "Chromobacterium violaceum infection: a clinical review of an important but neglected infection," *Journal of the Chinese Medical Association*, vol. 74, no. 10, pp. 435–441, 2011.

[2] J. I. Campbell, N. P. H. Lan, P. T. Qui, L. T. Dung, J. J. Farrar, and S. Baker, "A successful antimicrobial regime for *Chromobacterium violaceum* induced bacteremia," *BMC Infectious Diseases*, vol. 13, no. 1, article 4, 2013.

[3] E. Carter, K. Cain, and B. Rutland, "Chromobacterium violaceum cellulitis and sepsis following cutaneous marine trauma," *Cutis*, vol. 81, no. 3, pp. 269–272, 2008.

[4] R. J. Duma, "Aztreonam, the first monobactam," *Annals of Internal Medicine*, vol. 106, no. 5, pp. 766–767, 1987.

[5] S. K. Dhar and R. Johnson, "The oxidase activity of chromobacterium," *Journal of Clinical Pathology*, vol. 26, no. 4, pp. 304–306, 1973.

[6] G. Slesak, P. Douangdala, S. Inthalad et al., "Fatal Chromobacterium violaceum septicaemia in northern Laos, a modified oxidase test and post-mortem forensic family G6PD analysis," *Annals of Clinical Microbiology and Antimicrobials*, vol. 8, article 24, 2009.

[7] Clinical and Laboratory Standards Institute, "Performance standards for antimicrobial susceptibility testing," Twenty-Fourth Informational Supplement vol. 34, no. 1, Clinical and Laboratory Standards Institute, Wayne, Pa, USA, 2014.

[8] A. Søraas, A. Sundsfjord, I. Sandven, C. Brunborg, and P. A. Jenum, "Risk factors for community-acquired urinary tract infections caused by ESBL-producing enterobacteriaceae—a case-control study in a low prevalence country," *PLoS ONE*, vol. 8, no. 7, Article ID e69581, 2013.

[9] H. C. Scholz, A. Witte, H. Tomaso, S. Al Dahouk, and H. Neubauer, "Detection of *Chromobacterium violaceum* by multiplex PCR targeting the *prgI*, *spaO*, *invG*, and *sipB* genes," *Systematic and Applied Microbiology*, vol. 29, no. 1, pp. 45–48, 2006.

[10] B. Swain, S. Otta, K. K. Sahu, K. Panda, and S. Rout, "Urinary tract infection by Chromobacterium violaceum," *Journal of Clinical and Diagnostic Research*, vol. 8, no. 8, pp. DD01–DD02, 2014.

[11] A. Y. B. Teoh, M. Hui, K. Y. Ngo, J. Wong, K. F. Lee, and P. B. S. Lai, "Fatal septicaemia from *Chromobacterium violaceum*: case reports and review of the literature," *Hong Kong Medical Journal*, vol. 12, no. 3, pp. 228–231, 2006.

[12] J. A. Díaz Pérez, J. García, and L. A. Rodriguez Villamizar, "Sepsis by Chromobacterium violaceum: first case report from Colombia," *Brazilian Journal of Infectious Diseases*, vol. 11, no. 4, pp. 441–442, 2007.

[13] W. E. Farrar Jr. and N. M. O'Dell, "β-Lactamase activity in Chromobacterium violaceum," *Journal of Infectious Diseases*, vol. 134, no. 3, pp. 290–293, 1976.

Permissions

List of Contributors

Masato Kimura, Eichiro Kawai, Hisao Yaoita, Natsuko Ichinoi, Osamu Sakamoto, and Shigeo Kure
Department of Pediatrics, Tohoku University Graduate School of Medicine, Sendai, Miyagi 980-8574, Japan

Prasan K. Panda, Siddharth Jain, Rita Sood and Naval K. Vikram
Department of Internal Medicine, All India Institute of Medical Sciences, New Delhi 110029, India

Rajni Yadav
Department of Pathology, All India Institute of Medical Sciences, New Delhi 110029, India

Ali Ridha and Sarah Al-Abayechi
University of Arkansas for Medical Science, 4301West Markham Street, Little Rock, AR 72205, USA

Njideka Oguejiofor and Emmanuel Njoku
Chicago Medical School, Rosalind Franklin University of Medicine and Science, 3333 Green Bay Rd., North Chicago, IL 60064, USA

Raquel Sousa Almeida, Petra M. Pego, Maria João Pinto, and João Matos Costa
3rd Department of Internal Medicine, Hospital Distrital de Santar´em, Santar´em, Portugal

Eric R. Yoo
Department of Medicine, University of Illinois College of Medicine, Chicago, IL, USA

Ryan B. Perumpail and Aijaz Ahmed
Division of Gastroenterology and Hepatology, Stanford University School of Medicine, Stanford, CA, USA

George Cholankeril
Division of Gastroenterology and Hepatology, University of Tennessee Health Sciences Center, Memphis, TN, USA

Jackie Ho, Arash Heidari and Royce Johnson
Kern Medical, 1700 Mount Vernon Avenue, Bakersfield, CA 93306-4018, USA

Jeffrey C. Jolliff and Jeremiah Joson
Kern Medical, 1700 Mount Vernon Avenue, Bakersfield, CA 93306-4018, USA
University of the Pacific School of Pharmacy & Health Sciences, 3601 Pacific Avenue, Stockton, CA 95211-0109, USA

Negin Niknam, Thien Doan and Elizabeth Revere
Hofstra Northwell School of Medicine, Hempstead, NY, USA

Marjan Islam and Dennis Karter
Department of Medicine, Mount Sinai Beth Israel, New York, NY 10003, USA

Jerry Altshuler
Department of Pharmacy, Mount Sinai Beth Israel, New York, NY 10003, USA

Diana Altshuler
Department of Pharmacy, NYU Langone Medical Center, New York, NY 10016, USA

David Schwartz
Department of Medicine, NYU Langone Medical Center, New York, NY 10016, USA
NYU School of Medicine, New York, NY 10016, USA

Gianluca Torregrossa
Department of Cardiac Surgery, Mount Sinai Beth Israel, New York, NY 10003, USA

Murtaza Mazhar and Ijlal Akbar Ali
Department of Internal Medicine, Suite 6300, 800 Stanton L Young Boulevard, Oklahoma University Health Sciences Center, Oklahoma City, OK 73104, USA

Nelson Iván Agudelo Higuita
Department of Infectious Diseases, Suite 7300, 800 Stanton L Young Boulevard, Oklahoma University Health Sciences Center, Oklahoma City, OK 73104, USA

Sujeet Raina and Rajesh Sharma
Department of Medicine, Dr. RPGMC, Tanda, Kangra 176001, India

Ashish Sharma and Amit Bhardwaj
Department ofNeurology, Dr. RPGMC, Tanda, Kangra 176001, India

Louie Mar Gangcuangco
Department of Internal Medicine, Yale New Haven Health-Bridgeport Hospital, Bridgeport, CT, USA

Patricia Clark and Cynthia Stewart
Department of Microbiology, Yale New Haven Health-Bridgeport Hospital, Bridgeport, CT, USA

Goran Miljkovic and Zane K. Saul
Department of Internal Medicine, Yale New Haven Health-Bridgeport Hospital, Bridgeport, CT, USA
Internal Medicine and Infectious Disease Associates P.C., Stratford, CT, USA

Vassiliki Pitiriga, Georgia Vrioni and Athanassios Tsakris
Department of Microbiology, Medical School, National and Kapodistrian University of Athens, M. Asias 75, Goudi, 11527 Athens, Greece

John Dendrinos and Emanuel Nikitiadis
Metropolitan Hospital, EthnarchouMakariou 9 & El. Venizelou 1, N. Faliro, 18547 Athens, Greece

Gholamreza Pouladfar, Zahra Jafarpour, Bahman Pourabbas and Anahita Sanaei Babaei
Professor Alborzi Clinical Microbiology Research Center, Namazi Hospital, Shiraz University of Medical Sciences, Shiraz, Iran

Bita Geramizadeh
Transplant Research Center, Pathology Department, Shiraz University of Medical Sciences, Shiraz, Iran

Amir Hossein Babaei
Professor Alborzi Clinical Microbiology Research Center, Namazi Hospital, Shiraz University of Medical Sciences, Shiraz, Iran
Student Research Committee, Shiraz University of Medical Sciences, Neshat Street, Shiraz 71348 43638, Iran

Biswajit Dey and Debasis Gochhait
Department of Pathology, Jawaharlal Institute of Postgraduate Medical Education and Research (JIPMER), Pondicherry, India

Nagendran Prabhakaran, Laxmisha Chandrashekar and Biswanath Behera
Department of Dermatology, Jawaharlal Institute of Postgraduate Medical Education and Research (JIPMER), Pondicherry, India

Ueno Daisuke
Department of Digestive Surgery, Kawasaki Medical School, Kurashiki, Japan

Tomohiro Oishi and Kihei Terada
Department of Pediatrics, Kawasaki Medical School, Kurashiki, Japan

Kunikazu Yamane
Department of Public Health, Kawasaki Medical School, Kurashiki, Japan

Krunal Bharat Patel, James Benjamin Gleason and Nydia Martinez-Galvez
Department of Pulmonary & Critical Care Medicine, Cleveland Clinic Florida,Weston, FL, USA

Maria Julia Diacovo
Department of Pathology, Cleveland Clinic Florida,Weston, FL, USA

Masoud Doroodgar and Moein Doroodgar
School of Medicine, Shahid Beheshti University of Medical Sciences, Tehran, Iran

Abbas Doroodgar
Department of Medical Parasitology, Kashan University of Medical Sciences, Kashan, Iran

Onivola Raharolahy, Lala S. Ramarozatovo, Irina M. Ranaivo, Fandresena A. Sendrasoa, Malalaniaina Andrianarison and Fahafahantsoa Rapelanoro Rabenja
USFR Dermatologie, Centre Hospitalier Universitaire Joseph Raseta Befelatanana, 101 Antananarivo, Madagascar

Mala Rakoto Andrianarivelo
Centre d'Infectiologie Charles Mérieux, Université d'Antananarivo, 101 Antananarivo, Madagascar

Emmanuelle Cambau
APHP, Hôpital Lariboisière, Bactériologie, Centre National de Référence des Mycobactéries et de la Résistance des Mycobactéries aux Antituberculeux, 75475 Paris Cedex 10, France

Prabin Sharma and Laia Jimena Vazquez Guillamet
Department of Internal Medicine, Yale New Haven Health System, Bridgeport Hospital, Bridgeport, CT 06610, USA

Goran Miljkovic
Department of Infectious Diseases, Yale New Haven Health System, Bridgeport Hospital, Bridgeport, CT 06610, USA

Sevliya Öcal Demir, Serkan Atici, GülGen Akkoç, Nurhayat Yakut, Ahmet Soysal and Mustafa Bakir
Marmara University School of Medicine, Department of Pediatrics, Division of Pediatric Infectious Diseases, 34912 Istanbul, Turkey

Nilay Baş İkizoğlu
Marmara University School of Medicine, Department of Pediatrics, Division of Pediatric Pulmonology, 34912 Istanbul, Turkey

Luca T. Giurgea
Department of Medicine, Dartmouth-Hitchcock Medical Center, Lebanon, NH 03756, USA

Tim Lahey
Section of Infectious Disease and International Health, Department of Medicine, Dartmouth-Hitchcock Medical Center,
Lebanon, NH 03756, USA

Alexandros Makis, Aikaterini Perogiannaki and Nikolaos Chaliasos
Child Health Department, Faculty of Medicine, University of Ioannina, Ioannina, Greece

Onur Yazici
Department of Chest Disease, Adnan Menderes University, Aydın, Turkey

Mustafa Cortuk and Erdogan Cetinkaya
Department of Chest Disease, Karabuk University, Karabuk, Turkey

Hasan Casim
Department of Chest Disease, Karabuk University Training and Research Hospital, Karabuk, Turkey

Ali Mert
Department of Infectious Diseases, İstanbul Medipol University, İstanbul, Turkey

Ali Ramazan Benli
Department of Family Medicine, Karabuk University, Karabuk, Turkey

R. Zea-Vera and M. Sanchez
Universidad Peruana Cayetano Heredia, San Martin de Porres, Lima, Peru

E. Castañeda
Universidad Peruana Cayetano Heredia, San Martin de Porres, Lima, Peru
Cardiovascular Surgery Department, Hospital Cayetano Heredia, San Martin de Porres, Lima, Peru

L. Soto-Arquiñigo
Universidad Peruana Cayetano Heredia, San Martin de Porres, Lima, Peru
Infectious Disease Department, Hospital Cayetano Heredia, San Martin de Porres, Lima, Peru

Robert Ali, Julio Perez-Downes, Firas Baidoun, Bashar Al Turk and Carmen Isache
Department of Internal Medicine, University of Florida-Jacksonville, 655W8th Street, Jacksonville, FL 32209, USA

Girish Mohan and Charles Perniciaro
Department of Pathology, University of Florida-Jacksonville, 655W8th Street, Jacksonville, FL 32209, USA

Bryan H. Schmitt, Thomas E. Davis and Ryan F. Relich
Department of Pathology and Laboratory Medicine, Indiana University School of Medicine, Indianapolis, IN 46202, USA

Miguel A. Arroyo
Department of Pathology and Laboratory Medicine, Indiana University School of Medicine, Indianapolis, IN 46202, USA
U.S. Army Medical Department Center and School, Fort Sam Houston, TX 78234, USA

Annie Oh
Division of Hematology/Oncology, University of Illinois at Chicago, Chicago, IL 60612, USA

Karen Sweiss
Department of Pharmacy Practice, University of Illinois at Chicago, Chicago, IL 60612, USA
Cancer Center, University of Illinois, Chicago, IL 60612, USA

Damiano Rondelli and Pritesh Patel
Cancer Center, University of Illinois, Chicago, IL 60612, USA
Division of Hematology/Oncology, University of Illinois at Chicago, Chicago, IL 60612, USA

Mariana Meireles
Internal Medicine Department, Porto Hospital Centre, Porto, Portugal

Conceição Souto Moura
Pathological Anatomy Department, São João Hospital Centre, Porto, Portugal

Margarida França
Clinical Immunology Unit, Porto Hospital Centre, Porto, Portugal

Erika M. Carrillo-Casas and Margarita Leyva-Leyva
Departamento de Biología Molecular e Histocompatibilidad, Direccíon de Investigacíon, Hospital General "Dr. Manuel Gea González", 14080 Tlalpan, MEX, Mexico

Andrea Rangel-Cordero
Laboratorio de Microbiología Clínica, Instituto Nacional de Ciencias Médicas y Nutrición "Salvador Zubirán", 14080 Tlalpan, MEX, Mexico

Juan Xicohtencatl-Cortes
Departamento de Infectología, Hospital Infantil de México "Federico Gómez", Dr. Márquez 162, Cuauhtémoc, 06720 Ciudad de México, DF, Mexico

Roberto Arenas
Servicio de Micología, Hospital General "Dr. Manuel Gea González", 14080 Tlalpan, MEX, Mexico

Rigoberto Hernández-Castro
Departamento de Ecología de Agentes Patógenos, Hospital General "Dr. Manuel Gea González", 14080 Tlalpan, MEX, Mexico

Jorge García-Méndez
Departamento de Posgrado y Educación Médica Continua, Instituto Nacional de Cancerología, Mexico Departamento de Microbiología, Facultad de Medicina, UNAM, 04510 Coyoacán, MEX, Mexico

Wissam K. Kabbara
Department of Pharmacy Practice, School of Pharmacy, Lebanese American University (LAU), P.O. Box 36/F-37, Byblos, Lebanon

Aline T. Sarkis and Paola G. Saroufim
School of Pharmacy, Lebanese American University (LAU), Byblos, Lebanon

Berta Becerril Carral, Salvador López Cárdenas and Jesús Canueto Quintero
Unidad Clínica de Gestión de Enfermedades Infecciosas y Microbiología del Área Sanitaria del Campo de Gibraltar, Cádiz, Spain

Elvira Alarcón Manoja
Unidad Clínica de Gestión de Medicina Interna del Área Sanitaria del Campo de Gibraltar, Cádiz, Spain

Lukas Birkner
Department of Internal Medicine, Ev. KrankenhausWitten gGmbH, University of Witten/Herdecke, Pferdebachstr 27, 58455Witten, Germany

Zuhal Yesilbag
Department of Infectious Diseases and Clinical Microbiology, Bakirkoy Dr. Sadi Konuk Education and Research Hospital, Istanbul, Turkey

Asli Karadeniz
Department of Infectious Diseases and Clinical Microbiology, Maltepe University Faculty of Medicine, Istanbul, Turkey

Fatih Oner Kaya
Department of Internal Medicine, Maltepe University Faculty of Medicine, Istanbul, Turkey

Abdurrahman Aycan, İsmail Gulsen and Harun Arslan
Neurosurgery Department, Yuzuncu Yıl University Faculty of Medicine, 65040 Van, Turkey

Ozgür Yusuf Aktas, Feyza Karagoz Guzey, Azmi Tufan and Cihan Isler
Neurosurgery Department, Bagcilar Training and Research Hospital, Istanbul, Turkey

Nur Aycan
Pediatric Department, Private İstanbul Hospital, Van, Turkey

Lydia Tang and Shyam Kottilil
Institute of Human Virology, University of Maryland School of Medicine, 725West Lombard Street, Baltimore, MD 21201, USA

Kimberly L. Beavers
Division of Gastroenterology and Hepatology, Department of Medicine, Medical University of South Carolina, 114 Doughty Street Suite 249, MSC 702, Charleston, SC 29425, USA

Eric G. Meissner
Division of Infectious Diseases, Department of Medicine, Medical University of South Carolina, 135 Rutledge Avenue Suite 1209, MSC 752, Charleston, SC 29425, USA

Madelyne Bean
Division of Infectious Diseases, Department of Medicine, Medical University of South Carolina, 135 Rutledge Avenue Suite 1209, MSC 752, Charleston, SC 29425, USA
Department of Pharmacy Services, Medical University of South Carolina, 150 Ashley Avenue, Charleston, SC 29425, USA

Ye-sheng Wang, Qi-wei Li, Lin Zhou, Run-feng Guan, Xiang-ming Zhou, Ji-hong Wu and Shuang Zhu
Guangdong Province Key Laboratory for Biotechnology Drug Candidates, School of Biosciences and Biopharmaceutics, Guangdong Pharmaceutical University, Guangzhou, Guangdong 510006, China

Nan-yan Rao
Sun Yat-sen Memorial Hospital of Zhongshan University, Guangzhou, Guangdong 510120, China

Dominique Dilorenzo, Naganna Channaveeraiah, Patricia Gilford and Bruce Deschere
Orange Park Medical Center Family Medicine GME, 2021 Professional Center Drive, Suite 100, Orange Park, FL 32073, USA

Razieh Afrough and Setareh Sagheb
Department of Pediatrics, Tehran University of Medical Sciences, Tehran, Iran

Sayyed Shahabeddin Mohseni
Department of Dermatology, Tehran Medical Sciences Branch, Islamic Azad University, Tehran, Iran

Iordanis Romiopoulos, Charalampos Antachopoulos and Emmanuel Roilides
Infectious Diseases Unit, 3rd Department of Pediatrics, Faculty of Medicine, Aristotle University School of Health Sciences, Hippokration General Hospital, Thessaloniki, Greece

Anna Varouktsi, Elisavet Simoulidou and Asterios Karagiannis
2nd Propaedeutic Department of Internal Medicine, Faculty of Medicine, Aristotle University School of Health Sciences, Hippokration General Hospital, Thessaloniki, Greece

Konstantina Kontopoulou
Laboratory of Microbiology, Gennimatas General Hospital, Thessaloniki, Greece

Ekaterini Karantani
Laboratory of Microbiology, Hippokration General Hospital, Thessaloniki, Greece

Vivian Georgopoulou
Laboratory of Radiology, Hippokration General Hospital, Thessaloniki, Greece

Konstantinos Kitsios
Department of Medicine, Gennimatas Hospital, Thessaloniki, Greece

Apostolos Mamopoulos
3rd Department of Obstetrics and Gynecology, Faculty of Medicine, Aristotle University School of Health Sciences, Hippokration General Hospital, Thessaloniki, Greece

Felicia Ratnaraj, David Brooks, Mollie Walton, Arun Nagabandi and Mahmoud Abu Hazeem
CHI Health Creighton University Medical Center, Omaha, NE, USA

Praveen Sudhindra and Robert B. Nadelman
Division of Infectious Diseases, New York Medical College, Valhalla, NY 10595, USA

Guiqing Wang
Department of Pathology, New York Medical College, Valhalla, NY 10595, USA

Reem M. Hassan and Dina M. Bassiouny
Department of Clinical and Chemical Pathology, Faculty of Medicine, Cairo University, Cairo, Egypt

Yomna Matar
Department of Psychiatry, Faculty of Medicine, Cairo University, Cairo, Egypt

Murat Özer
Department of Pediatrics, Hacettepe University Faculty of Medicine, Ankara, Turkey

Yasemin Özsürekci and Ali Bülent Cengiz
Pediatric Infectious Diseases, Hacettepe University Faculty of Medicine, Ankara, Turkey

Nagehan Emiralioğlu and Deniz Doğru
Pediatric Chest Diseases, Hacettepe University Faculty of Medicine, Ankara, Turkey

Kader Karh Oğuz and Onur Akça
Department of Radiology, Hacettepe University Faculty of Medicine, Ankara, Turkey

Özgür Özkayar
Department of Pathology, Hacettepe University Faculty of Medicine, Ankara, Turkey

Abdalla Khalil, Asem Saleh and Rasha Ali
Internal Medicine Department, International Medical Center (IMC) Hospital, Jeddah, Saudi Arabia

Musaad Qurash
Radiology Department, IMC Hospital, Jeddah, Saudi Arabia

Mohamed Elwakil
Emergency Medicine Department, IMC Hospital, Jeddah, Saudi Arabia

Vishnu Kaniyarakkal, Shabana Orvankundil, Saradadevi Karunakaran Lalitha, Raji Thazhethekandi and Jahana Thottathil
Government Medical College Kozhikode, Kozhikode, India

Index

www.ingramcontent.com/pod-product-compliance
Lightning Source LLC
Chambersburg PA
CBHW050456200326
41458CB00014B/5197